Point-of-Care Tests for Severe Hemorrhage

Marco Ranucci • Paolo Simioni
Editors

Point-of-Care Tests for Severe Hemorrhage

A Manual for Diagnosis and Treatment

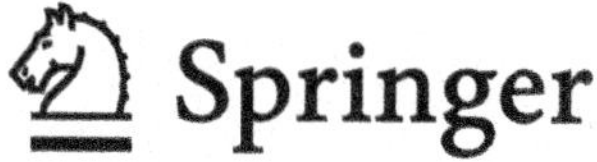

Editors
Marco Ranucci, MD, FESC
Department of Anaesthesia
and Intensive Care
IRCCS Policlinico San Donato
San Donato Milanese
Italy

Paolo Simioni, MD, PhD
Department of Medicine
Hemorrhagic and Thrombotic
Diseases Unit
University of Padua Medical School
Padua
Italy

ISBN 978-3-319-79680-2 ISBN 978-3-319-24795-3 (eBook)
DOI 10.1007/978-3-319-24795-3

Springer Cham Heidelberg New York Dordrecht London

Softcover reprint of the hardcover 1st edition 2016

Printed on acid-free paper

Springer International Publishing AG Switzerland is part of Springer Science+Business Media (www.springer.com)

Preface

At the end of 2013, a group of Italian clinicians sharing a common interest in hemostasis and coagulation in critically ill patients began meeting periodically (first in Padua, then in different locations). During these meetings, the group agreed that there was a growing interest in point-of-care (POC) coagulation tests, as well as a great need for acquiring knowledge and expertise from various clinicians involved in patient care in different fields, such as cardiac surgery, intensive care unit, postpartum hemorrhage, liver surgery, trauma, and other disciplines. At the beginning of 2014, this group was officially formed and named "INTACT" (the Italian Network to Address Coagulopathy Treatment). To fulfill its educational role, the group decided it was time to join efforts to create a single textbook addressing the use of POC coagulation tests in different clinical scenarios. It was in fact clearly evident that the information in this field was quite sparse and that all interested clinicians were forced to navigate through published articles, textbook chapters, meeting sessions, and the Internet to find the information they needed. Conversely, the INTACT group aimed to compile all relevant information about POC coagulation tests in a single textbook, written both from a technical standpoint and a clinical point of view in regard to different clinical scenarios.

The present textbook *Point-of-Care Tests for Severe Hemorrhage: A Manual for Diagnosis and Treatment* is the result of the INTACT group's dedicated efforts toward this end. Each of the various chapters' contributors are clinicians who are involved daily in the clinical management of severe hemorrhage in different areas, and while the content of this manual is based primarily on existing evidence, it also includes valuable personal points of view based on the authors' daily clinical practice. For each clinical scenario, the authors provide introductory notes on the specific aspects of the coagulopathy involved in severe hemorrhage determination, followed by the possible POC coagulation test applications as a guide for both diagnosis and treatment.

The manual contains basic information on the general pathophysiology of hemostasis and coagulation, as well as the historical and technical aspects of practically all existing POC coagulation tests, with specific reference to viscoelastic tests and platelet function tests.

Five clinical scenarios are addressed in individual chapters: intensive care unit, cardiovascular surgery, postpartum hemorrhage, trauma, and liver surgery. Additionally, the treatment strategies (blood derivatives and prohemostatic drugs) are discussed and the effects of antithrombotic drugs assessed. Lastly, the manual offers valuable insights into clinical cases drawn from the authors' actual experiences.

We thank all those who contributed to this manual and hope that the INTACT group's efforts have fulfilled its aim of successfully contributing to a better understanding of this evolving topic.

San Donato Milanese, Milan, Italy — Marco Ranucci, MD, FESC
Padua, Italy — Paolo Simioni, MD, PhD

Members of the Intact Group

Vanessa Agostini, Cesena
Ekaterina Baryshnikova, Milano
Gianni Biancofiore, Pisa
Lucio Bucci, Milano
Elena Campello, Padova
Dionisio Colella, Roma
Andrea De Gasperi, Milano
Lesley De Pietri, Modena
Guido Di Gregorio, Padova
Paolo Feltracco, Padova
Maria Grazia Frigo, Roma
Alberto Grassetto, Mestre
Dorela Haxhiademi, Massa
Blanca Martinez, Udine
Massimo Micaglio, Firenze
Giuseppe Nardi, Roma
Rita Paniccia, Firenze
Daniele Penzo, Trento
Domenico Prisco, Firenze
Marco Ranucci, Milano
Peter Santer, Brunico
Paolo Simioni, Padova
Luca Spiezia, Padova
Vincenzo Tarzia, Padova

Contents

Contributors

Vanessa Agostini, MD Transfusion Medicine Cesena/Forlì and Blood Establishment, Clinical Pathology Department-Cesena Azienda U.S.L Romagna, Romagna, Italy

Ekaterina Baryshnikova, PhD Department of Cardiothoracic-Vascular Anesthesia and ICU, IRCCS Policlinico San Donato, San Donato Milanese, Milan, Italy

Gianni Biancofiore, MD Liver Transplant Anaesthesia and Critical Care, Azienda Ospedaliera Universitaria Pisana, Pisa, Italy

Maria Lucia Bindi, MD Liver Transplant Anaesthesia and Critical Care, Azienda Ospedaliera Universitaria Pisana, Pisa, Italy

Agostino Brizzi, MD Department of Anesthesia and Intensive Care, Santa Maria Hospital, Bari, Italy

Lucio Bucci, MD ICU "Bozza" – 1st Service Anesthesia and Intensive Care, A.O. Niguarda Ca' Granda Hospital, Milan, Italy

Elena Campello, MD Department of Medicine, University of Padua Medical School, Padua, Italy

Emiliano Cingolani, MD Shock and Trauma Center, S. Camillo-Forlanini Hospital, Roma, Italy

Dionisio Colella, MD, PhD Department of Cardiac Anesthesia, Policlinico Tor Vergata, University of Rome Tor Vergata, Rome, Italy

Andrea De Gasperi, MD 2nd Service Anesthesia Critical Care Medicine, Ospedale Niguarda Ca' Granda, Milan, Italy

Lesley De Pietri, MD Division of Anaesthesiology and Intensive Care Unit, Azienda Ospedaliero-Universitaria di Modena-Policlinico, Modena, Italy

Guido Di Gregorio, MD Anesthesia and Intensive Care Unit, Department of Medicine, Padua University Hospital, Padua, Italy

Paolo Feltracco, MD Department of Medicine, Anesthesia and Intensive Care Unit, Padova University Hospital, Padova, Italy

Maria Grazia Frigo, MD Obstetric Anesthesia, Fatebenefratelli Hospital Isola Tiberina Rome, Rome, Italy

Alberto Grassetto, MD UOC Anestesia e Rianimazione, Dipartimento Emergenza Urgenza, Ospedale dell'Angelo di Mestre, Venice, Italy

Dorela Haxhiademi, MD Anesthesia and Intensive Care, G. Pasquinucci Hospital, G. Monasterio Foundation, Massa, Italy

Sara Maggiolo, MD Department of Medicine, University of Padua Medical School, Padua, Italy

Blanca Martinez, MD Department of Anesthesia and Intensive Care Medicine, University Hospital of Udine, Udine, Italy

Massimo Micaglio, MD Department of Anesthesia and Intensive Care, Careggi University Hospital, Florence, Italy

Luca Monastra, MD UOC Anesthesia and Intensive Care, A.O. Ospedale dei Colli Presidio Monaldi, Naples, Italy

Giuseppe Nardi, MD Shock and Trauma Center, S. Camillo-Forlanini Hospital, Roma, Italy

Rita Paniccia, MSc Department of Experimental and Clinical Medicine, University of Florence; Careggi University Hospital, Florence, Italy

Concetta Pellegrini, MD U.O.C. Anesthesia and Intensive Care, M.Rummo Hospital, Benevento, Italy

Daniele Penzo, MD 2nd Service Anesthesia Critical Care Medicine, S. Chiara Hospital, Trento, Italy

Domenico Prisco, MD, PhD Department of Experimental and Clinical Medicine, University of Florence; Careggi University Hospital, Florence, Italy

Maria Pia Rainaldi, MD Department of Obstetrics and Gynecology, Sant'Orsola Malpighi University Hospital, University of Bologna, Bologna, Italy

Marco Ranucci, MD, FESC Department of Cardiothoracic-Vascular Anesthesia and ICU, IRCCS Policlinico San Donato, San Donato Milanese, Milan, Italy

David Sacerdoti, MD, PhD Department of Medicine, University of Padua Medical School, Padua, Italy

Peter Santer, MD Clinical Pathology Laboratory, Brunico Hospital, Brunico, Italy

Marco Senzolo, MD Multivisceral Transplant Unit, Gastroenterology, Department of Surgery, Oncology and Gastroenterology, Padua University Hospital, Padua, Italy

Paolo Simioni, MD, PhD Department of Medicine, Hemorrhagic and Thrombotic Diseases Unit, University of Padua Medical School, Padua, Italy

Luca Spiezia, MD Department of Medicine, University of Padua Medical School, Padua, Italy

Vincenzo Tarzia, MD Division of Cardiac Surgery, Department of Cardiac, Thoracic and Vascular Sciences, University of Padua, Padua, Italy

1 Pathophysiology of Coagulation

Paolo Simioni and Elena Campello

Hemostasis preserves vascular integrity by balancing the physiologic processes that maintain blood in a fluid state under normal circumstances and prevent excessive bleeding after vascular injury. Preservation of blood fluidity depends on an intact vascular endothelium and a complex series of regulatory pathways that maintains platelets in a quiescent state and keeps the coagulation system in equilibrium. In contrast, arrest of bleeding requires rapid formation of hemostatic plugs at sites of vascular injury to prevent exsanguination. Perturbation of hemostasis can lead to bleeding or thrombosis. Bleeding will occur if there is failure to seal vascular leaks either because of defective hemostatic plug formation or because of premature breakdown of the plugs [1–3].

The normal hemostatic system comprises four compartments: the vasculature and platelets (primary hemostasis), the coagulation proteins (secondary hemostasis), and the fibrinolytic system. When a blood vessel is injured, all four components interact in a coordinated manner to prevent blood loss by forming a clot and localizing this to the area of injury (Fig. 1.1) [4–7].

P. Simioni, MD, PhD (✉)
Department of Medicine,
Hemorrhagic and Thrombotic Diseases Unit,
University of Padua Medical School, Padua, Italy
e-mail: paolo.simioni@unipd.it

E. Campello, MD
Department of Medicine,
University of Padua Medical School, Padua, Italy

1.1 Primary Hemostasis

The term "primary hemostasis" encompasses all aspects of platelet adhesion and aggregation. Apart from platelets, components of the vessel wall – subendothelial matrix components in particular – and von Willebrand factor (vWF) are involved in this process (Fig. 1.2) [3, 8, 9].

1.1.1 Vascular Endothelium

A monolayer of endothelial cells lines the intimal surface of the circulatory tree and separates the blood from the prothrombotic subendothelial components of the vessel wall. Rather than serving as a static barrier, the healthy vascular endothelium is a dynamic organ that actively regulates hemostasis by inhibiting platelets, suppressing coagulation, promoting fibrinolysis, and modulating vascular tone and permeability. Defective vascular function can lead to bleeding if the endothelium becomes more permeable to blood cells, if vasoconstriction does not occur, or if premature degradation of hemostatic plug opens seals in the vasculature [3, 10].

1.1.2 Platelets

Ordinarily platelets circulate in a quiescent state, near the endothelial cells lining the blood vessels

M. Ranucci, P. Simioni (eds.), *Point-of-Care Tests for Severe Hemorrhage: A Manual for Diagnosis and Treatment*, DOI 10.1007/978-3-319-24795-3_1

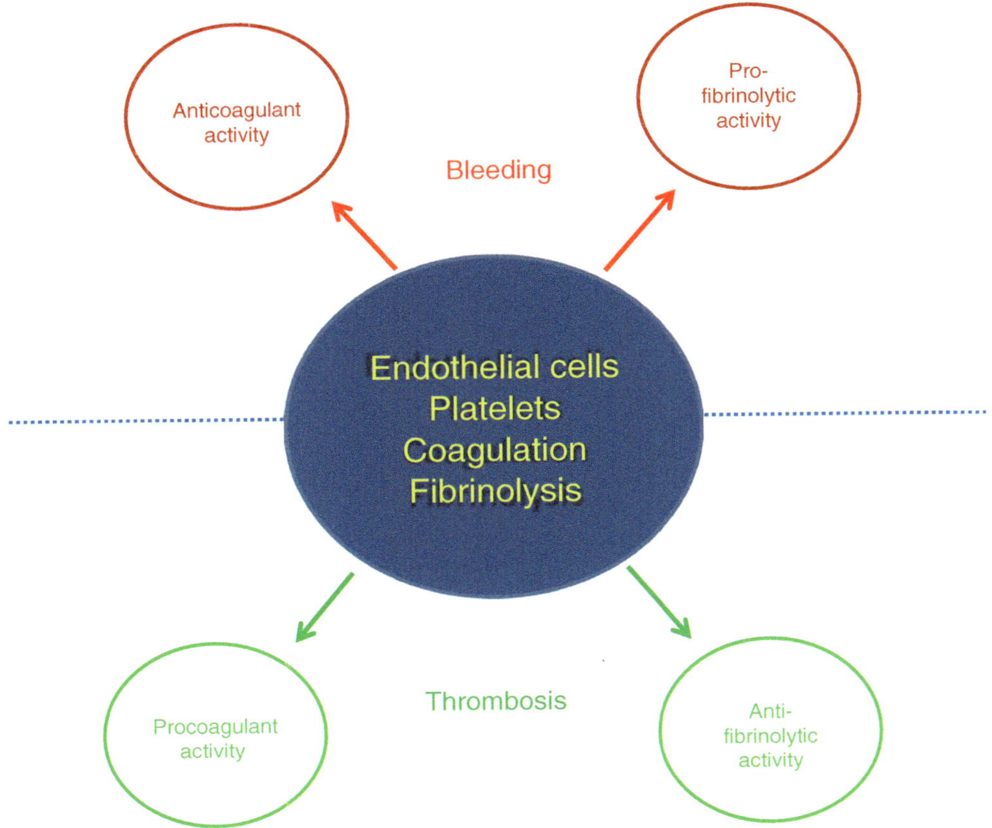

Fig. 1.1 In healthy individuals, cellular and protein components of prohemostasis and antihemostasis pathways have adequate capacities to adapt to acute physiologic stresses

without forming stable adhesions. However, after breaches of the vasculature, a number of highly reactive subendothelial matrix proteins become exposed including vWF, collagen, fibrinogen, and fibronectin. Damage to the intimal lining of the vessel exposes the underlying subendothelial matrix. Platelets home to sites of vascular disruption and adhere to the exposed matrix proteins. Initial platelet adhesion is mediated principally by platelet surface receptors interacting with their cognate ligands. Initial platelet-adhesive interactions are mediated by platelet surface glycoproteins (GPs) including GPVI and GPIbα interacting with endothelial-bound collagen and VWF, respectively. Adherent platelets undergo activation and not only release substances that recruit additional platelets to the site of injury but also promote thrombin generation and fibrin formation. The excretion of the content of the platelets' α- and δ-granules leads to the release of a variety of components (e.g., coagulation factors, calcium, ADP) and modulators of hemostasis, such as thromboxane A2 and platelet-activating factor, both of which are potent platelet activators and promote vasoconstriction. Upon activation, platelets also exhibit a more thrombogenic surface by exposing a negatively charged phospholipid layer, providing the catalytic surface for the binding of coagulation factors and, thus, the process of fibrin formation and stabilization. Furthermore, externalization, clustering, and activation of receptors on the platelets' surface occur, allowing for a complex and intense interaction of platelets with matrix proteins and other platelets. In this process, platelets aggregate by cross-linking the highly expressed GP IIb/IIIa

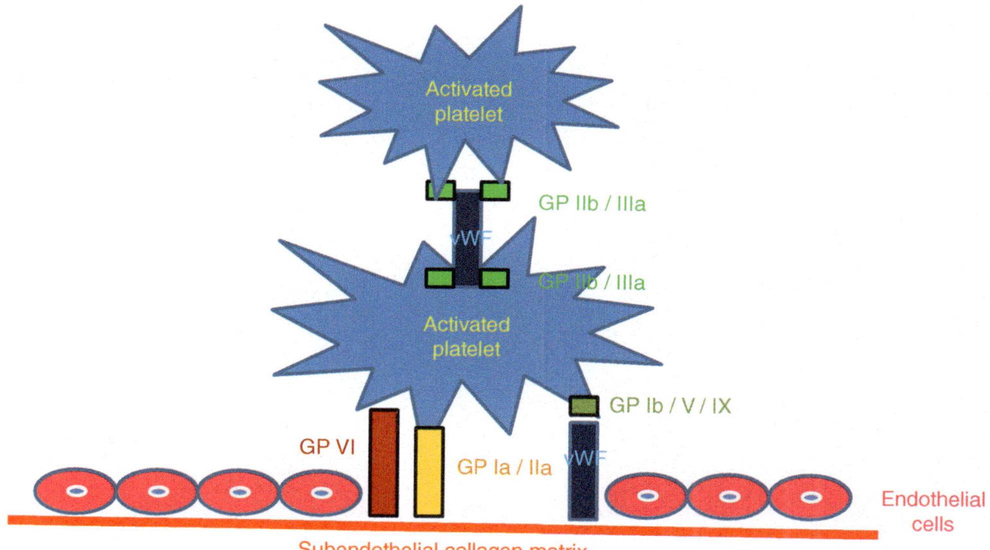

Fig. 1.2 Schematic view of platelet adhesion and aggregation. Following endothelial injury, platelets adhere to collagen by interaction of the receptor glycoprotein (*GP*) Ib/V/IX with von Willebrand factor which is bound to collagen. This adhesion is stabilized by direct interaction of platelet collagen receptors GP Ia/IIa and GP VI with collagen. Following activation of the aggregation receptors GP IIb/IIIa, platelets aggregate, mediated by von Willebrand factor or fibrinogen (Adapted from: Sucker and Zotz [8])

aggregation receptors on the platelet surfaces via vWF or fibrinogen. As a result of primary hemostasis, a primary platelet plug forms on the injured endothelium, mainly consisting of platelets and vWF. This platelet clot is further modified and stabilized by cross-linking of fibrin [8, 11–16].

1.2 Secondary Hemostasis

The secondary hemostasis process involves multiple enzymatic steps, resulting in the generation of thrombin, which converts soluble fibrinogen to fibrin. Coagulation occurs through the action of discrete enzyme complexes, which are composed of a vitamin K-dependent enzyme and a nonenzyme cofactor, and assemble on anionic phospholipid membranes in a calcium-dependent fashion. Each enzyme complex activates a vitamin K-dependent substrate that becomes the enzyme component of the subsequent complex. Together these complexes generate a small amount of thrombin, which amplifies its own generation by activating the nonenzyme cofactors and platelets, which then provide an anionic surface on which the complexes assemble [3–7, 17–20]. General characteristics of factors relevant for coagulation are reported in Table 1.1.

The three enzyme complexes involved in thrombin generation are (Fig. 1.3):

Extrinsic Tenase: it forms upon exposure of tissue factor-expressing cells on the blood. Tissue factor (TF) is an integral membrane protein that serves as a receptor for factor VIIa. With TF exposure on anionic cell surfaces, factor VIIa binds a calcium-dependent fashion to form the extrinsic tenase complex, which is a potent activator of factors IX and X. After being activated, factor IXa and Xa serve as the enzyme components of intrinsic and prothrombinase, respectively [21, 22].

Intrinsic Tenase: Factor IXa binds to factor VIIIa on anionic cell surfaces in a calcium-dependent fashion to form intrinsic tenase, which activated factor X. Absence of the membrane of

Table 1.1 Factors relevant for coagulation

Name		Function	Molecular weight (kDA)	Mean concentration (μg/ml)	Reference range (IU/ml)	t 1/2 (h)
Fibrinogen	FI	Substrate of coagulation: forms fibrin	340	3000	n.a.	72–100
Prothrombin	FII	Serine protease (VKD): multiple targets	72	100	0.60–1.40	60
Labile factor	FV	Cofactor to FX	330	10	0.60–1.40	15
Stable factor	FVII	Serine protease (VKD): activates FX (and FIX)	50	0.5	0.60–1.40	5
Antihemophilic factor	FVIII	Cofactor to FIX	185	0.1	0.50–2.0	12
Christmas factor	FIX	Serine protease (VKD): activates FX	56	5	0.60–1.40	18
Stuart-Prower factor	FX	Serine protease (VKD): activates FII	56	10	0.60–1.40	30
Plasma thromboplastin antecedent	FXI	Serine protease: activates FIX	160	5	0.60–1.40	45
Hageman factor	FXII	Serine protease: activates FXI	80	30	0.60–1.40	
Fibrin-stabilizing factor	FXIII	Cross-links soluble fibrin monomers to insoluble fibrin strand	320	60	0.50–1.50	216
von Willebrand factor	vWF	Mediates platelet adhesion to collagen; stabilizes and transports FVIII	225xn	10	0.50–2.0	10
Tissue factor	TF	Main initiator of coagulation in vivo: cofactor to FVII/FVIIa	45	n.a.	n.a.	n.a.

Plasma half-life (t½) is intended under physiological conditions; it may be considerably shorter in the presence of bleeding

Tissue factor, the main initiator of coagulation in vivo, is principally a membrane-bound protein expressed on subendothelial cells. Under pathophysiological conditions, it may: (1) circulate bound to microparticles or monocytes, (2) circulate in truncated form as a free protein, or (3) be ectopically expressed on endothelial and other cells

VKD vitamin K dependent

factor VIIIa almost completely abolishes enzymatic activity. Because this complex activates factor X at a rate 50- to 100-fold faster than extrinsic tenase, it plays a critical role in the amplification of factor Xa and subsequent thrombin generation.

Prothrombinase: Factor Xa binds to factor Va, its activated cofactor, on anionic phospholipid membrane surfaces to form the prothrombinase complex. Prothrombin binds to the prothrombinase complex, where it undergoes conversion to thrombin [23].

Fibrinogen and fibrin formation: Fibrinogen is the first coagulation factor to be discovered, and it plays a key role in perioperative hemostasis because it is the first coagulation factor to reach critical levels in massive bleeding. Fibrinogen, synthesized in the liver, is an abundant plasma protein with concentrations typically ranging

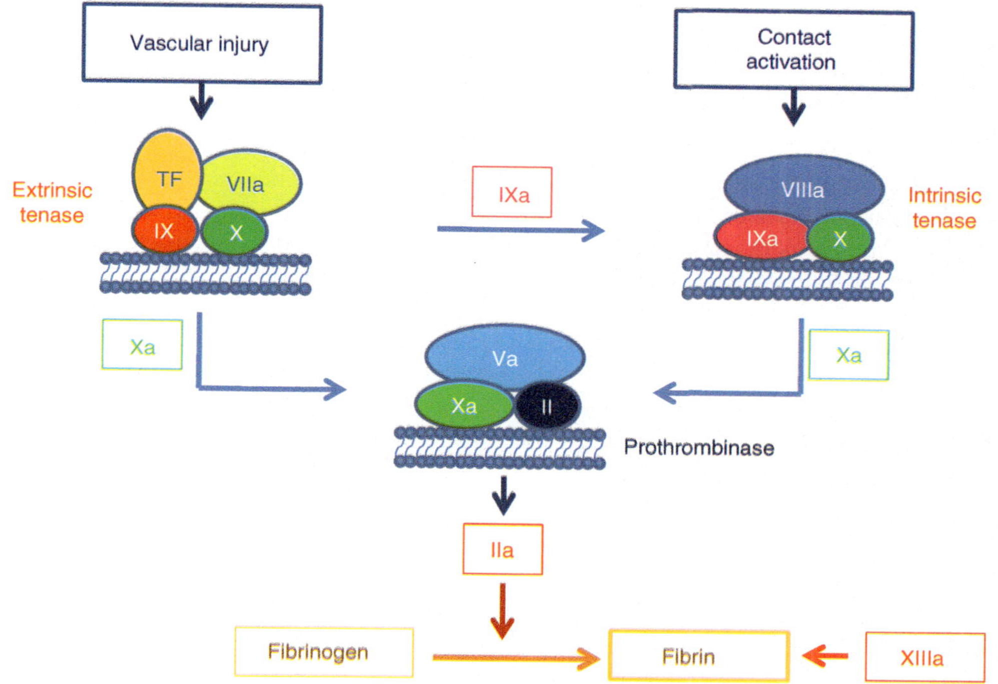

Fig. 1.3 Coagulation system. Coagulation occurs through the action of discrete enzyme complexes, which are composed of a vitamin K-dependent enzyme and a nonenzyme cofactor. These complexes assemble on anionic phospholipid membranes in a calcium-dependent fashion. Vascular injury exposes tissue factor (*TF*), which binds factor VIIa to form extrinsic tenase. Extrinsic tenase activates factors IX and X. Factor Ixa binds to factor VIIIa to form intrinsic tenase, which activates factor X. Factor Xa binds to factor Va to form prothrombinase, which convert prothrombin (II) to thrombin (IIa). Thrombin then converts soluble fibrinogen into soluble fibrin

between 1.5–4.0 g/l and 6–13 μmol/l. It is a dimeric molecule, each half of which is composed of three polypeptide chains – the Aα, Bβ, and γ chains. Fibrinogen circulates in an active form. Thrombin converts soluble fibrinogen into insoluble fibrin. Thrombin binds to the amino terminal of the Aα and Bβ chains of fibrinogen, where it cleaves specific peptide bonds to release fibrinopeptide A and B and generates fibrin monomer. Non-covalently linked fibrin protofibrils are unstable. The stability of the fibrin network is enhanced by platelets and procoagulant cells. Platelets bind fibrin via GPIIb/IIIa and promote the formation of a dense fibrin networks, but they also release factor XIII. FXIII stabilizes the fibrin in a calcium-dependent fashion and renders it relatively resistant to degradation, by covalently cross-linking the α- and γ-chains of adjacent fibrin monomers [24–26].

Fibrinogen has at least four major biological functions: (i) it is a substrate of coagulation; (ii) it is a cross-linker in platelet aggregation; (iii) it is a coagulation inhibitor as "antithrombin I"; (iv) and it is a substrate for interaction with other proteins [27–31].

(i) Most other coagulation factors are serine proteases capable of specifically recognizing target molecules and activating many of them. For example, one activated thrombin molecule can activate more than 1000 molecules of fibrinogen. Indeed, enzymatically active coagulation factors can continue to interact with many other target molecules, while fibrinogen, in its role as substrate, will be consumed. One activated molecule of fibrinogen will give rise to one molecule of fibrin in the resulting clot.

(ii) Fibrinogen's second role is that of the cross-linker in platelet aggregation. Once platelets have been activated "outside," an "inside" activation will occur that leads to an altered structure of the glycoprotein IIb/IIIa receptor on the platelet surface. This structural change permits the interaction of one fibrinogen molecule with several GP IIb/IIIa receptors on several platelets, leading to the formation of platelet aggregates.

(iii) The third role involves fibrinogen's ability to bind thrombin.

(iv) Finally, FXIII is reported to covalently link α2-plasmin inhibitor on to fibrinogen; this reaction is important for the stability of the resulting fibrin clot.

Contact Pathway: current thinking is that tissue factor exposure represents the sole pathway for activation of coagulation and that the contact system – which includes factor XII, prekallikrein, and high molecular kininogen – is unimportant for hemostasis because patients deficient in these factors do not have bleeding problems. However, the contact pathway cannot be ignored because coronary catheters and other blood-contacting medical devices, such as stents or mechanical valves, likely trigger clotting through this mechanism. Factor XII bound to the surface of catheters or devices undergoes a conformational change that results in its activation. Factor XIIa propagates coagulation by activating factor XI.

1.3 Fibrinolytic System

The fibrinolytic system allows for the lysis of a fibrin clot. Fibrinolysis initiates when plasminogen activators convert plasminogen to plasmin, which then degrades fibrin into soluble fragments. Blood contains two immunologically and functionally distinct plasminogen activators, t-PA and u-PA. t-PA mediates intravascular fibrin degradation, whereas u-PA activates cell-bound plasminogen. Regulation of fibrinolysis occurs at two levels: PAI-1 (and to a lesser extent PAI-2) inhibits the plasminogen activators (both t-PA and u-PA) and α2-antiplasmin inhibits plasmin. Finally, thrombin-activated fibrinolysis inhibitor (TAFI) also modulates fibrinolysis cleaving lysine residues from degrading fibrin (binding sites for plasminogen, plasmin, and t-PA) (Fig. 1.4). TAFI are activated by thrombin–thrombomodulin complex. Notably, fibrinolytic capacity differs significantly among different tissues, with high activities in the genitourinary tract and the oral mucosa. This tissue-dependent variability of fibrinolytic capacity provides an explanation of the bleeding pattern in patients with pathologically enhanced fibrinolysis (hyperfibrinolysis) [1, 3].

1.4 Modeling Hemostasis

The process of hemostasis is complex. A model is a way of conceptualizing and understanding a complicated system. A good model should be simple enough to understand, yet complicated enough to accurately reflect the process it was designed to represent. A "cascade" or "waterfall" model was a great advance in the understanding of coagulation and was originally proposed by two groups nearly simultaneously. This model was subsequently refined to the scheme described above as more was learned about the biochemistry of the coagulation factors. The cascade model of coagulation resulted from work that was aimed at elucidating the identity, function, and interactions of the individual procoagulant proteins. It accurately represents the overall structure of the coagulation process as a series of proteolytic reactions. Each protease cleaves and activates the subsequent protease in the series. The cascade model also included the recognition that anionic phospholipid, especially phosphatidylserine, was required for the assembly and optimal function of most of the coagulation complexes. This information was absolutely critical to understanding the coagulation reactions. However, the viewpoint that is implicit in this concept of coagulation is that the role of cells, especially platelets, is primarily to provide anionic phospholipid for coagulation complex assembly [32–35].

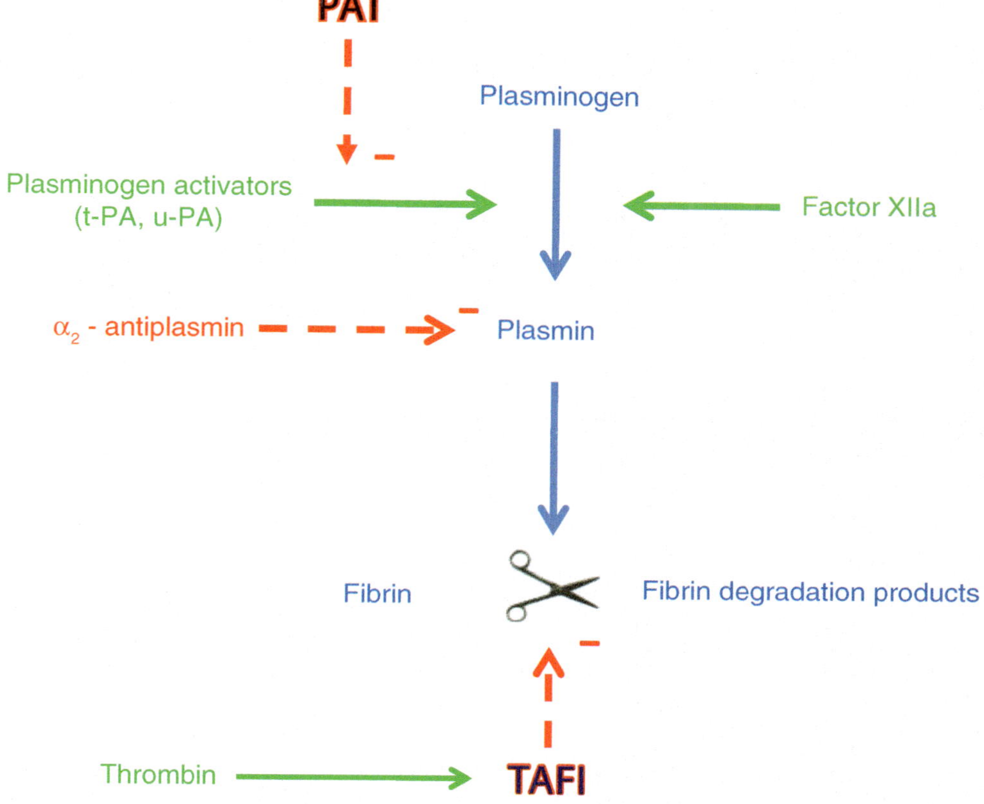

Fig. 1.4 Fibrinolytic system. Plasminogen is converted to plasmin by plasminogen activators, mainly tissue-type plasminogen activator (*t-PA*) or urokinase-type plasminogen activator (*u-PA*). Plasmin cleaves fibrin to fibrin degradation products. The system is strictly regulated by inhibitors such as α2-antiplasmin, plasminogen activator inhibitor (*PAI*), and thrombin-activatable fibrinolysis inhibitor (*TAFI*)

1.4.1 The Cell-Based Model of Hemostasis

This model views hemostasis as occurring in three (overlapping) phases. The *initiation* of coagulation takes place on TF-bearing cells, such as the fibroblast illustrated in Fig. 1.5. If the procoagulant stimulus is sufficiently strong, enough factors Xa, IXa, and thrombin are formed to successfully initiate the coagulation process. *Amplification* of the coagulant response occurs as the "action" moves from the TF-bearing cell to the platelet surface. The procoagulant stimulus is amplified as platelets adhere, are activated, and accumulate activated cofactors on their surfaces. Finally, in the *propagation* phase, the active proteases combine with their cofactors on the platelet surface – the site best adapted to generate hemostatic amounts of thrombin. The activity of the procoagulant complexes produces the burst of thrombin generation that results in fibrin polymerization (Fig. 1.5).

Inappropriate coagulation is prevented by several mechanisms. The inactivation and propagation steps are localized on different cell surfaces. The plasma protease inhibitors localize the reactions to cell surfaces by inhibiting active proteases that diffuse into the fluid phase. Finally, endothelial cells express active antithrombotic features that prevent coagulation from being initiated in the intact endothelium [36–41].

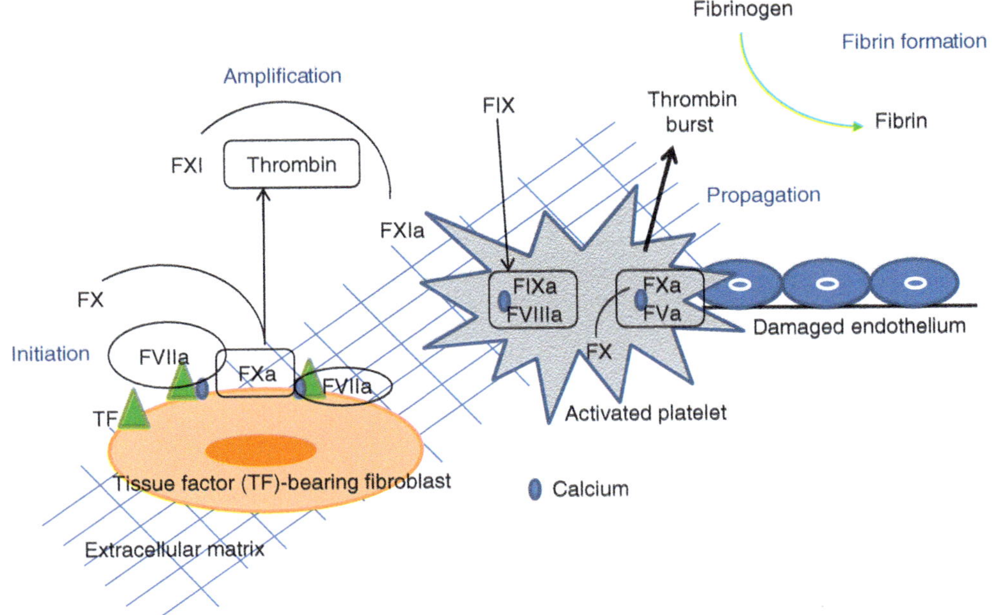

Fig. 1.5 Cell-based model of coagulation. Initiation phase: the complex of tissue factor (*TF*) and factor VII activates factor VII to factor VIIa. The complex of TF/factor VIIa activates factors IX and X, resulting in the generation of thrombin (IIa) by means of the complex of factor Xa and its cofactor, factor Va (activated by factor Xa). Amplification phase: thrombin activates platelets, which then present a thrombogenic surface. On this catalytic surface, other coagulation factors such as V and XI are activated, and factor VIII is released by its carrier, von Willebrand factor. Factor XIa activates factor IX. Activated platelets bind factors Va, VIIIa, and IXa on their surface. Propagation phase: factor VIIIa/IXa complex activates factor X on the catalytic platelet surfaces, and factors Xa/Va activate prothrombin (factor II), resulting in a massive generation of thrombin (factor IIa) – a "thrombin burst." This burst is able to convert fibrinogen to fibrin and, in addition, to activate factor XIII to XIIIa, which cross-links the fibrin fibers and stabilizes the fibrin clot

1.4.2 Initiation

TF is the primary physiologic initiator of coagulation. It is structurally unrelated to the rest of the coagulation proteins and is an integral membrane protein. Therefore, TF remains localized to the membrane of the cell in which it was synthesized. It is expressed on a variety of extravascular cells under normal conditions and can also be expressed by blood monocytes and endothelial cells in inflammatory states. There are now data suggesting that TF-containing membrane vesicles may bind to platelet surfaces in an evolving thrombus [42]. The source and physiologic role of such vesicles remain uncertain, but it is clear that normal circulating unactivated platelets neither contain nor express TF. It is important that the initiating and propagating steps are normally sequestered to different cell surfaces to limit the undesired activation of coagulation. Bringing factor VIIa/TF activity into close proximity to activated platelet surfaces is a key step in effective initiation of hemostatic coagulation (or thrombosis). During the process of hemostasis, a break in the vessel wall allows plasma to come into contact with TF-bearing extravascular cells. Factor VII in plasma binds tightly to cellular TF and is rapidly activated by coagulation and non-coagulation proteases. The factor VIIa/TF complex activates both factor X and factor IX. Factor Xa can activate plasma factor V, as can non-coagulation cellular proteases. The factor X activated by the factor VIIa/TF complex is rapidly inhibited by TFPI or ATIII if it leaves the protected environment of the cell surface. However, the factor Xa that remains on the cell surface can combine with factor Va to produce small amounts of thrombin which plays an important role in subsequently activating platelets and factor VIII during the amplification phase.

1.4.3 Amplification

Damage to the vasculature allows platelets as well as plasma to come into contact with extravascular tissues. Platelets adhere to extravascular matrix components at the site of injury. The process of binding to matrix proteins partially activates platelets, as well as localizing them near a site of TF exposure. Small amounts of thrombin generated on TF-bearing cells amplify the initial procoagulant signal by enhancing platelet adhesion, fully activating platelets and activating factors V, VIII, and XI. Thus, thrombin acts on the platelet surface to "set the stage" for procoagulant complex assembly. Thrombin is a potent platelet activator via its protease-activated receptors (PAR). During activation, platelets release factor V from alpha granules onto their surfaces in a partially activated form. Factor V(a) is then fully activated by thrombin or factor Xa. Some of the thrombin bound to non-PAR receptors, such as GPIb/IX, remains active and can activate other coagulation factors on the platelet surface. vWF/factor VIII binds to platelets and is efficiently cleaved by thrombin to activate factor VIII and release it from vWF. The factor VIIIa remains bound to the platelet surface. Now that the platelets have been activated and have activated cofactors V and VIII bound to their surfaces, assembly of the procoagulant complexes and large-scale thrombin generation begins.

1.4.4 Propagation

During the propagation phase, the "tenase" and "prothrombinase" complexes are assembled on the platelet surface, and large-scale thrombin generation takes place. Platelets express high affinity binding sites for factor IX(a), factor X(a), and factor XI. These receptors play important roles in coordinating assembly of the coagulation complexes. The "tenase" (factor VIIIa/IXa) complexes assemble when factor IXa reaches the platelet surface. The factor IXa can diffuse to platelet surfaces from its site of activation on TF-bearing cells, since it is not rapidly inhibited by ATIII or other plasma protease inhibitors. In addition, plasma factor XI can bind to activated platelets, facilitating its activation by thrombin. The factor XIa can then provide additional factor IXa directly on the platelet surface. The factor IXa/VIIIa complexes activate factor X on the platelet surface where the resulting factor Xa can move directly into a complex with its cofactor, factor Va, as illustrated in Fig. 1.3. The platelet surface factor Xa/Va complexes can now produce the burst of thrombin necessary to form a hemostatic fibrin clot.

1.5 Hemostatic Disorders

Bleeding can occur if there is abnormal platelet plug formation or reduced thrombin generation and subsequent fibrin clot formation at the site of vascular injury: disorders of primary and secondary hemostasis, respectively. Bleeding also can occur if the platelet or fibrin clot is prematurely degraded because of excessive fibrinolysis: disorder of tertiary hemostasis. The features distinguishing disorders of primary, secondary, and tertiary hemostasis are outlined in Table 1.2 [3, 43–46].

1.5.1 Disorders of Primary Hemostasis

Platelet plug formation, the first step in the arrest of bleeding at sites of injury, requires three key components: (1) an adequate number of functional platelets; (2) vWF, the molecular glue that mediates platelet adhesion to the damaged vessel wall; and (3) a normal blood vessel that constricts in response to injury. Because the platelet plug provides the first line of defense against bleeding, patients with these disorders often present with immediate bleeding after injury and petechiae, pinpoint hemorrhages, may be noted. In addition

Table 1.2 Comparison of the features of disorders of primary, secondary, or tertiary hemostasis

Features	Primary	Secondary	Tertiary
Components involved	Platelets, vWF, and vessel wall	Coagulation	Fibrinolytic factors
Site of bleeding	Skin and mucocutaneous and soft tissues	Muscles, joints, and deep tissues	Wounds and genitourinary tract
Physical findings	Petechiae and ecchymoses	Hematomas and hemarthroses	Hematuria and menorrhagia
Timing of bleeding	Immediate	Delayed	Delayed
Inheritance	Autosomal dominant	Autosomal or X-linked recessive	Autosomal recessive

vWF von Willebrand factor

they may manifest mucocutaneous bleeding (epistaxis, bleeding gums, hematochezia, excessive menstrual bleeding).

- Thrombocytopenia or congenital or acquired disorders of platelet function are common causes of bleeding. Thrombocytopenia can be the result of: (1) decreased production (failure, infiltration, or fibrosis of the bone marrow), (2) increased platelet destruction (immune, nonimmune mechanisms or consumption because of activation of coagulation, such as disseminated intravascular coagulation), and (3) abnormal distribution (platelet pooling in the spleen).
- Platelet function disorders include congenital disorders of platelet: (1) adhesion (von Willebrand disease and Bernard–Soulier syndrome), (2) aggregation (Glanzmann thrombasthenia), or (3) procoagulant activity (Scott syndrome) in which the platelets fail to support clotting factor complex assembly. Acquired disorders of platelet function can occur in patients taking drugs that impair platelet function, such as aspirin, nonsteroidal anti-inflammatory drugs, or in patients with uremia, paraproteins, or myelodysplastic or myeloproliferative disorders.
- Bleeding can also occur with inflammation (Henoch–Schonleinpurpura, vasculitis, systemic lupus erythematosus) or malformations of the blood vessels (hereditary hemorrhagic telangiectasia) or abnormalities of the connective tissue supporting the blood vessels (Marfan syndrome, Ehlers–Danlos syndrome).

Table 1.3 Disorders of secondary hemostasis

Components affected	Causes
Coagulation factors	Congenital deficiency, autoantibodies, increased consumption, drugs that attenuate thrombin generation or thrombin activity
Fibrinogen	1. Decreased production 2. Increased consumption or synthesis of an abnormal protein 3. Impaired fibrin polymerization because of fibrin(ogen) degradation products or paraproteins
Fibrin cross-linking	Congenital or acquired factor XIII deficiency

1.5.2 Disorders of Secondary Hemostasis

Secondary hemostasis depends on rapid generation of sufficient amounts of thrombin to generate a fibrin mesh that not only consolidates the platelet aggregates but is also stable enough to provide a barrier that prevents leakage of blood from the damaged vessel. Secondary hemostasis can be compromised by: (1) impaired thrombin generation because of congenital or acquired deficiencies of coagulation factors or cofactors or intake of drugs that inhibit one or more steps in the coagulation pathways, (2) congenital or acquired fibrinogen deficiency or dysfunction, and (3) impaired cross-linking of fibrinogen because of congenital or acquired deficiency of factor XIII (Table 1.3).

- Congenital inherited deficiencies of coagulation factors include hemophilia A and B, deficiencies of factor VIII and factor IX, respectively. Because of redundancy in the coagulation system, only patients with a factor VIII or factor IX level <1 % have severe disease characterized by spontaneous bleeding or bleeding with minimal trauma. Whereas those with factor levels between 1 and 5 % have an intermediate phenotype, patients with levels >5 % usually have mild disease and bleed only with trauma or surgery. Congenital deficiencies of prothrombin (factor II), factors V, VII, X, or XI or fibrinogen are less common causes of bleeding. In contrast, deficiencies of components of the contact pathway are not associated with bleeding. Acquired deficiencies of coagulation factors can result from decreased synthesis because of severe liver disease, vitamin K deficiency, or intake of drugs that can interfere with vitamin K metabolism, consumption because of excessive activation of coagulation (i.e., disseminated intravascular coagulation), or accelerated clearance caused by adsorption by paraproteins or amyloid or caused by autoantibodies that shorten the half-life or attenuate or abolish clotting factor activity.
- Congenital disorders of fibrinogen include absence or low levels of fibrinogen (afibrinogenemia and hypofibrinogenemia, respectively) or synthesis of a dysfunctional protein (dysfibrinogenemia). Acquired hypofibrinogenemia is thus a frequently observed problem in massively bleeding patients. Hiippala's pioneering work identified the clinical relevance of fibrinogen in massively bleeding patients. He studied 60 massively bleeding patients and measured platelet counts and coagulation factor levels. Based on "critical levels," or thresholds, which he took from a prominent coagulation textbook of the time, he observed that the fibrinogen threshold of 1.0 g/l was reached at 142 % of blood loss. Other parameters he monitored only fell below their respective thresholds considerably later: platelet count at 230 %, factor II at 201 %, factor V at 229 %, and factor VII at 236 % [31]. Others corroborated the finding that fibrinogen will be the first factor to reach critical levels in massive bleeding. A less frequent problem is acquired dysfibrinogenemia; this may occur in end-stage liver cirrhosis as a consequence of an altered glycosylation of fibrinogen molecules that interferes with the plasma assembly of fibrin monomers. The laboratory hallmark of this disorder is longer thrombin time and a reduced ratio of functional to antigenic fibrinogen tests (<0.7).
- Stabilization of fibrin requires cross-linking of the α- and γ-chains of adjacent fibrin monomers to yield a polymer that is resistant to premature breakdown. Factor XIIIa, a transglutaminase, performs this function by catalyzing the condensation of lysine residues on one chain with glutamic acid residues on another chain. Congenital or acquired deficiency of factor XIII can impair cross-linking, resulting in bleeding. The hallmarks of severe factor XIII deficiency include umbilical stump bleeding in the neonatal period, intracranial hemorrhage with little or no trauma, recurrent soft tissues hemorrhages, and recurrent spontaneous miscarriages in women.

1.5.3 Disorders of Tertiary Hemostasis

Tertiary hemostasis depends on the generation of plasmin, which degrades fibrin and restores blood flow in damaged vessels. Premature lysis of fibrin in hemostatic plugs can lead to bleeding; this can occur systematically or can be localized (Table 1.4). Systemic fibrinolysis that occurs in the absence of activation of coagulation, so-called primary hyperfibrinolysis, is rare but can occur with (1) inherited deficiency of PAI-1 or α_2-antiplasmin, the inhibitors of the plasminogen activators and plasmin, respectively; (2) advanced liver disease; and (3) snake bites. More com-

Table 1.4 Disorders of tertiary hemostasis

Components affected	Causes
Plasminogen activators	Increased t-PA or u-PA release in the genitourinary tract or other tissues
Plasmin	Deficiency of PAI-1 or α_2-antiplasmin, resulting in an increased plasmin concentration
Plasminogen activation	Enhanced plasminogen activation secondary to activation of coagulation by procoagulants, such as cancer cells, artificial surfaces, or snake venoms

PAI-1 plasminogen activator inhibitor 1, *t-PA* tissue plasminogen activator, *u-PA* urokinase-type plasminogen activator

monly, systemic hyperfibrinolysis is secondary to activation of coagulation by procoagulants, such as tissue factor (i.e., trauma, metastatic cancer) or artificial surfaces (i.e., in cardiopulmonary bypass or with cardiac heart devices). Examples of localized hyperfibrinolysis include menorrhagia or hematuria after prostatectomy triggered by excessive plasmin generation induced by the high concentration of t-PA and u-PA in the uterus and genitourinary tract, respectively.

1.6 Laboratory Testing of Hemostasis

Early on, clotting assays that were sensitive to components of the coagulation system were developed and were used to define the enzymatic pathways leading to clot formation. The two most important of these, the prothrombin time (PT) developed by Quick and the partial thromboplastin time (PTT) developed by Langdell et al. and later modified by Rapaport, continue to be used by coagulation laboratories throughout the world.

1.6.1 Sample Collection

The accuracy of hemostasis tests depends on the sample quality. Pre-analytical variables strongly influence hemostasis test results, and particular attention should be paid to blood collection, sample transportation, and storage. Blood collection must be as thorough as possible in order to obtain reliable results: samples should be obtained from a peripheral vein using an atraumatic puncture, away from any intravenous perfusion line. Tubes containing 3.2 % (0.109 M) sodium citrate are recommended as other anticoagulants may yield invalid results. These tubes must be carefully filled to predetermined levels in order to respect the blood-to-anticoagulant ratio and then gently inverted five times to mix them together. The first few milliliters of blood collected after the puncture should be discarded [47].

1.6.2 The PT and APTT

The PT is the in vitro clotting time measured after addition of PT reagent, which contains thromboplastin (phospholipids with tissue factor) and calcium to citrated plasma. The PT detects important deficiencies (and rarely inhibitors) of factors II, V, VII, X, and fibrinogen. The APTT is the in vitro clotting time measured after addition of calcium, an intrinsic pathway activator and the APTT reagent, which contains phospholipid (a platelet, also called "partial thromboplastin" as it lacks tissue factor) to plasma. The APTT detects bleeding disorders due to deficiencies of factors II, V, VIII, IX, X, XI, XII, and fibrinogen and inhibitors including lupus anticoagulant and therapeutic anticoagulants.

Prolongation of the PT and/or APTT only indicates a problem with the quantity and/or quality of single or multiple factors within the relevant pathways. Further specific coagulation tests are required to characterize the actual cause [48, 49].

Prolonged PT, associated with prolonged APTT, can be due to:

- Deficiencies in factors II, V, and X or fibrinogen
- Presence of factor inhibitors
- VKA treatment
- Direct thrombin inhibitor
- Vitamin K deficiency, malabsorption
- Liver disease
- Disseminated intravascular coagulation

- Dilutional coagulopathy
- Hemorrhage

Another assay, thrombin time (TT), detects an insufficient conversion of fibrinogen to fibrin upon stimulation by exogenous thrombin. This assay is used to diagnose an absence, deficiency, or dysfunction of fibrinogen but also factors inhibiting or disturbing the action of thrombin on fibrinogen, such as heparin or thrombin inhibitors [49].

The causes of prolonged PT and APTT, whether or not they predispose to bleeding, are summarized in Table 1.5.

Both the PT and the APTT are also subject to a number of important limitations [4]. These include:

1. Artifact due to sample collection or contamination (i.e., inadequate volume, difficult or traumatic phlebotomy causing coagulation activation, prolonged storage, and failure to adjust for high hematocrit causing an increase in citrate to plasma volume and artifactual prolongation of PT and APTT).
2. Derivation of normal range whereby 2.5 % of otherwise normal individuals are considered to be out with the upper limit of normal.
3. Intensity to clinically important bleeding disorders with normal PT and APTT (i.e., mild von Willebrand disease or hemophilia A, factor XIII and α_2-antiplasmin deficiency).
4. Detection of conditions not associated with bleeding, i.e., the lupus anticoagulant which can prolong both the PT and APTT, factor XII deficiency which prolongs APTT.
5. The same blood sample tested in different laboratories can give variable results; mainly due to differences in commercial reagents having different responsiveness to coagulation factor deficiencies and inhibitors and, to a lesser extent, the automated instrument.

1.6.3 Fibrinogen

Fibrinogen is the most abundant clotting protein in plasma (2–4 g/l). As mentioned above, fibrinogen abnormalities can be either qualitative (dysfibrinogenemia) or quantitative (total lack, afibrinogenemia, or partial deficiency, hypofibrinogenemia). Fibrinogen measurement is usually performed using a functional qualitative method (von Clauss chronometric assay); when a high concentration of thrombin is added to diluted plasma, the clotting time is proportional to the level of clottable fibrinogen. Fibrinogen activity levels can also be estimated using a prothrombin time-based kinetic assay, which is a rapid, inexpensive, automated assay, although less specific of fibrinogen activity. Immunoassays for fibrinogen antigen quantification are also available, but are not used for screening tests. These immunological assays measure the protein concentration rather than the functional activity of fibrinogen. Fibrinogen measurement is indicated in cases of apparent bleeding symptoms or in cases of suspicion of disseminated intravascular coagulation, hepatic insufficiency, or hyperfibrinolysis (Table 1.6) [49].

1.6.4 Platelet Count

Platelet count is measured using an automated counter, on blood drawn in EDTA anticoagulated samples. In cases of thrombocytopenia (<150 G/l), platelet clumps have to be considered; if clumps are identified, platelet count should be assessed on blood collected in citrate-anticoagulated tubes. The normal platelet count range for adults is 150–400 G/l. Platelet count, of course, does not evaluate their qualitative performance.

1.7 The Clinical Context for Testing

The PT and the APTT are among the most commonly requested laboratory assays. Typical indications include anticoagulant monitoring, routine perioperative screening, and bleeding. In addition to the limitations already described, the clinician needs to be aware of specific issues related to each of these clinical indications for testing [4, 50–52].

Table 1.5 Routine coagulation assays distinguishing defects related or not related to bleeding

PT	APTT	TT	Defect related to bleeding	Defect not related to bleeding
Normal	Normal	Normal	Factor XIII deficiency von Willebrand disease (mild)	
Prolonged	Normal	Normal	Factor VII deficiency Vitamin K antagonist/deficiency Liver disease	
Normal	Prolonged	Normal	Factor VIII deficiency (hemophilia A) Factor IX deficiency (hemophilia B) Factor XI deficiency von Willebrand disease Acquired hemophilia	Lupus anticoagulant Factor XII deficiency HMWK deficiency Prekallikrein deficiency
Prolonged	Prolonged	Normal	Factor II deficiency Factor V deficiency Factor X deficiency Combined deficiencies	
Normal/prolonged	Prolonged	Prolonged	Treatment with heparin, hirudin, argatroban	
Normal/prolonged	Normal/prolonged	Prolonged	Afibrinogenemia Hypofibrinogenemia Hemorrhagic dysfibrinogenemia Heparin-like defects Inhibitors of fibrin polymerization	Thrombotic dysfibrinogenemia

Adapted from Sucker and Zotz [8]
Bleeding with normal screening assay and platelet count results can be caused by mild von Willebrand disease, factor XIII deficiency, platelet defects or medication, low molecular weight heparin, hypothermia, acidosis, and hypocalcemia
Low platelet counts with normal screening assays are found in cases of pseudothrombocytopenia, idiopathic thrombocytopenic purpura, and hereditary platelet disorders (e.g., Bernard–Soulier syndrome, gray platelet syndrome)
Low platelet counts with prolonged APTT/PT are found in cases of disseminated intravascular coagulation, hemodilution, and liver disease

Table 1.6 Causes of abnormal fibrinogen levels

Reduced fibrinogen levels	Increased fibrinogen levels
Disseminated intravascular coagulation	Age
Dilutional coagulopathy	Pregnancy, oral contraception, postmenopausal
Liver disease with decreased synthesis	Inflammatory syndrome
Inherited deficiencies	Malignancy
Thrombolytic therapy	
High doses of corticosteroids	

Adapted from Bonhomme and Fontana [49]

1.7.1 Anticoagulant Monitoring

The problems associated with PT and APTT for monitoring vitamin K antagonists (VKA) and unfractionated heparin (UFH) relate mainly to the varying responsiveness of test reagent to single and/or multiple defect deficiencies and inhibitors. There is considerably variability in the PT thromboplastin reagent to the coagulation defect caused by VKA. Therefore, to allow PT results from different laboratories to be comparable, the calibration system that compares PT results to a WHO standard expressed as the International normalized ratio (INR) was developed. However, the INR is only valid for patients stabilized on VKA. This means that they are neither reliable nor reproducible for patients with prolonged PT for other reasons, i.e., liver disease, disseminated intravascular coagulation, and congenital factor deficiency. The INR is accurate only for values within 1.5–4.5 range, as only patient samples with INRs within this range were used for calibration. This means that INR values >4.5 may no longer observe the linear relationship demonstrated for those with INRs of 1.5–4.5. In contrast, no such standardization exists for APTT reagent, resulting in marked variation in the sensitivity of different reagents to coagulation factor deficiencies and inhibitors. To standardize the APTT used to monitor UFH use, individual laboratories should develop their own therapeutic range corresponding with accepted therapeutic UFH levels. The APTT is generally not sensitive to low molecular weight heparin. Although the new oral anticoagulants have been developed without the need for routine monitoring, these may be required in special circumstances (i.e., bleeding and perioperatively). All the new oral agents affect the APTT and PT but similar to VKA and UFH, different PT and APTT reagents show varying responsiveness. Results cannot be used for drug level monitoring or standardized across different laboratories.

1.7.2 Investigation of Bleeding

When the PT and APTT are used in the context of a patient with bleeding, the clinician should have a clear and systematic approach to the clinical and laboratory diagnosis. A detailed bleeding history including drug and family history, followed by careful examination can help to compartmentalize the hemostatic defect and direct laboratory investigations in a logical manner. However, bleeding histories in patients with mild bleeding disorders are challenging as many patients report mild bleeding symptoms, which are common in and overlap with the normal population. More recently, structured bleeding assessment tools to objectively quantify bleeding symptoms in a standardized manner have been developed. These bleeding assessment tools have shown with good negative predictive value, and their greatest clinical utility presently may lie in identifying patients who do not require further testing but validation for bleeding disorders outside von Willebrand disease is still needed. If the predictive value of the structured bleeding assessment tools is confirmed in prospective studies, this approach is likely to be extremely valuable in standardizing and improving the specificity of determining abnormal bleeding that requires further investigations.

1.7.3 Routine Preoperative Screening

Perhaps the most controversial indication for coagulation testing is in routine preoperative screening. Both the PT and APTT were designed as diagnostic tests to confirm the clinical suspicion of bleeding. This is different from their use as screening tests in otherwise healthy preoperative patients, where the prevalence of bleeding disorders is extremely low. Their use in populations with low pretest probability will invariably detect a high degree of normal results. Even when the results are abnormal, these are more likely to result from false positives or the detection of disorders not associated with bleeding, e.g., FXII deficiency and lupus anticoagulant, which have relatively high prevalence in an otherwise normal population. These false-positive results cause potentially unnecessary further investigations that generate delay, anxiety, cost, and harm. Additionally, 30–95 % of abnormal results from screening tests are either not documented or followed up, potentially increasing the risk of litigation. Similarly, given that the PT and APTT may not detect some clinically significant disorders, a normal result can give false reassurance. Accordingly, preoperative assessments should start with a structured bleeding history and coagulation screening performed only if there is a concern about a bleeding tendency or risk arising from the history. The majority of patients with congenital bleeding disorders are aware of their diagnosis either through a positive family history and/or a personal history of bleeding. Similarly, patients with acquired bleeding risk or disorders will give a personal history of bleeding, relevant comorbidity or anti-hemostatic medication. In the absence of an abnormal bleeding history, the utility of the coagulation screen in detecting previously unidentified individuals with a bleeding disorder is likely to be extremely low and should not be performed.

An ideal haemostatic assay would not only be capable of testing the overall function of the entire hemostatic system but also be able to define the qualitative and/or quantitative contribution of each compartment accurately and precisely. Until such a test is developed and validated for use, appropriate use of coagulation screens must involve consideration of the clinical context, disease prevalence, and laboratory limitations of the tests including performance characteristics, cost, and potential impact of false-positive and false-negative results.

References

1. White GC II, Marder VJ, Shulman S, Aird WC, Bennett JS (2013) Overview of basic coagulation and fibrinolysis. In: Marder VJ, Aird WC, Bennett JS, Schulman S, White GC II (eds) Hemostasis and thrombosis: basic principles and clinical practice. Lippincott, Williams & Wilkins, Philadelphia, pp 103–109
2. Davidson CJ, Tuddenham EG, McVey JH (2003) 450 million years of hemostasis. J Thromb Haemost 1:1487–1494
3. Weitz JI (2012) Overview of hemostasis and thrombosis. In: Hoffman R, Benz EJ Jr, Silberstein LE, Heslop HE, Witz JI, Anastasi J (eds) Hematology: basic principles and practice. Elsevier Saunders, Philadelphia, pp 1774–1783
4. Chee YL (2014) Coagulation. J R Coll Physicians Edinb 44:42–45
5. Versteeg HH, Heemskerk JWM, Levi M, Reitsma PH (2013) New fundamentals in hemostasis. Physiol Rev 93:327–358
6. Stassen JM, Arnout J, Deckmyn H (2004) The hemostatic system. Curr Med Chem 11:2245–2260
7. Arnout J, Hoylaerts MF, Lijnen HR (2006) Haemostasis. Handb Exp Pharmacol 176:1–41
8. Sucker C, Zotz RB (2015) The cell-based coagulation model. In: Marcucci CE, Schoettker P (eds) Perioperative hemostasis, 1st edn. Springer, Berlin, pp 3–11
9. Berndt MC, Metharom P, Andrews RK (2014) Primary haemostasis: newer insights. Haemophilia 20(Suppl 4):15–22
10. van Hinsbergh VW (2012) Endothelium: role in regulation and coagulation and inflammation. Semin Immunopathol 34:93–106
11. McFadyen JD, Kaplan ZS (2015) Platelets are not just for clots. Transfus Med Rev 29:110–119
12. Andrews RK, Berndt MC (2004) Platelet physiology and thrombosis. Thromb Res 114:447–453
13. Shattil SJ, Bennett JS (1981) Platelets and their membranes in hemostasis: physiology and pathophysiology. Ann Intern Med 94:108–118
14. Heemskerk JW, Bevers EM, Lindhout T (2002) Platelet activation and blood coagulation. Thromb Haemost 88:186–193
15. Lenting PJ, Pegon JN, Groot E, de Groot PG (2010) Regulation of von Willebrand factor-platelet interactions. Thromb Haemost 104:449–455
16. Broos K, Feys HB, De Meyer SF, Vanhoorelbeke K, Deckmyn H (2011) Platelets at work in primary hemostasis. Blood Rev 25:155–167
17. Hawiger J (1987) Formation and regulation of platelet and fibrin hemostatic plug. Hum Pathol 18:111–122

18. Smith SA, Travers RJ, Morrissey JH (2015) How it all starts: initiation of the clotting cascade. Crit Rev Biochem Mol Biol 28:1–11
19. Hoffman M, Pawlinski R (2014) Hemostasis: old system, new players, new directions. Thromb Res 133(Suppl 1):S1–S2
20. Brass LF, Wannemacher KM, Ma P, Stalker TJ (2011) Regulating thrombus growth and stability to achieve an optimal response to injury. J Thromb Haemost 9(Suppl 1):66–75
21. Mackman N, Tilley RE, Key NS (2007) Role of the extrinsic pathway of blood coagulation in hemostasis and thrombosis. Arterioscler Thromb Vasc Biol 27:1687–1693
22. Nemerson Y (1987) Tissue factor and the initiation of blood coagulation. Adv Exp Med Biol 214:83–94
23. Davie EW, Kulman JD (2006) An overview of the structure and function of thrombin. Semin Thromb Hemost 32(Suppl 1):3–15
24. Laurens N, Koolwijk P, de Maat MP (2006) Fibrin structure and wound healing. J Thromb Haemost 4:932–939
25. Hoppe B (2014) Fibrinogen and factor XIII at the intersection of coagulation, fibrinolysis and inflammation. Thromb Haemost 112:649–658
26. Weisel JW, Litvinov RI (2013) Mechanisms of fibrin polymerization and clinical implications. Blood 121:1712–1719
27. Saldanha C (2013) Fibrinogen interaction with the red blood cell membrane. Clin Hemorheol Microcirc 53:39–44
28. Levy JH, Szlam F, Tanaka KA, Sniecienski RM (2012) Fibrinogen and hemostasis: a primary hemostatic target for the management of acquired bleeding. Anesth Analg 114:261–274
29. Lowe GD, Rumley A, Mackie IJ (2004) Plasma fibrinogen. Ann Clin Biochem 41:430–440
30. Asmis LM (2015) Coagulation factor concentrates. In: Marcucci CE, Schoettker P (eds) Perioperative hemostasis. Springer, Berlin, pp 177–204
31. Hiippala ST, Myllyla GJ, Vahtera EM (1995) Hemostatic factors and replacement of major blood loss with plasma-poor red cell concentrates. Anesth Analg 81:360–365
32. Izaguirre Avila R (2005) The centennial of blood coagulation doctrine. Arch Cardiol Mex 75(Suppl 3):118–129
33. MacFarlane RG (1964) An enzyme cascade in the blood clotting mechanism, and its function as a biochemical amplifier. Nature 202:498–499
34. Douglas AS (1999) Historical review: coagulation history. Oxford 1951–1953. Br J Haematol 107:22–32
35. Davie EW, Ratnoff OD (1964) Waterfall sequence for intrinsic blood clotting. Science 145:1310–1312
36. Hoffman M, Monroe DM 3rd (2001) A cell-based model of hemostasis. Thromb Haemost 85:958–965
37. McMichael M (2012) New models of hemostasis. Top Companion Anim Med 27:40–45
38. Walsh PN (2004) Platelet coagulation-protein interactions. Semin Thromb Hemost 30:461–471
39. Barkhan P, Silver MJ, Da Costa PB, Tocantins LM (1958) Phosphatidyl serine and blood coagulation. Nature 182:1031–1032
40. Dahlback B, Villoutreix BO (2005) Regulation of blood coagulation by the protein C anticoagulant pathway: novel insights into structure-function relationships and molecular recognition. Arterioscler Thromb Vasc Biol 25:1311–1320
41. Bombeli T, Mueller M, Haeberli A (1997) Anticoagulant properties of the vascular endothelium. Thromb Haemost 77:408–423
42. Owens AP 3rd, Mackman N (2011) Microparticles in hemostasis and thrombosis. Circ Res 108:1284–1297
43. Eby C (2009) Pathogenesis and management of bleeding and thrombosis in plasma cell dyscrasias. Br J Haematol 145:151–163
44. de Maat MP, Verschuur M (2005) Fibrinogen heterogeneity: inherited and non-inherited. Curr Opin Hematol 12:377–383
45. Goodnight SH Jr, Hathaway WE (2001) Disorders of hemostasis and thrombosis, a clinical guide. McGraw-Hill, New York
46. Nurden A, Nurden P (2011) Advances in our understanding of the molecular basis of disorders of platelet function. J Thromb Haemost 9(Suppl 1):76–91
47. Lippi G, Salvagno GL, Montagnana M, Lima-Oliveira G, Guidi GC, Favaloro EJ (2012) Quality standards for sample collection in coagulation testing. Semin Thromb Hemost 38:565–575
48. Kamal AH, Tefferi A, Pruthi RK (2007) How to interpret and pursue an abnormal prothrombin time, activated partial thromboplastin time, and bleeding time in adults. Mayo Clin Proc 82:864–873
49. Bonhomme F, Fontana P (2015) Laboratory testing of hemostasis. In: Marcucci CE, Schoettker P (eds) Perioperative hemostasis. Springer, Berlin, pp 13–24
50. Marlar RA (2013) Hemostasis test validation, performance, and reference intervals: international recommendations and guidelines. In: Kitchen S, Olson D, Preston FE (eds) Quality in laboratory hemostasis and thrombosis. Wiley Blackwell, Oxford, pp 12–21
51. Haas T, Fries D, Tanaka KA, Asmis L, Curry NS, Schöchl H (2015) Usefulness of standard plasma coagulation tests in the management of perioperative coagulopathic bleeding: is there any evidence? Br J Anaesth 114:217–224
52. Watson HG, Greaves M (2008) Can we predict bleeding? Semin Thromb Hemost 34:97–103

General Aspects of Viscoelastic Tests

2

Alberto Grassetto, Rita Paniccia,
and Gianni Biancofiore

2.1 Introduction

In recent years, a growing interest toward point-of-care tests (POCTs) and haemostasis has resulted in many scientific publications on viscoelastic tests (VETs) and, particularly, on thromboelastography and thromboelastometry. Although the development of thromboelastography took place at the end of the 1940s, only in the last decade its potential has been finally expressed.

One reason for this renewed popularity was the introduction in the market of new devices more suitable to be used on the "field", as the definition of point of care implies itself. Then, we assisted to the migration of those instruments from the laboratory to the intensive care unit and operating room, in order to achieve rapid information about the haemostatic asset, especially during bleeding emergencies.

Standard laboratory exams, like prothrombin time (PT) and activated partial thromboplastin time (aPTT), have generally too long turnaround times to be really useful when minutes count and fast decisions are needed. Moreover, they have never been validated for addressing treatment of perioperative bleeding [1]. Some initial results of thromboelastography and thromboelastometry are available in few minutes, giving the opportunity to make decisions in "real time" [2].

Another important difference between VETs and standard coagulation assays is that they can be performed using whole blood, thus giving a more complete picture of haemostasis. It is clear that any test that misses the interaction with platelet, fibrinogen, FXIII and blood cells, is far from answering a simple however important question: does this clot plug?

PT and PTT substantially give one piece of information that is whether the thrombin generation has started, however, no information of what happens afterwards. It has been said that the value of PT or PTT is something like opening a book fable to a child, reading the first lines "Once upon a time…" and then closing the book. VETs give an "in vitro" picture of the growth of the clot and a measure of its stability until its physiological or pathological lysis. According to some authors, thromboelastography is better than PT, aPTT and activated clotting time (ACT) in detecting clotting abnormalities after hypothermia, hemorrhagic shock and resuscitation [3]; for others, it may even replace conventional coagulation exams in the emergency department when "time is blood" [4].

A. Grassetto, MD (✉)
UOC Anestesia e Rianimazione, Dipartimento Emergenza Urgenza, Ospedale dell'Angelo di Mestre, Venice, Italy
e-mail: alberto.grassetto@gmail.com

R. Paniccia, MSc
Department of Experimental and Clinical Medicine, University of Florence, Careggi University Hospital, Florence, Italy

G. Biancofiore, MD
Liver Transplant Anaesthesia and Critical Care, Azienda Ospedaliera Universitaria Pisana, Pisa, Italy

M. Ranucci, P. Simioni (eds.), *Point-of-Care Tests for Severe Hemorrhage: A Manual for Diagnosis and Treatment*, DOI 10.1007/978-3-319-24795-3_2

Moreover, the reader should consider that PT and aPTT fundamentally represent tests to monitor anticoagulation (warfarin and heparin, respectively) and isolated congenital or acquired coagulation deficits. However, they have been never validated to predict the risk of bleeding or to guide transfusions. Substantially, we have continued to use them on a routine basis, due to the lack of something better. Paradigmatic is the case of the cirrhotic patients in which PT doesn't reflect the risk of bleeding, because it only measures the activity of the procoagulants and not of the anticoagulants, whose activity is reduced too, producing a sort of equilibrium at a lower level [5].

On the other hand, the reader should not forget that VETs, as well as all the coagulation tests we use, do not represent exactly what really happens "in vivo". Activation of coagulation is done using reagents that speed the reaction, and the whole picture misses the contribution of important components like endothelium and the shear stress.

Finally, the results of these tests should be always correlated with the clinical situations, bearing clearly in mind that numbers must always be interpreted.

2.2 Thromboelastography and Thromboelastometry

2.2.1 How They Work

Blood clot may be ideally considered as a Maxwell body, thus with viscous and elastic properties. Thromboelastography and thromboelastometry are based on the same concept, described by Hartert in 1948, and measure the "shear modulus" of the clot, which represents its tendency to deform by the action of opposing forces. The shear modulus is defined as the ratio between shear stress and shear strain. Every material has its own typical shear modulus; however, in the case of blood, this is not constant and changes along with the process of clotting. The SI unit (Système International d'Unitès) of shear modulus is dyne/cm^2 (gigapascal).

In the classical thromboelastography (TEG, Haemoscope Corp., Niles, IL), a blood sample is injected in a heated cylindrical sample cup which rotates slowly back and forth through an arc of 4.45°, every 5 s, along the longitudinal axis. A free pin, suspended on a wire, is immersed in the blood and, as long as the coagulation process begins, it detects the variation of strength between the pin and the cup's wall (Fig. 2.1). This measure is electromechanically transduced and converted into the classical thromboelastographic tracing (Fig. 2.2).

In ROTEM (TEM International GmbH, Munich, Germany), the mechanism is the opposite, as it is the pin which moves through an arc of 4.75°, while the cup is fixed. As the coagulation starts and the first strands of fibrin are formed, the pin's free rotation is restricted proportionally to the increasing strength of the clot (Fig. 2.1). This reduction of movement is detected by an optical system and the generated electrical signal expressed as a graphical representation (Fig. 2.2).

Table 2.1 summarises the main principal features of TEG and ROTEM.

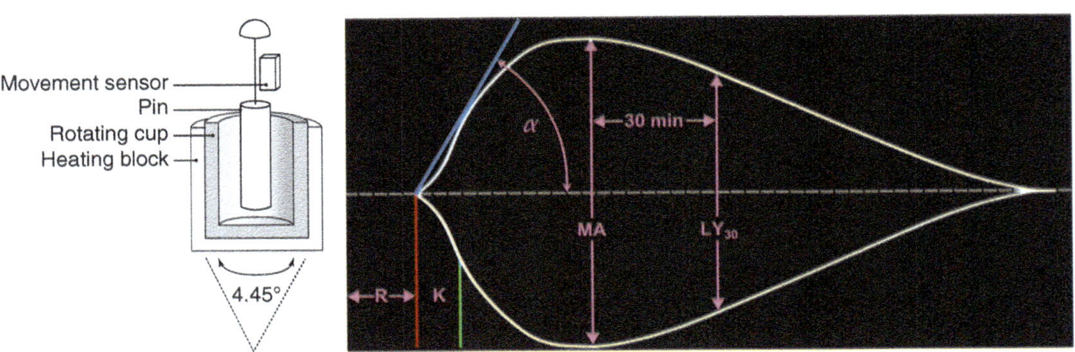

Fig. 2.1 TEG mechanism and curve

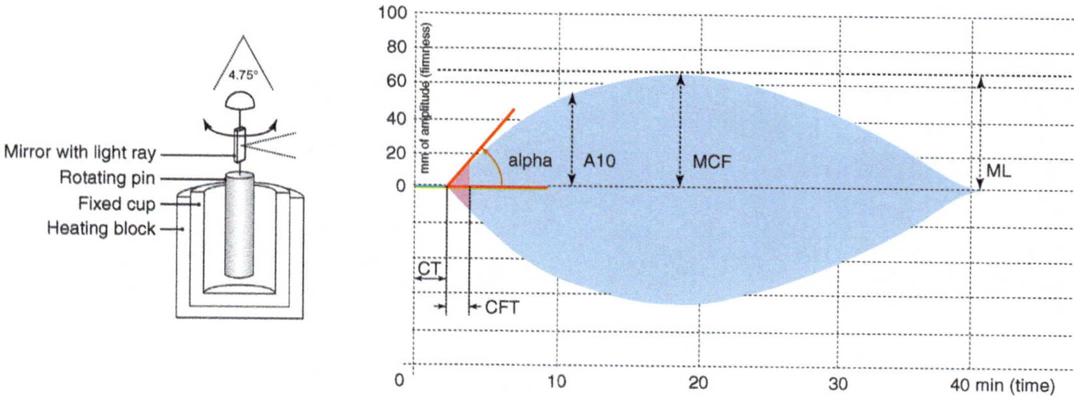

Fig. 2.2 ROTEM mechanism and curve

Table 2.1 Tecnical features of TEG and ROTEM

	TEG	ROTEM
Manufacturer	Haemoscope Corp., Niles, IL	Tem International, Munich, Germany
Description	2-channel unit, separate computer and printer, barcode (optional), network remote connection	4-channel unit, integrated pc, touch screen monitor, separated printer, barcode, network remote connection
Mechanism	Torsion wire connected by spring to electromechanic transducer	Rotating pin connected to an optical detector
Pipettes/blood sample	Manual pipettes (automatic optional)/340 μL per test, citrated or native blood	Automatic pipette, step-by-step procedure through graphic user interface/300 μL, citrated or native blood (if NATEM used)
Reagents/assays	Single-use vials/Kaolin, Rapid-TEG®, Functional Fibrinogen. Heparinase cuvette for heparin effect. Platelet mapping for platelet function analysis	Single-use or liquid multi-use vials/ EXTEM, INTEM, FIBTEM, HEPTEM, APTEM. Optional module ROTEM® *platelet* for platelet function analysis
Temperature	Direct measure for every channel, possibility to set	Possibility to set on service panel
Calibration/quality controls	12/24 h quality check (level positioning and machine check) QC weekly quality control (level I and/or Level II)	Constantly running QC test, weekly formal control (ROTROL N or ROTROL P)
Marks/approbation	CE/FDA	CE/FDA

2.2.2 TEG and ROTEM Parameters

The TEG and ROTEM tracings represent a picture which starts from the very beginning of clot formation throughout its lysis. Measured parameters and their meaning are summarised in Table 2.2.

2.2.3 The Reagents

In both TEG and ROTEM, the blood sample can be tested without any reagent, the so-called native, or after recalcification if the sample is taken in a citrate tube. Even the presence of citrate may influence the results; however, it is the most suitable way to test the sample if it cannot be immediately processed. Storage in a citrate tube has shown enough stability of the sample up to 2 h at least [6]. Repeated sampling from the same tube may result in activation of platelets as well as coagulation factors and therefore should be avoided if possible [7]. In general, VETs use different kind of activators to speed up the initiation of coagulation or to focus on some

Table 2.2 Main parameters measured on TEG and ROTEM and their meanings

	TEG	ROTEM	Meaning
Time to reach to 2 mm amplitude	*R* – reaction time	CT – clotting time	Time needed for initiation of clotting, thrombin generation, start of fibrinogen polymerisation
Time to reach 20 mm amplitude	*K*	CFT – clot formation time	Estimation of clot growth kinetic by fibrin polymerisation, thrombocytes and FXIII
Angle formed by tangent line from baseline to 20 mm	*α*	*α*	Same meaning as *K* and CFT
Amplitude at 10–20 min	*not available*	A10–A20	Estimation of clot strength at fixed times, strongly correlated with MCF
Higher amplitude reached	MA – maximum amplitude	MCF – maximum clot firmness	Final clot strength given by its stabilisation
Lysis %	LY-30	ML – maximum lysis	Measure of fibrinolysis

aspects of the hemostatic process (e.g. contribution of fibrinogen or platelets). Each device has its panel of reagents, and a comparative analyses can be done running several tests in parallel.

2.2.3.1 ROTEM Reagents

EXTEM: this assay explores the extrinsic coagulation pathway and use thromboplastin (tissue factor) as activator.

INTEM: this assay explores the intrinsic coagulation pathway and use ellagic acid as activator.

FIBTEM: this assay explores the contribution of fibrinogen on the clot amplitude and use tissue factor as activator, the same of EXTEM, and cytochalasin D to block platelets' function.

HEPTEM: this assay is the same as INTEM, but has heparinase inside. It can be used to confirm a heparin effect when compared to INTEM.

APTEM: this assay is the same as EXTEM, but has an antifibrinolytic, aprotinin, inside. It can be used to confirm a fibrinolysis when compared to EXTEM.

ECATEM: this assay is sensitive for thrombin inhibitors: it contains ecarin, a purified metalloprotease from *Echis carinatus*.

2.2.3.2 TEG Reagents

KAOLIN: this assay explores the intrinsic coagulation pathway and use kaolin as activator.

RAPID-TEG: this assay uses tissue factor and kaolin as activator, thus accelerating the coagulation initiation for quicker results.

FF (functional fibrinogen): this assay explores the contribution of fibrinogen on the clot amplitude and use abciximab to block platelet function.

HEPARINASE: in TEG, a heparin effect can be confirmed or excluded using not properly a reagent but a cuvette with heparinase. Then, all the assays can be run with or without a heparinase cuvette.

2.3 Interpretation of TEG and ROTEM Tracings

Generally, a prolongation of CT/R is due to a coagulation initiation defect, while a reduced MCF/MA is due to a substrate deficit (e.g. fibrinogen, platelets, FXIII). On the contrary, a shortened CT/R or increased MA/MCF is due to an acceleration of coagulation initiation or increased substrates levels, respectively. CFT/K express the kinetic of clot formation and fundamentally depend on substrates, mainly fibrinogen and platelets. Clot lysis is a physiological phenomenon, but, when enhanced above normal levels, it can severely impair clot stability and then the hemostatic competence. Hypocoagulable and hypercoagulable features of thromboelastographic tracings are summarised in Table 2.3.

CT/R are affected by factor activity, so they are sensitive to acquired or inherited factor deficit and to anticoagulation drugs (see next paragraph for details) and better represent the balance

Table 2.3 Typical features of hypo and hypercoagulable phenotypes

	Hypercoagulable	Hypocoagulable
Clotting time	↓	↑
Clot strength	↑	↓
Rate of clot formation	↑	↓
Lysis	=	↑

between procoagulant and anticoagulant factor activity than PT and aPTT. In vitro studies showed that after 30 % hemodilution with saline, PT and aPTT tend to prolong, while CT/R shorten, probably because the dilution of anticoagulants activity has, at least initially, the major weight; further hemodilution obviously produces a CT/R prolongation [8]. Moreover, being functional assays, thromboelastometry and thromboelastography are sensitive not only to quantitative, but also to qualitative alterations of factors and substrates. For example, colloids interfere with coagulation initiation and fibrinogen polymerisation, so they typically prolong CT/R and reduce MCF/MA even after minor hemodilution [9]. Other pre-analytical and analytical factors that influence CT/R and MCF/MA are discussed in the next paragraph.

ROTEM and TEG curves should be considered as a whole: despite a normal amplitude, a prolongation of CT/R will determine itself a hemostatic impairment; the same happens when clotting time is normal but amplitude is reduced.

Evaluation of MCF generally needs time, so, routinely, for clinical purpose, amplitude at 10 min (A10) is considered, given the good correlation between them.

The use of different reagents and multiple channels enables the identification of different pathways and specific contributors to the thromboelastometric/thromboelastographic tracing. Table 2.4 summarises the available tests and reference ranges.

2.3.1 Extrinsic/Intrinsic Pathways

With ROTEM, defects of extrinsic or intrinsic pathways may be evaluated through EXTEM and INTEM, respectively. An isolated prolongation of CT in INTEM may subtend an intrinsic pathway defect (factors XII, XI, IX, VIII), while an isolated prolongation of CT in EXTEM may subtend an extrinsic pathway defect (factor VII plus tissue factor). If CT is prolonged in both tests, a common pathway coagulation deficit (factors X-V-II) or a multifactorial deficit has to be considered.

2.3.2 Heparin Effect

Both ROTEM and TEG can discriminate if a CT or R prolongation is due to heparin. This aspect can be particularly useful to confirm a complete heparin reversal after protamine administration. When a "heparin effect" is suspected, a double test is performed with ROTEM: INTEM and HEPTEM. For a heparin concentration of 0.3 U/mL, CT in INTEM is prolonged over 240 s and other parameters are not affected. Above a concentration of 1 U/mL, CT is usually longer than 15 min. If CT in INTEM is longer than in HEPTEM, a heparin effect can be confirmed, while, if no difference exists, a heparin effect can be excluded. It should be noted that one-shot reagents r-EXTEM and r-FIBTEM, differently from the same liquid reagents, are heparin sensitive, so before performing these tests, a heparin effect should be excluded or reversed. With TEG, a heparinase cuvette is used, comparing the result with a test performed without heparinase. Figures 2.3 and 2.4 show how heparin influences ROTEM and TEG curves.

2.3.3 Fibrinogen Contribution to Clot Firmness

Being the main contributor to clot firmness, specific tests to evaluate fibrinogen are available, helping to differentiate the causes of altered clot strength. FIBTEM and FF inhibit platelet function giving a picture of the fibrin component of the clot (see next paragraph for details). Moreover, many studies showed that FIBTEM and FF better reflect the hemostatic impairment than Clauss

Table 2.4 Commercially available tests for TEG and ROTEM and reference ranges

Device	Activator/inhibitor	Effect
TEG	Kaolin	Intrinsic activator: coagulation time (*r*-value) is increased by aprotinin, sensitive to heparin
	Kaolin + heparinase	Cup coated with heparinase; neutralises heparin effects
	Kaolin + tissue factor	r-TEG yields results 50 % faster than conventional TEG
	Activator F (reptilase-factor XIIIa mixture); adenosine diphosphate, arachidonic acid	Platelet mapping: platelet functioning. Measures clot strength and MA. Sensitive to diminution in platelet function in response to aspirin and clopidogrel
	Lyophilized tissue factor and platelet inhibitor (abciximab)	Functional fibrinogen level. Reagent inhibits GPIIb/IIa receptors on platelets, eliminating their contribution to clot strength (MA) and reflecting functional fibrinogen activity

Reference values for TEG

	r- time reaction time (min)	*K* time (min)	α-angle	MA maximum amplitude (mm)	LY lysis (%)
Whole blood	4–8 min	1–4 min	47–74°	55–73 mm	
Citrated blood + kaolin	3–8 min	1–3 min	55–78°	51–69 mm	
r-TEG	0–1 min	1–2 min	66–82°	54–72	0.0–7.5
Citrated blood + kaolin and heparinase	Comparison with kaolin test: a shortening in CT in kaolin and heparinase indicates the presence of heparin or heparin-like substances				

Device	Activator/inhibitor	Effect
ROTEM	EXTEM (tissue factor)	Extrinsic activator (tissue factor); not affected by aprotinin, sensitive to heparin; fast assessment of clot formation
	INTEM (contact activator)	Intrinsic activator; sensitive to heparin; assessment of clot formation and fibrin polymerisation
	HEPTEM (contact activator + heparinase)	Neutralises heparin effects; specific detection of heparin
	FIBTEM (tissue factor + platelet antagonist cytochalasin D)	Pharmacologic inactivation of platelet cytoskeleton by cytochalasin D; FIBTEM represents the strength of the clot under platelet inhibition
	APTEM (tissue factor + aprotinin)	Inhibition of premature lysis by the addition of aprotinin; fast detection of fibrinolysis when compared at the same time to EXTEM
	ECATEM (ecarin)	Used in the management of direct thrombin inhibitors

Reference ranges for ROTEM

	CT Clotting time (s)	CFT Clot formation time (s)	A 10 Amplitude 10 min after CT (mm)	MCF Maximum clot firmness (mm)	ML Maximum lysis (% of MCF)
INTEM	100–240 s	30–110 s	44–66	50–72 mm	<15 %
EXTEM	38–79 s	34–159 s	43–65	50–72 mm	<15 %
FIBTEM			8–24	9–25 mm	
APTEM	Comparison with EXTEM: a stable MCF confirms hyperfibrinolysis				
HEPTEM	Comparison with INTEM: a shortening in HEPTEM CT indicates the presence of heparin or heparin-like substances				

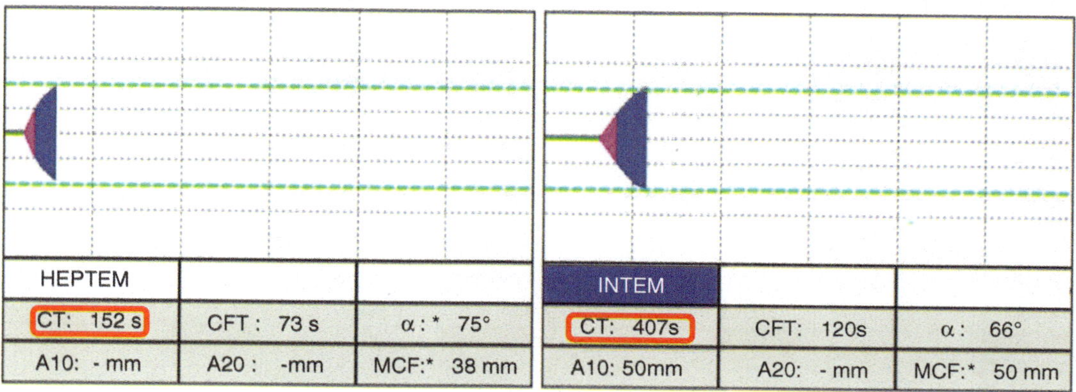

Fig. 2.3 Heparin effect on ROTEM. CT INTEM is prolonged, but normalised in HEPTEM

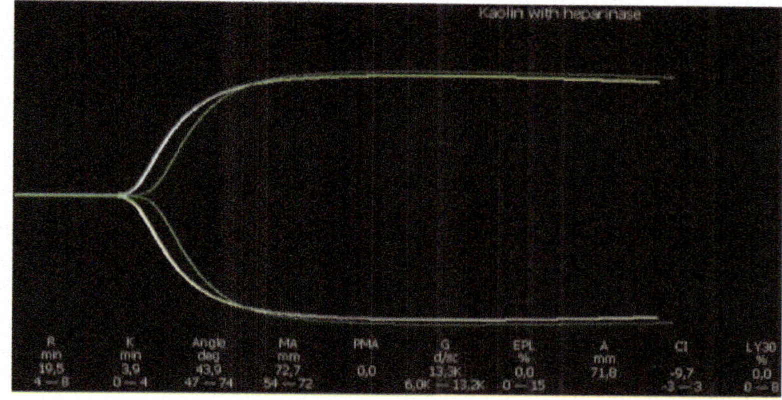

Fig. 2.4 Heparin effect on TEG. *R* is normalised in Kaolin with heparinase

fibrinogen [10]. Fibrinogen contribution affects primarily clot firmness, but when fibrinogen levels are very low also a prolongation of clotting time may be seen (as it happens with PT and aPTT that are unreliable under a fibrinogen concentration below 1 g/L). Some studies showed how fibrinogen administration produces an exponential increase on clot firmness and can eventually compensate a platelet deficit [11]. Figure 2.5 shows all the possible combinations of EXTEM/FIBTEM tracings and their meaning.

2.3.4 Hyperfibrinolysis

Hyperfibrinolysis is defined as a premature, supraphysiological lysis of the clot. With ROTEM/TEG, lysis is usually defined as the ratio between MCF/MA and the amplitude at 30 or 60 min and normal values are below 7.5 % or 15 %, respectively. Hyperfibrinolysis was shown to correlate with mortality in bleeding patients in many different settings, especially in trauma where it is included in the mechanism of trauma-induced coagulopathy [12]. ROTEM/TEG hyperfibrinolysis should be intended as a systemic type of fibrinolysis and its absence does not exclude that a local hyperfibrinolysis, not identifiable by ROTEM/TEG, may play a role in some situations. APTEM test is usually performed to confirm hyperfibrinolysis. Figures 2.6 and 2.7 show typical hyperfibrinolysis tracings on ROTEM and TEG, respectively.

a
EXTEM
FIBTEM
b
EXTEM
FIBTEM
c
EXTEM
FIBTEM
d
EXTEM S
FIBTEM S
e
EXTEM
FIBTEM
f
EXTEM
FIBTEM

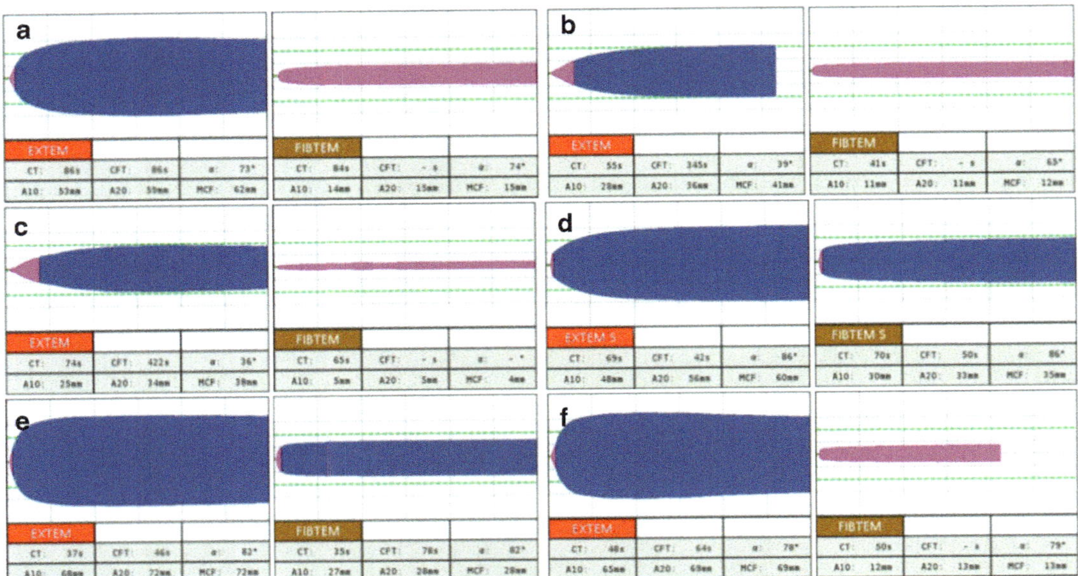

Fig. 2.5 (**a**) Normal profile, (**b**) platelet deficit, (**c**) fibrinogen and platelet deficit, (**d**) compensated platelet deficit, (**e**) hyperfibrinogenemia (pregnancy), (**f**) thrombocytosis

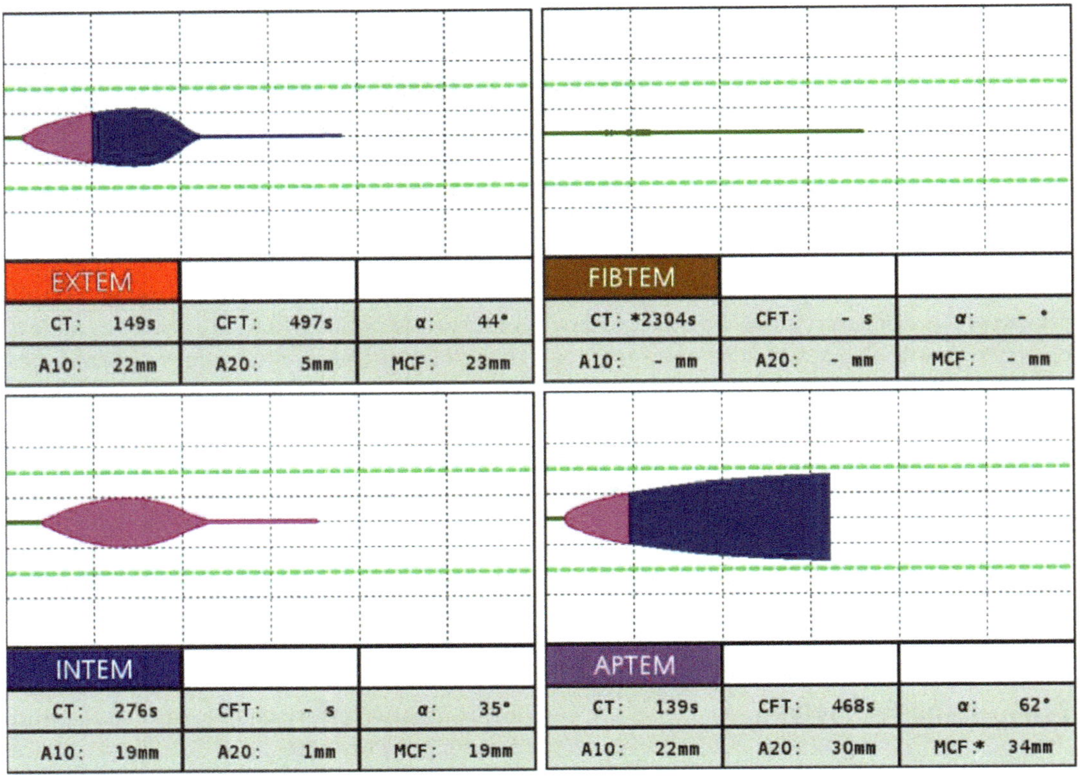

EXTEM
CT: 149s
CFT: 497s
α: 44°
A10: 22mm
A20: 5mm
MCF: 23mm
FIBTEM
CT: *2304s
CFT: - s
α: - °
A10: - mm
A20: - mm
MCF: - mm
INTEM
CT: 276s
CFT: - s
α: 35°
A10: 19mm
A20: 1mm
MCF: 19mm
APTEM
CT: 139s
CFT: 468s
α: 62°
A10: 22mm
A20: 30mm
MCF:* 34mm

Fig. 2.6 ROTEM – fulminant hyperfibrinolysis

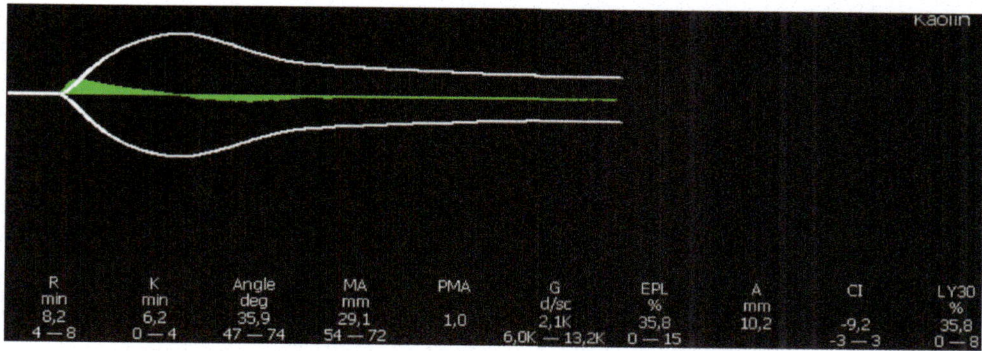

Fig. 2.7 TEG – hyperfibrinolysis

2.4 Substantial Differences between TEG and ROTEM and Limits of Their Measurement

Despite the fact that TEG and ROTEM are based on the same concept, we have just mentioned that their results are not interchangeable. It does not depend only on mechanical differences of the instruments, but also on the different mechanism of action of reagents [13]. In one study regarding trauma patients, the best agreement between the two machines was found to be on the MA/MCF variable, while R/CT showed poor correlation [14]. The same was noted in cardiac surgery [15].

The main difference between the two systems is that ROTEM uses stronger activators than classical TEG with kaolin: ellagic acid (INTEM) and tissue factor (EXTEM) are stronger in initiating the coagulation process than kaolin, thus ROTEM tracing may theoretically be less sensitive to detect the effect of low molecular weight heparins, anticoagulants, and antiplatelet drugs. However, these differences may also subtend a different philosophy, including the aim of obtaining quicker results. The introduction of Rapid-TEG has represented the TEG answer to this need, and one study in trauma patients has reported a strong correlation between rapid thromboelastography and conventional thromboelastography in terms of overall clot strength [16].

The contribution of fibrinogen on clot firmness is measured in TEG and ROTEM by FF (functional fibrinogen) and by FIBTEM, respectively. FF uses abciximab, a glycoprotein IIb/IIIa inhibitor to blunt the platelet contribution to clot firmness; FIBTEM is based on cytochalasin D, a strong inhibitor of platelet cytoskeleton, to achieve the same effect.

FF MA values have been reported to be generally higher than FIBTEM MCF, and TEG functional fibrinogen may lead to an overestimation of fibrinogen levels [17]. This depends principally on the different capacity of the two reagents to block platelets, as well as on the intrinsic difference between the two instruments. Lang and co-workers have reported lower whole-blood maximum clot elasticity when using both agents compared with either agent alone [18]. Similarly, other studies have reported that a new experimental ROTEM assay, FIBTEM PLUS, which contains cytochalasin D and tirofiban, provides a greater inhibition of platelets than FIBTEM; however, this effect is not significant on patients with low platelet count [19]. From a clinical point of view, a proper platelet inhibition ensures a more accurate assessment of the fibrinogen contribution to clot firmness and therefore the need for fibrinogen supplementation therapy [20].

An important consideration is that nor ROTEM nor TEG gives information of primary haemostasis; thus, defects of primary haemostasis (e.g. von Willebrand disease) cannot be identified by these instruments. Moreover, the reagents used induce a burst of thrombin generation, therefore activating the platelets downstream via PAR1 and PAR4 receptors, overcoming and masking an eventual platelet inhibition. That is the reason why ROTEM and TEG have a poor sensitivity for aspirin and thienopyridine effects and a low one for GPIIb/IIIa receptor antagonists [21].

Regarding the anticoagulant activity detection, two similar studies on vitamin K antagonist-treated patients monitored with TEG and ROTEM have shown a prolongation tendency of R and CT however remaining within the normal reference range in some patients, despite an INR at therapeutic level [22, 23]. Conversely, at supratherapeutic anticoagulant, levels both TEG/ROTEM easily show a significant prolongation of clotting times [24].

A prolongation of CT/R has also been shown in in vitro studies considering the new oral anticoagulants like the direct thrombin inhibitor dabigatran [25] and the Xa inhibitors [26]. However, the capacity to identify patient within therapeutic range of these drugs remains controversial. Recently, a new ROTEM test, using ecarin, has been found to be a more sensitive assay for direct thrombin inhibitors [27]. The effects of low molecular weight heparins (LMWH) are generally detected by TEG, comparing kaolin with kaolin/heparinase, and an overdose is assumed to be detected also with ROTEM, comparing INTEM with HEPTEM [28].

It must be stressed that at this time, despite all these promising results, VETs are not intended to monitor the effect of anticoagulant drugs with the possible exception of heparin reversal.

2.5 Factors Influencing the Thromboelastographic/Thromboelastometric Curve

2.5.1 Age, Gender and Particular Conditions

Elderly patients tend to have shorter CT/R and an increase in amplitude (MCF/MA). The same happens, to a lesser extent, in females vs. males [11]. For children, some authors have suggested a dedicated reference range [29]. During pregnancy, the hemostatic changes are well depicted by TEG and ROTEM with a sort of "prothrombotic phenotype" (e.g. shorter CT/R, increase in MCF/MA mostly due to high fibrinogen levels). Recently, appropriate reference ranges for pregnancy have been proposed [30].

2.5.2 Haematocrit

Many authors have investigated the role of haematocrit and its impact on viscoelastic variables. Haematocrit has shown to inversely correlate with ROTEM MCF in a group of sideropenic anaemia patients [31]. The same was noticed with high haematocrit in cyanotic congenital heart disease patients using TEG [32]. The contribution to clot formation by red blood cells should be taken into account when considering tests that are performed on whole blood. Some authors believe this to be more of an advantage than a limit, for example, when considering FIBTEM instead of plasma fibrinogen concentration. However, in diluted conditions, which are a common situation in the bleeding patients, this effect appears negligible.

2.5.3 Temperature

TEG/ROTEM are usually performed at 37 °C. The setting of the temperature is possible with both instruments (directly with TEG, on the service panel with ROTEM). As the temperature is set under 37 °C, a proportional prolongation of R/CT is seen with decreasing temperature [33]. The clot amplitude is probably less affected by temperature than CT/R and different studies have shown conflicting results in MCF/MA [34]. However, from a clinical point of view, the benefit of setting the temperature remains debatable: during haemorrhage, severe hypothermia should always be corrected, independently from ROTEM/TEG results, and adding this variable may be potentially misleading.

2.5.4 Acidosis

It represents a well-known contributor to coagulopathy and its effect on ROTEM/TEG tracings have been investigated by many authors. In one study with ROTEM, acidosis was shown to synergistically impair coagulation when mixed with hypothermia, whereas without hypothermia, its effects were not significant [35].

2.5.5 Alcohol

Few studies with TEG reported some issue in identifying coagulopathy in patients with elevated blood alcohol levels. It is not clear if the shown impaired clot formation constitutes an artefact or not and further investigation is needed [36].

2.6 Evidence of TEG and ROTEM Feasibility and Usefulness in Various Settings

As previously highlighted, a growing body of literature, especially in cardiac surgery [37–39], liver transplant [40, 41], trauma [42–46] and post-partum haemorrhage [47, 48], led to an increasing interest in these instruments. However, the real contribution of a monitoring device "per se" is difficult to demonstrate, when considering, for example, blood products or cost sparing, or reduction of morbidity and mortality, which basically depend on treatment algorithms. Monitoring, with the exception of observational studies, often implicates a therapy (including the "not to treat" option of course). Unfortunately, the literature shows a wide range of different approaches in different countries and different institutions (e.g. concentrate-based or fresh frozen plasma-based hemostatic resuscitation). Such heterogeneity is perhaps the main confounding factor in the search for "evidence" and the result is conflicting recommendations. The recent European guidelines on management of bleeding and coagulopathy following major trauma recommend, with a Grade 1C level, that VETs are performed to assist in characterising the coagulopathy and in guiding haemostatic therapy [49]. On the other side, a recent review by The Cochrane Collaboration, analysing the accuracy of TEG and ROTEM in identifying trauma patients with trauma-induced coagulopathy, has concluded that these tests should only be used for research [50]. This apparent contradiction may be smoothed by a critical approach, taking into account limits and strengths of these instruments.

2.7 Standardisation, Quality Assurance and Quality Control of TEG and ROTEM

In 2010, the UK National External Quality Assessment Scheme (NEQAS) for Blood Coagulation undertook a series of exercises evaluating the provision of External Quality Assessment (EQA) material for TEG and ROTEM. The precision of the tests varied greatly for both devices ranging from 7.1 to 39.8 for TEG and 83.6 % for ROTEM [51]. The next year, a different group compared again TEG and ROTEM with the aim of a standardisation of the methodology. Among the measured parameters, the coefficient of variation for R/CT and MA/MCF was less than 20 % [52]. These results may seem discouraging, however, for guiding clinical decisions accuracy may be sometime more important than precision itself. Of course these machines need quality checks, quality controls and proper training.

2.8 The Sonoclot

The Sonoclot Analyzer (Sienco Inc., Arvada, CO) was introduced first in 1975 [53]. To start a measurement, a hollow, open-ended disposable plastic probe is mounted on the transducer head. Then, a whole-blood sample is added to the cuvette containing different coagulation activators/inhibitors. After an automated mixing procedure, the probe is immersed into the sample to a fixed depth where it oscillates vertically at a distance of 1 μm at a frequency of 200 Hz.

The blood sample exerts a viscous drag on the probe, mechanically impending its free vibration (Fig. 2.8). The drag increases as the sample clots and fibrin strands form on the probe's tip and

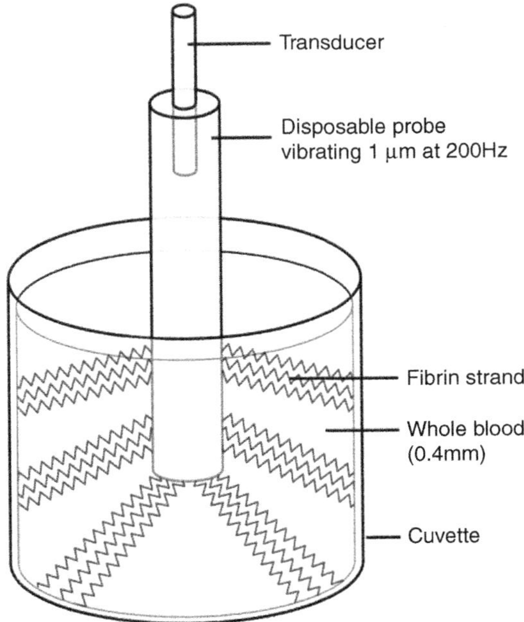

Fig. 2.8 Sonoclot mechanism

between the probe and the cuvette's wall effectively increasing the mass of the probe. The increasing impedance to the probe's vibration as the blood clots is detected by the devices' electronic circuits and converted to an output signal on a paper or digital chart. The Sonoclot Analyzer provides information on the entire haemostasis process both on a qualitative graph, known as the Sonoclot Signature and as quantitative results: the activated clotting time (ACT), the clot rate (CR) and the platelet function (PF). The Sonoclot Signature is shown in Fig. 2.9.

2.8.1 Interpreting the Sonoclot Signature

2.8.1.1 Activated Clotting Time (ACT)

This is the period from the beginning of the test when the sample is still a liquid until the point where fibrinogen begins to convert into a fibrin

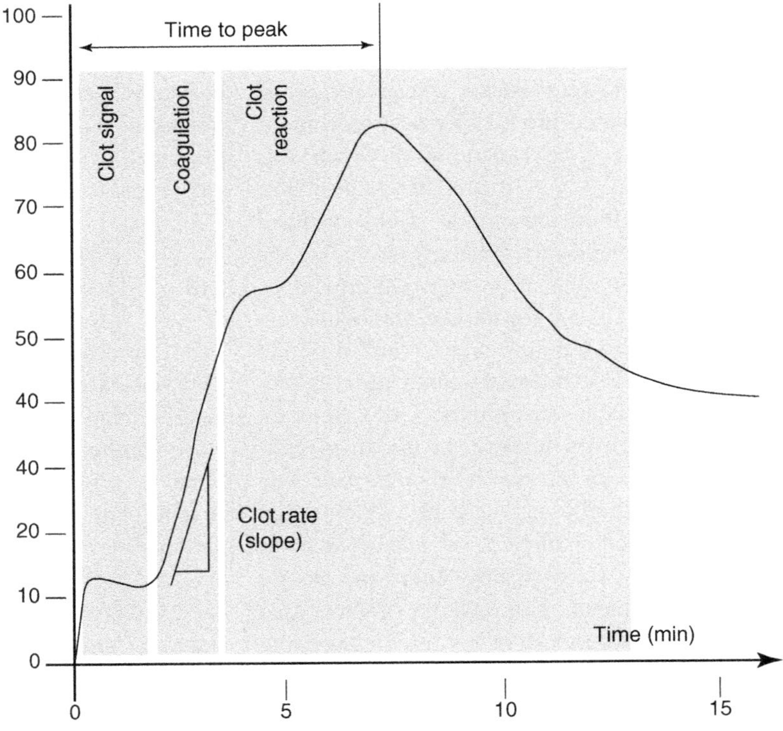

Fig. 2.9 Sonoclot curve

gel, thus increasing the viscosity of the sample. The Sonoclot Analyzer produces an automated result as the onset or activated clotting time. This is the point where the viscosity measurement rises by 1.0 clot signal unit on the Sonoclot Signature.

Therefore, ACT is the time from the activation of the sample until the beginning of a fibrin formation. ACT reflects initial fibrin formation, whereas R/CT reflects a more developed, and later, stage of initial clot formation.

2.8.1.2 Fibrin Gel Formation

This is the period during which fibrinogen forms a fibrin gel and is represented by the first rise in the Sonoclot Signature. The Sonoclot Analyzer produces an automated result called the clot rate. The clot rate is the maximum slope of the Sonoclot Signature during initial gel formation.

2.8.1.3 Clot Retraction

Clot retraction causes a peak or peaks on the Sonoclot Signature. Historically, platelet function has been characterised by several graphical indicators such as the time-to-peak. When run using Signature Viewer Software, the Sonoclot produces an automated result called "platelet function" (PF). The platelet function number quantifies the quality of the clot retraction. The nominal range of values for the PF goes from 0, representing no PF (no clot retraction and flat Sonoclot Signature after fibrin formation) to approximately 5, representing strong PF (clot retraction occurs sooner and is very strong, with clearly defined, sharp peaks in the Sonoclot Signature after fibrin formation).

The Sonoclot Analyzer has been criticised because its results were influenced by age, sex and platelet count [54]. Additionally, studies have shown poor reproducibility of some of the measured variables, especially CR and PF [55, 56].

However, others have found the Sonoclot Analyzer to be valuable and reliable in patients undergoing cardiac surgical procedures [57, 58]. Only few studies are available on the use of the Sonoclot Analyzer in hepatic surgery and liver transplantation. However, this technique has been found to be useful in the perioperative coagulation management of these patients [59, 60].

Finally, the Sonoclot Analyzer has also been shown to reliably detect pharmacological GPIIb/IIIa inhibition [61] and anticoagulation [62].

References

1. Haas T, Fries D, Tanaka KA, Asmis L, Curry NS, Schöchl H (2015) Usefulness of standard plasma coagulation tests in the management of perioperative coagulopathic bleeding: is there any evidence? Br J Anaesth 114:217–224
2. Cotton BA, Faz G, Hatch QM et al (2011) Rapid thromboelastography delivers real-time results that predict transfusion within 1 hour of admission. J Trauma 71:407–414
3. Martini WZ, Cortez DS, Dubick MA, Park MS, Holcomb JB (2008) Thrombelastography is better than PT, aPTT, and activated clotting time in detecting clinically relevant clotting abnormalities after hypothermia, hemorrhagic shock and resuscitation in pigs. J Trauma 65:535–543
4. Holcomb JB, Minei KM, Scerbo ML et al (2012) Admission rapid thrombelastography can replace conventional coagulation tests in the emergency department. Ann Surg 256:476–486
5. Tripodi A, Mannucci PM (2011) The coagulopathy of chronic liver disease. N Engl J Med 365:147–156
6. Theusinger OM, Nürnberg J, Asmis LM, Seifert B, Spahn DR (2010) Rotation thromboelastometry (ROTEM) stability and reproducibility over time. Eur J Cardiothorac Surg 37:677–683
7. Zambruni A, Thalheimer U, Leandro G, Perry D, Burroughs AK (2004) Thromboelastography with citrated blood: comparability with native blood, stability of citrate storage and effect of repeated sampling. Blood Coagul Fibrinolysis 15:103–107
8. Schlimp CJ, Cadamuro J, Solomon C, Redl H, Schöchl H (2013) The effect of fibrinogen concentrate and factor XIII on thromboelastometry in 33% diluted blood with albumin, gelatine, hydroxyethyl starch or saline in vitro. Blood Transfus 11:510–517
9. Fenger-Eriksen C, Tønnesen E, Ingerslev J, Sorensen B (2009) Mechanisms of hydroxyethyl starch-induced dilutional coagulopathy. J Thromb Haemost 7:1099–1105
10. Urwyler N, Theiler L, Hirschberg M, Kleine-Brueggeney M, Colucci G, Greif R (2012) Standard vs. point-of-care measurement of fibrinogen: potential impact on clinical decisions. Minerva Anestesiol 78:550–555

11. Lang T, von Depka M (2006) Possibilities and limitations of thrombelastometry/-graphy. Hamostaseologie 26(3 Suppl 1):S20–S29
12. Theusinger OM, Wanner GA, Emmert MY et al (2011) Hyperfibrinolysis diagnosed by rotational thromboelastometry (ROTEM) is associated with higher mortality in patients with severe trauma. Anesth Analg 113:1003–1012
13. Solomon C, Sørensen B, Hochleitner G, Kashuk J, Ranucci M, Schöchl H (2012) Comparison of whole blood fibrin-based clot tests in thrombelastography and thromboelastometry. Anesth Analg 114:721–730
14. Hagemo JS, Næss PA, Johansson P et al (2013) Evaluation of TEG(®) and RoTEM(®) interchangeability in trauma patients. Injury 44:600–605
15. Venema LF, Post WJ, Hendriks HG, Huet RC, de Wolf JT, de Vries AJ (2010) An assessment of clinical interchangeability of TEG® and RoTEM® thromboelastographic variables in cardiac surgical patients. Anesth Analg 111:339–344
16. Lee TH, McCully BH, Underwood SJ, Cotton BA, Cohen MJ, Schreiber MA (2013) Correlation of conventional thrombelastography and rapid thrombelastography in trauma. Am J Surg 205:521–527
17. Ågren A, Wikman AT, Östlund A, Edgren G (2014) TEG® functional fibrinogen analysis may overestimate fibrinogen levels. Anesth Analg 118:933–935
18. Lang T, Toller W, Gütl M et al (2004) Different effects of abciximab and cytochalasin D on clot strength in thrombelastography. J Thromb Haemost 2:147–153
19. Solomon C, Rahe-Meyer N, Schöchl H, Ranucci M, Görlinger K (2013) Effect of haematocrit on fibrin-based clot firmness in the FIBTEM test. Blood Transfus 11:412–418
20. Schlimp CJ, Solomon C, Ranucci M, Hochleitner G, Redl H, Schöchl H (2014) The effectiveness of different functional fibrinogen polymerization assays in eliminating platelet contribution to clot strength in thromboelastometry. Anesth Analg 118:269–276
21. Gorlinger K, Jámbor C, Hanke A et al (2007) Perioperative coagulation management and control of platelet transfusion by point-of-care platelet function analysis. Transfus Med Hemother 34:396–411
22. Spiezia L, Bertini D, Salmaso L, Simioni P (2008) Whole blood rotation thrombelastometry in subjects undergoing vitamin K antagonist treatment: hypo- or hypercoagulable profiles? Thromb Res 122:568–569
23. Dunham CM, Rabel C, Hileman BM et al (2014) TEG® and RapidTEG® are unreliable for detecting warfarin-coagulopathy: a prospective cohort study. Thromb J 12:4
24. Schmidt DE, Holmström M, Majeed A, Näslin D, Wallén H, Ågren A (2015) Detection of elevated INR by thromboelastometry and thromboelastography in warfarin treated patients and healthy controls. Thromb Res 35:1007–1011
25. Solbeck S, Meyer MAS, Johansson PI et al (2014) Monitoring of dabigatran anticoagulation and its reversal in vitro by thrombelastography. Int J Cardiol 176:794–799
26. Eller T, Busse J, Dittrich M et al (2014) Dabigatran, rivaroxaban, apixaban, argatroban and fondaparinux and their effects on coagulation POC and platelet function tests. Clin Chem Lab Med 52:835–844
27. Schaden E, Schober A, Hacker S, Kozek-Langenecker S (2013) Ecarin modified rotational thrombelastometry: a point-of-care applicable alternative to monitor the direct thrombin inhibitor argatroban. Wien Klin Wochenschr 125:156–159
28. Harenberg J (2009) Thrombelastometer and low molecular weight heparin. Anaesthesia 64:920–921
29. Oswald E, Stalzer B, Heitz E et al (2010) Thromboelastometry (ROTEM) in children: age-related reference ranges and correlations with standard coagulation tests. Br J Anaesth 105:827–835
30. de Lange NM, van Rheenen-Flach LE, Lancé MD et al (2014) Peri partum reference ranges for ROTEM thromboelastometry. Br J Anaesth 112:852–829
31. Spiezia L, Radu C, Marchioro P et al (2008) Peculiar whole blood rotation thromboelastometry (Rotem) profile in 40 sideropenic anaemia patients. Thromb Haemost 100:1106–1110
32. Westbury SK, Lee K, Reilly-Stitt C, Tulloh R, Mumford AD (2013) High haematocrit in cyanotic congenital heart disease affects how fibrinogen activity is determined by rotational thromboelastometry. Thromb Res 132:e145–e151
33. Rundgren M, Engström M (2008) A thromboelastometric evaluation of the effects of hypothermia on the coagulation system. Anesth Analg 107:1465–1468
34. Ramaker AJ, Meyer P, van der Meer J et al (2009) Effects of acidosis, alkalosis, hyperthermia and hypothermia on haemostasis: results of point of care testing with the thromboelastography analyser. Blood Coagul Fibrinolysis 20:436–439
35. Dirkmann D, Hanke AA, Gorlinger K, Peters J (2008) Hypothermia and acidosis synergistically impair coagulation in human whole blood. Anesth Analg 106:1627–1632
36. Howard BM, Kornblith LZ, Redick BJ et al (2014) The effects of alcohol on coagulation in trauma patients: interpreting thrombelastography with caution. J Trauma Acute Care Surg 77:865–871
37. Weber CF, Gorlinger K, Meininger D et al (2012) Point-of-care testing: a prospective, randomized clinical trial of efficacy in coagulopathic cardiac surgery patients. Anesthesiology 117:531–547
38. Tanaka KA, Bolliger D, Vadlamudi R, Nimmo A (2012) Rotational thromboelastometry (ROTEM)-based coagulation management in cardiac surgery and major trauma. J Cardiothorac Vasc Anesth 26:1083–1093
39. Girdauskas E, Kempfert J, Kuntze T et al (2010) Thromboelastometrically guided transfusion protocol during aortic surgery with circulatory arrest: a prospective, randomized trial. J Thorac Cardiovasc Surg 140:1117–1124
40. Trzebicki J, Flakiewicz E, Kosieradzki M et al (2010) The use of thromboelastometry in the assessment of hemostasis during orthotopic liver transplantation

reduces the demand for blood products. Ann Transplant 15:19–24
41. Mallett SV, Chowdary P, Burroughs AK (2013) Clinical utility of viscoelastic tests of coagulation in patients with liver disease. Liver Int 33:961–974
42. Schöchl H, Voelckel W, Grassetto A, Schlimp CJ (2013) Practical application of point-of-care coagulation testing to guide treatment decisions in trauma. J Trauma Acute Care Surg 74:1587–1598
43. Da Luz L, Nascimento B, Shankarakutty A, Rizoli S, Adhikari NK (2014) Effect of thromboelastography (TEG®) and rotational thromboelastometry (ROTEM®) on diagnosis of coagulopathy, transfusion guidance and mortality in trauma: descriptive systematic review. Crit Care 18:518
44. Meyer ASP, Meyer MAS, Sørensen AM et al (2014) Thrombelastography and rotational thromboelastometry early amplitudes in 182 trauma patients with clinical suspicion of severe injury. J Trauma Acute Care Surg 76:682–690
45. Schöchl H, Nienaber U, Hofer G et al (2010) Goal-directed coagulation management of major trauma patients using thromboelastometry (ROTEM®)-guided administration of fibrinogen concentrate and prothrombin complex concentrate. Crit Care 14:R55
46. Johansson PI, Stissing T, Bochsen L, Ostrowski SR (2009) Thrombelastography and tromboelastometry in assessing coagulopathy in trauma. Scand J Trauma Resusc Emerg Med 17:45
47. Jámbor C, Kozek-Langenecker SA, Frietsch T, Knels R (2008) Thrombelastography should be included in the algorithm for the management of postpartum hemorrhage. Transfus Med Hemother 35:391–392
48. de Lange NM, Lancé MD, de Groot R, Beckers EA, Henskens YM, Scheepers HC (2012) Obstetric hemorrhage and coagulation: an update. Thromboelastography, thromboelastometry, and conventional coagulation tests in the diagnosis and prediction of postpartum hemorrhage. Obstet Gynecol Surv 67:426–435
49. Spahn DR, Bouillon B, Cerny V et al (2013) Management of bleeding and coagulopathy following major trauma: an updated European guideline. Crit Care 17:R76
50. Hunt H, Stanworth S, Curry N et al (2015) Thromboelastography (TEG) and rotational thromboelastometry (ROTEM) for trauma-induced coagulopathy in adult trauma patients with bleeding. Cochrane Database Syst Rev (2):CD010438
51. Kitchen DP, Kitchen S, Jennings I, Woods T, Walker I (2010) Quality assurance and quality control of thrombelastography and rotational Thromboelastometry: the UK NEQAS for blood coagulation experience. Semin Thromb Hemost 36:757–763
52. Chitlur M, Sørensen B, Rivard GE et al (2011) Standardization of thromboelastography: a report from the TEG-ROTEM working group. Haemophilia 17:532–537
53. Von Kaulla KN, Ostendorf P, von Kaulla E (1975) The impedance machine: a new bedside coagulation recording device. J Med 6:73–88
54. Horlocker TT, Schroeder DR (1997) Effect of age, gender, and platelet count on Sonoclot coagulation analysis in patients undergoing orthopedic operations. Mayo Clin Proc 72:214–219
55. McKenzie ME, Gurbel PA, Levine DJ, Serebruany VL (1999) Clinical utility of available methods for determining platelet function. Cardiology 92:240–247
56. Ekback G, Carlsson O, Schott U (1999) Sonoclot coagulation analysis: a study of test variability. J Cardiothorac Vasc Anesth 13:393–397
57. Miyashita T, Kuro M (1998) Evaluation of platelet function by Sonoclot analysis compared with other hemostatic variables in cardiac surgery. Anesth Analg 87:1228–1233
58. Yamada T, Katori N, Tanaka KA, Takeda J (2007) Impact of Sonoclot hemostasis analysis after cardiopulmonary bypass on postoperative hemorrhage in cardiac surgery. J Anesth 21:148–155
59. Chapin JW, Becker GL, Hulbert BJ et al (1989) Comparison of Thromboelastograph and Sonoclot coagulation analyzer for assessing coagulation status during orthotopic liver transplantation. Transplant Proc 21:3539
60. Bindi ML, Biancofiore GD, Consani G et al (2001) Coagulation monitoring during liver transplantation: Sonoclot analysis and laboratory tests. Minerva Anestesiol 67:359–369
61. Tucci MA, Ganter MT, Hamiel CR, Klaghofer R, Zollinger A, Hofer CK (2006) Platelet function monitoring with the Sonoclot analyzer after in vitro tirofiban and heparin administration. J Thorac Cardiovasc Surg 131:1314–1322
62. Nilsson CU, Engström M (2007) Monitoring fondaparinux with the Sonoclot. Blood Coagul Fibrinolysis 18:619–622

3 General Aspects of Platelet Function Tests

Rita Paniccia, Blanca Martinez,
Dorela Haxhiademi, and Domenico Prisco

3.1 Introduction

Human platelets are involved in both normal hemostasis and pathological hemorrhage and thrombosis. These cells promote the vessel wall contraction and repair and contribute to the host defense [1, 2]. In addition, platelets interlocking with endothelial, white, or smooth muscle cells play a critical role in inflammation, in promotion of atherosclerosis, in tumor growth, and in metastasis [3–7]. Despite different roles carried out by the platelets, the main platelet function methods investigate mostly the alterations related to the hemostatic process [8]. Initially, these assays have been employed for the identification and management of patients with or at risk of bleeding rather than those at risk of thrombosis [9].

In normal primary hemostasis, human platelets keep blood fluidity through the maintenance of vascular integrity and the blockade of hemorrhage following blood vessel wound. At the site of vascular injury, platelets promptly adhere to the subendothelium, and, following the rapid activation and release of platelet/clotting compounds and adhesive proteins, aggregate each another forming a hemostatic platelet plug with the exposure of a procoagulant surface. These different proper actions get the activated platelets to form a hemostatic plug that blocks the site of vascular damage to prevent blood loss [10]. In presence of a dropped platelet count and/or platelet dysfunction, an increased risk of hemorrhage could arise. On the other hand, an increase in platelet count or reactivity could prompt unsuitable thrombus formation. Indeed, along atherosclerotic lesions, platelets adhere, activate, and aggregate developing an occluding arterial thrombus that may result in thromboembolic disease such as myocardial infarction or stroke, two of the main causes of morbidity and mortality in the Western world [11–14].

To date, platelet function may be consistently assessed by using a variety of methodologies employed in specialized laboratories as tests of second or third level. Platelet function tests may be used to study inherited or acquired platelet dysfunctions in order to identify patients with hemorrhagic problems [15–18]. In addition, the monitoring of antiplatelet therapy by using these tests has become a useful tool for the identification of hyper- or hyporesponder patients at risk of both thrombosis or hemorrhage [19–22].

In this scenario, the development of new, simpler devices for the study of platelet function at the point of care (POC) or bedside has allowed to investigate platelet function testing not only in specialized clinical or research laboratories but also in general laboratories and in different

R. Paniccia, MSc (✉) • D. Prisco, MD, PhD
Department of Experimental and Clinical Medicine, University of Florence, Careggi University Hospital, Florence, Italy
e-mail: rita.paniccia@unifi.it

B. Martinez, MD
Department of Anesthesia and Intensive Care Medicine, University Hospital of Udine, Udine, Italy

D. Haxhiademi, MD
Anesthesia and Intensive Care, G. Pasquinucci Hospital, G. Monasterio Foundation, Massa, Italy

M. Ranucci, P. Simioni (eds.), *Point-of-Care Tests for Severe Hemorrhage: A Manual for Diagnosis and Treatment*, DOI 10.1007/978-3-319-24795-3_3

clinical setting. Indeed, the growing number of patients on antiplatelet drugs, with an increased risk of bleeding, principally during trauma and surgical procedures, has motivated the use of platelet function POC testing (POCT) in the perioperative setting as useful tools for the prediction of hemorrhage and for monitoring the efficacy of different prohemostatic therapies [23–27]. In addition, the evaluation of hemostasis during the different phases of platelet banking (concentrates, transfusions, and evaluation of donor platelet function) is gaining strength in predicting bleeding and assessing the efficacy of prohemostatic treatments [15, 28, 29].

This chapter attempts to describe the different available POC methods and the pertinent instrumentation for studying platelet function in different clinical settings. Different methodologies are dedicated both to the diagnosis of inherited and acquired bleeding disorders and to the monitoring of residual platelet reactivity of patients on antiplatelet treatment.

3.2 The Past of Platelet Function Testing and the Digest of New Methodologies

The bleeding time (BT) by the Duke procedure (1910) [30] was the first test for investigating ex vivo the ability of platelets to form a plug. This technique has been a long time considered a useful screening test to identify both congenital and acquired platelet disorders [31].

In the 1960s, the cornerstone of the assessment of platelet function was the light transmission aggregometry (LTA) according to Born's studies [32]. This methodology evaluates in vitro the phenomenon of platelet aggregation induced by external aggregating agents – agonists: i.e., adenosine diphosphate (ADP), arachidonic acid (AA), collagen, epinephrine (EPI), and others – in the particular milieu of platelet-rich plasma (PRP) [33]. This method has been and continues to be considered the reference method for the assessment of platelet function in clinical research and for the diagnosis of bleeding disorders [17, 34].

In the 1970s, Wu and Hoak [35] firstly described a method for investigating circulating platelet aggregates fixed by formalin. Grotemeyer improved this test comparing platelet counts performed within two blood EDTA tubes (EDTA alone and EDTA plus fixative) [36, 37]. The assessment in vitro of platelet adhesion and retention of platelets exposed to foreign surfaces was developed originally by Hellem [38]. Further modifications of this test were the O'Brien filterometer [39], the Homburg retention test [40], and the platelet adhesion assay [41]. Over the years, different prototype instruments have been developed such as the thrombotic status analyzer [42] and the clot signature analyzer [43], but they are no longer available. However, some of these methods opened the door to the new POC devices such as the platelet function analyzer –100 (PFA-100) (Siemens AG, Munich, Germany) [44], Plateletworks system (Helena Biosciences, Beaumont, Texas) [45], and the global thrombosis test (GTT) (Montrose Diagnostics Ltd, London, UK) [46].

In the 1980s, new platelet function assays, based on different operating principles, have become available for being employed in clinical research or specialized laboratories. Impedance platelet aggregometry performed in whole blood (WB), the study of activated platelets ex vivo by flow cytometry technique, the measurement of specific compounds released by platelets, and the assessment of platelet nucleotides have become available [47–49]. However, these laboratory methods can investigate one by one the different facets of platelet (dys)function – i.e., platelet adhesion/aggregation and/or measurement of granule content/release. In this manner, there was no one pivotal screening test for the diagnosis and management of patients suffering from hemorrhagic problems [19]. In addition, these different methodologies are labor intensive, costly, time consuming, and require a fair degree of expertise and experience. These drawbacks have restricted their extensive clinic use. Actually, these assays are available only in specialized clinical laboratories dedicated to the studies of pathophysiological processes of hemostasis and thrombosis.

As the assessment of platelet function might have a key position in the management of severe bleeding, improved skills to assess platelet function in a timely and efficient mode is necessary. During the last two decades, platelet function POC testing (POCT) has been proposed. These new systems can be used within nonspecialized laboratories or directly at the bedside of patients at high risk of bleeding or thrombotic complications. With the improvement of the diagnostic panel, the development of informatics, and the amelioration of patient outcome, the study of platelet function by using POCT has become more easy to perform and often mandatory in different clinical settings. Indeed, platelet function POCT is now used for the identification of patients with bleeding disorders, for monitoring the response to antiplatelet treatment, in the assessment of perioperative hemostasis, in obstetrical illnesses and in trauma-emerging coagulopathies, and in the transfusion medicine setting [15, 23–29].

Platelet POC devices are based on different operating principles, and available devices may be based on the assessment of platelet adhesion and aggregation such as platelet aggregation performed in WB by using the Multiplate apparatus (Multiplate Electrode Aggregometry, MEA) (Dynabyte, Roche Diagnostics, Germany) [50], the VerifyNow system (ITC, Edison, USA) [51], or the Plateletworks system. In addition, available instruments including the updated Innovance PFA-200 device [52], the Impact-R-cone and plate(let) technology- analyzer (IMPACT) (DiaMed, Cressier sur Morat, Switzerland) [53], and the GTT measure platelet adhesion and aggregation under conditions of high shear, in an attempt to simulate in vivo primary hemostatic mechanisms. Moreover, new platelet tests have been added to the new viscoelastic assays, i.e., the thromboelastography (TEG) that employs the Thrombelastograph TEG® 5000 (Haemonetics Corporation, Braintree, MA) and thromboelastometry that employs the ROTEM delta device (TEM Innovation, Munich, Germany) [54]. The "TEG platelet mapping" system is a modification of the original TEG and has been developed for monitoring antiplatelet therapy [55]. "Rotem Platelet" is a novel impedance aggregometer directly applied to the ROTEM delta device [56].

The different platelet function POC assays are grouped by the different method principles in Table 3.1. Normal ranges of each method has not been reported, because for POCT local (in house) normal ranges development is suggested.

In Table 3.2, advantages and disadvantages of each platelet function POC methodology are indicated.

3.3 Assays Based on Platelet Aggregation

Platelet aggregation assays at POC are derived from LTA, that is still thought as the reference method – the gold standard test – for platelet function testing. Notwithstanding this chapter is addressed to the assessment of platelet function by using POCT, a paragraph was dedicated to LTA in order to explain the basis of in vitro-induced platelet activation.

3.3.1 Light Transmission Platelet Aggregometry on Platelet-Rich Plasma

LTA [32, 57] assesses in vitro the phenomenon of platelet aggregation. A wide panel of agonists is used to activate different platelet pathways allowing to obtain a great number of information about platelet function and biochemistry [33, 34]. In this test, PRP is used as milieu in which agonists are added and the platelet-to-platelet clump formation occurs in a glycoprotein (GP) IIb/IIIa-dependent manner. The principle of method is based on the measurement of the increase of light transmission through the optically dense sample of PRP after the addition of exogenous platelet agonists that are able to activate the platelets to form aggregates. The dropping of the platelet clumps causes a decrease in the optical density of PRP that develops into platelet-poor plasma (PPP) with the concomitant increase of plasma brightness and light transmission. The instrument records the rate and maximal percentage of this

Table 3.1 Different methodologies for the assessment of platelet function

Assay	Sampling	Operating principle	Area of applicability
Bleeding time[a]	Native WB	In vivo measurement of bleeding block	Screening for bleeding tendency (obsolete)
Tests based on platelet aggregation			
LTA	Citrated PRP	Photo-optical detection of light transmission increase after addition of agonists	Screening for bleeding tendency Diagnostic for platelet defects Monitoring of antiplatelet treatment
Impedance aggregation	Citrated WB	Electrical impedance increase detection after agonist-induced aggregation	Screening for bleeding tendency Diagnostic for platelet defects Monitoring of antiplatelet treatment
Lumiaggregometry[a]	Citrated WB	Platelet aggregometry combined with simultaneous luminescence	Detection of storage/release disorders
Plateletworks	Citrated WB	Platelet counting before and after agonist-induced aggregation	Monitoring of antiplatelet treatment
Tests based on platelet adhesion under shear stress			
PFA-100 Innovance PFA-200	Citrated WB	WB flow block by high shear- and agonist-induced platelet plug formation	Screening for bleeding tendency Searching of severe platelet dysfunctions, revealing of VWD
Impact-R -cone and plate(let)- analyzer	Citrated WB	Platelet adhesion-aggregation on specific surface	Screening of primary hemostasis
GTT	Native WB	WB flow ending by low shear-induced platelet plug formation	Evaluation of platelet function and thrombolysis
Platelet function methods combined with viscoelastic test			
TEG/platelet mapping system	Citrated WB	Evaluation of clot formation based on low shear induced and agonist addition	Evaluation of hemostasis activation plus monitoring of antiplatelet therapy
ROTEM *platelet*	Citrated WB	Assessment of electrical impedance increase	Evaluation of hemostasis activation plus monitoring of antiplatelet therapy
Platelet analysis based on flow cytometry[a]			
Flow cytometry	Citrated WB, PRP, W-Plt	Laser-based detection of fluorescent-labeled platelets	Platelet counting and activation detection
Evaluation of thromboxane metabolites[a]			
RIA or ELISA	Serum, urine, plasma	Ligand-binding assays	Measurement of platelet-derived compounds (TxA2 metabolites, beta-TG, PF4, soluble P-Selectin)[a]

Abbreviations: Beta-Tg Beta Thromboglobulin, *ELISA* Enzyme Linked-ImmunoSorbent Assays, *GTT* global thrombosis test, *LTA* light transmission aggregometry, *RIA* radio immune assays, *PFA* platelet function analyzer, *PRP* platelet-rich plasma, *PF4* platelet factor 4, *TEG* Thrombelastography, *TxA2* thromboxane A2, *WB* whole blood, *W-plt* washed platelets

[a]Assays not considered in this issue

increase from 0 % (maximal optical density of PRP) to 100 % (no optical density of autologous PPP) by a photometer. This detection is transformed automatically in a graphic curve that parallels with the increase of light transmission during the platelet aggregation (Fig. 3.1). Among the different parameters recognized by the evaluation of the aggregation curve – lag phase, shape change, primary and secondary aggregation, and slope – the maximal extent of platelet aggregation, measured as %, is used as expression of results [58].

In specialized laboratories, this methodology is deemed the first step in the flowchart for the

Table 3.2 Advantages and disadvantages of platelet function POC tests

Assay	PROS	CONS
MEA system	Diagnostic method Flexible Different platelet pathways investigated Sensitive to antiplatelet therapy	Limited HCT and platelet count range
PFA-100; Innovance PFA-200	In vitro standardized BT Sensitive to severe platelet defects	Rigid system Platelet count – HCT dependent Not sensitive to platelet secretion defects
VerifyNow system	Waived No WB processing Easy, quick	Nonflexible Expensive Dedicated only to monitor antiplatelet therapy Limited HCT and platelet count
Plateletworks	No WB processing Easy, rapid screening test	Required additional platelet count Indirect assay
Impact-R -cone and plate(let)- analyzer	Global platelet method Small sample volume	Expensive Experienced staff Not widely available
GTT	Global platelet method Small sample volume	Lacking of clinical studies Not widely available
TEG platelet mapping	Global hemostasis test	Measure clot properties Indirect assay More studies are needed
ROTEM *platelet*	Global hemostasis test plus true WB platelet aggregometry	Very low platelet count (only for platelet system) Lacking of clinical studies

Abbreviations: GTT global thrombosis test, *HCT* hematocrit, *MEA* multiplate electrode aggregometry, *PFA* platelet function analyzer, *plt* platelet, *POC* point-of-care, *TEG* Thrombelastography

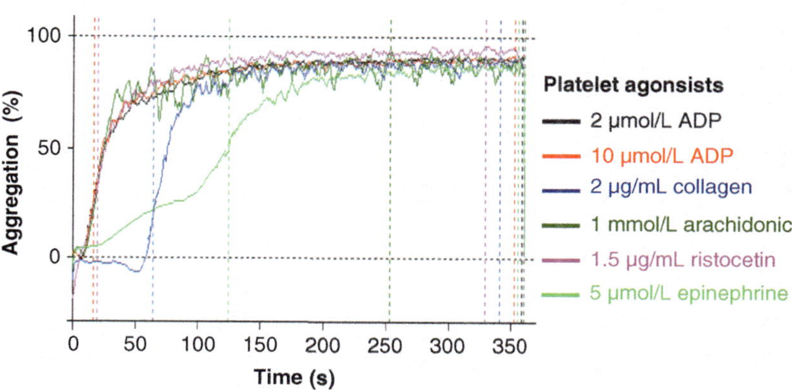

Fig. 3.1 Light transmission platelet aggregation tracings from a healthy subject in response to different agonists; final agonist concentrations are reported

study of hemorrhagic patient with inherited or acquired platelet dysfunctions and for monitoring antiplatelet therapies. In addition to routinely used agonists – ADP, AA, collagen, and epinephrine – other agonists should be utilized when signs of congenital/acquired bleeding disorders are revealed. These "third-level" agonists, such as thrombin receptor-activating peptide (TRAP), thromboxane A2 (TXA2) mimetic U46619, and ristocetin, allow a differential analysis to exclude/include the defective pathways of platelet activation [34, 59–63].

Recently, LTA has acquired the clinical value of useful tool for monitoring antiplatelet therapies, i.e., aspirin and thienopyridine. The high residual platelet reactivity on treatment defined by ADP- and AA-induced LTA or both has been associated with the occurrence of major adverse cardiovascular events (MACE) both in acute coronary syndrome (ACS) patients and in those with stable coronary artery disease (CAD) [21, 22, 64–66]. The assessment of a discriminating cutoff value has been a decisive support for the identification of hypo- or hyperresponders to antiplatelet agents and at high risk of MACE [67]. Nevertheless LTA testing is incorporated into clinical practice to stratify response to antiplatelet therapy, definitive data from randomized trials supporting a routine approach are still lacking [68–70].

Although LTA is still considered the most effective diagnostic platelet assay, this test presents some peculiar aspects and problems. First, it is quite nonphysiological, because separated platelets are stirred under low shear conditions and are not in relation with the white and red cells that are in WB. In these conditions, platelets do not accurately mimic the platelet adhesion upon vessel wall injury. Second, the technique may be affected by different pre-analytical and methodological conditions (i.e., type of anticoagulant, hemolysis, PRP handling, different concentrations of agonists), and the laboratory staff should have a high degree of skillfulness in performing the test and experience and expertise for interpreting LTA results. Indeed, this methodology is constantly verified by an ongoing standardization process [60, 71, 72], and recent specific guidelines for LTA that want to stabilize/normalize the correct procedure have been published [73–76].

Thus, different alternative POC tests are now available that assess platelet or that attempt to simulate primary hemostasis aggregation in citrated WB.

3.3.2 Multiple Electrode Aggregometry (MEA)

The concept of impedance aggregometry in WB was introduced in the 1980s by Cardinal and Flower [47]. Since then, platelet function testing in WB has been performed as a laboratory test. Only during the last years, the introduction in the clinical practice of a new methodology, the Multiplate Electrode Aggregometry (MEA), has allowed to assess WB platelet aggregation by using the new aggregometer Multiplate analyzer (Dynabyte, Roche Diagnostics, Germany). The technical peculiarities of this new device made possible the use of impedance platelet aggregometry as an assay at the point of care [50]. Indeed, this device consists of a computerized five-channel system and an automated pipetting. Moreover, it is equipped by disposable cuvettes ready to use with two independent sensor units: each unit is constituted by two silver-coated fixed distance electrodes. Also agonists and diluents for MEA are ready to use. With these essential advantages, MEA has achieved a high clinical value like that of LTA.

While in their resting state, platelets are nonthrombogenic, in the presence of soluble agonists, they get activated, expose their receptors, and can be attached not only on vascular injuries but even on artificial surfaces. This is the fundamental principle on which WB impedance aggregometry is based. MEA is assessed in duplicate by using separately each sensor unit, and the electrical resistance, or impedance, between the two electrodes is continuously recorded in Ohms. As platelets aggregate after the agonist addition, they create a growing layer stuck to the electrodes, and the impedance signal between them increases. This increase is turned into a graph similar to that of LTA. By MEA, impedance, measured in Ohms, is expressed in arbitrary aggregation units (AU). Three parameters can be calculated with this system: maximal aggregation (in AU), velocity (in AU/min), and area under curve (AUC) (AU × min). In the early reports about this method, AUC was shown to be the parameter with the highest diagnostic power [50] and is nowadays used in clinical settings.

Several specific test reagents are available for stimulation of different receptors or activation of signal transduction pathways of platelets (Fig. 3.2): ASPItest, in which is present in the AA, the substrate for cyclooxygenase (COX) which forms TXA2, a potent platelet agonist – this test is used to investigate COX-dependent aggregation pharmacologically

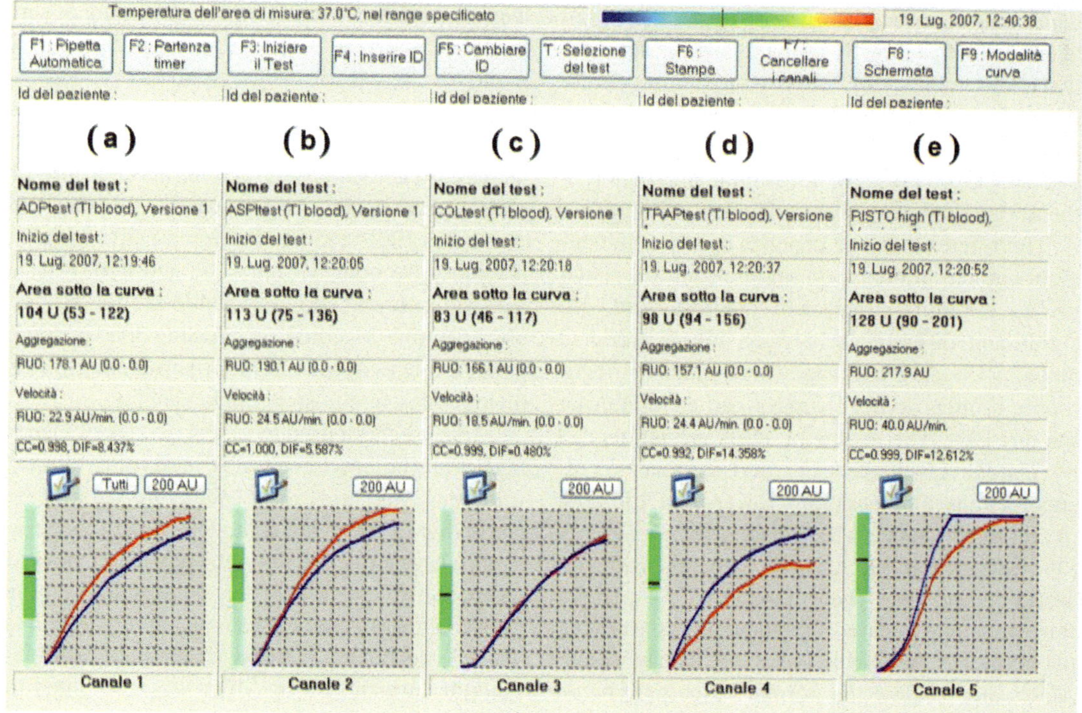

Fig. 3.2 Multiplate electrode aggregometry (MEA) screen tracings from a healthy subject in response to different agonists. (**a**) ADPtest, ADP; (**b**) ASPItest, arachidonic acid; (**c**) COLtest, collagen; (**d**) TRAPtest; thrombin receptor agonist peptide-6 (TRAP) (**e**) RISTOtest, ristocetin. Specifications: *Nome del test, Test name; Area sotto la curva, area under curve*

antagonized by aspirin, NSAIDs, and other COX inhibitors; COLtest, that uses as agonist the collagen, which activates the collagen receptor (GPIa/IIa), leading to the release of endogenous AA and resulting in platelet activation via TXA2 stimulation; ADPtest, in which ADP activates platelet by stimulation of ADP receptors; and ADPtest HS (ADP plus PgE1) in which, the stimulation of ADP receptors in the presence of the endogenous platelet inhibitor PGE1 makes it more sensitive toward the effects of P2Y12 inhibitors. In addition to these tests, also the TRAPtest and RISTOtest can be performed. In the first, TRAP-6 as agonist stimulates the thrombin receptors PAR1 and PAR4. Because thrombin is the most potent platelet activator, it is not sensible to aspirin and COX inhibitors and has little or not at all sensibility to P2Y12 receptor inhibitors. In the second, the antibiotic ristocetin, used as agonist at two different concentrations, binds to the platelet receptor glycoprotein (GpIb). This test is sensitive to disorders of VWF, particularly type IIb VWD.

The most important differences between MEA and LTA stay at two important modalities of method execution. The first is the surface on which platelets aggregate: in LTA, platelets aggregate with each other in the liquid phase, whereas in MEA, they aggregate on the surface of the electrodes. Although on artificial surfaces, aggregation in MEA is closer to in vivo platelet aggregation, which occurs on vascular surfaces. The second is the milieu in which the test is run: LTA uses plasma (PRP and PPP), and different centrifugation steps are required for carrying out this assay. MEA employs WB, the physiological environment where platelet function takes place in vivo. By using WB, the assessment of platelet function occurs in the presence of other cellular components that contribute to platelet aggregation: red blood cells (that directly promote platelet aggregation) and monocytes (that induce transcellular prostanoid formation). In addition, MEA, using a small quantity of WB (in which all subpopulations of platelets are present), needs no manipulation of the sample (avoiding pretest platelet activation).

The reference range depends on the anticoagulant applied in the blood sample (hirudin, heparin, or sodium citrate) and the test used. No significant differences between blood group O and non-O individuals can be noted, and aggregometric profiles do not change significantly during the day [77]. The results of MEA are influenced by platelet count. Stissing and associates [78] suggest that platelet counts lower than 150,000/μL might influence MEA results. Other authors [79] found that MEA measurements using all available agonists were indicative of platelet function alone in case of platelet counts 100,000/μL or more. For lower levels of platelet count, AUC values below the normal range may be an indicator of decreased overall platelet aggregability regardless of whether due to a low platelet count or impaired platelet function. They suggested the use of MEA in the perioperative settings to assess the overall platelet aggregability of that blood sample, not only the platelet function alone.

MEA shows a high sensitivity toward the effects of antiplatelet drugs, such as ASA, clopidogrel, and GPIIb/IIIa receptor inhibitors [80–83]. It has been used for individualizing the dual antiplatelet therapy after PCI [84] and for identifying patient-specific factors that determine thienopyridine resistance and platelet function recovery rate at drug suspension [85]. MEA has been shown to detect the risk for bleeding and thrombosis in patients on antiplatelet therapy. Sibbing and associates [86, 87] reported the use of MEA for the identification of patients on antiplatelet therapy at risk for stent thrombosis. Cutoff values are also set for the risk of hemorrhagic complications in patients on dual antiplatelet therapy after PCI procedures [83]. Many papers report the use of preoperative MEA in patients on P2Y12 receptor inhibitors that undergo cardiac surgery for the identification of those at risk for postoperative bleeding [88, 89]. In this clinical setting, they propose MEA to determine the timing of surgery. In particular, Ranucci and associates [89] found that in cardiac surgery patients on thienopyridine, a cutoff value of 31 U obtained by MEA ADP assay discriminated those patients at increased postoperative bleeding and needing of platelet transfusion. More recently, Ranucci and associates [90] studied the preoperative platelet reactivity by both MEA, ADP, and TRAP tests and set a combined cutoff value for the risk of postoperative bleeding, suggesting that residual platelet reactivity to thrombin stimulation limits the risk of severe postoperative bleeding.

MEA has been used to assess the risk of bleeding and thrombosis even in several other clinical situations. The most robust literature regards the predictive value of MEA in identifying preoperatively platelet dysfunction related to an increased postoperative bleeding and its management by the use of increased platelet transfusion requirements [91–93]. In trauma patients, an impaired platelet function investigated by MEA was associated to an increased early and late mortality [94, 95]. Davies and associates [96] found reduced platelet function with MEA to be significantly associated with morbidity and mortality in sepsis and SIRS patients. MEA has been used for the diagnosis of HIT [97]. Acquired von Willebrand syndrome in patients with aortic stenosis [98] and congenital von Willebrand disease have been detected with MEA as well [99]. Low platelet aggregation induced by TRAP has been shown to be an independent factor for intramyocardial hemorrhage of patients with myocardial infarction [100].

MEA, overwhelming the disadvantages of LTA, allows to timely evaluate the platelet function without the need of a specialized laboratory. This POC system needs minimal technical skill and training, its procedure is automatically completed, and only interpretation data are required. In the future, MEA would achieve a clinical value similar to that of LTA.

3.3.3 VerifyNow System

The VerifyNow system (ITC, Edison, USA), originally, was developed for monitoring the effect of platelet GPIIb/IIIa antagonists (abciximab, eptifibatide, or tirofiban) in cardiovascular patients undergoing percutaneous coronary intervention (PCI) [51]. Formerly, it was named Ultegra rapid platelet function analyzer (RPFA) [101]. This locked platelet POCT was specifically conceived for monitoring the different antiplatelet therapies in emergency cath lab or in perioperative setting without appealing to specialized laboratories and cannot be used for any other purpose [67, 102].

The system is made of a machine plus a system of different cartridge diagnostics containing fibrinogen-coated beads and platelet agonists (Fig. 3.3). Platelet aggregation occurs in the WB and is revealed by a turbidimetric-based optical detection exploiting the ability of activated platelets to bind upon the fibrinogen-coated beads within the assay cartridge in proportion of the number of the activated GPIIb/IIIa receptors. By using this fully automated system, no blood manipulation, instrument handling, neither pipetting are necessary. Actually, the methodology is so waived that citrated WB tubes are just get on the cartridge system (agonist plus fibrinogen-coated beads) previously inserted into the device.

Three different assays each sensitive to targeted drugs are available. VerifyNow IIb/IIIa Test, sensitive to GP IIb/IIIa antagonists, employs as agonist the thrombin receptor-activating peptide (4 μmol/L iso-TRAP), that greatly stimulates platelet aggregation and its results are expressed as platelet aggregation units (PAU) computed as rate and degree of aggregation [103]. VerifyNow Aspirin Test, which uses AA (1 mmol/L) as agonist, is sensitive to aspirin therapy and its results are expressed as aspirin reaction units (ARU). A cutoff value below 550 ARU was designed to identify "true" responder patients to ASA therapy [104]. VerifyNow PRUTest, that uses as agonists 20 μmol/L ADP plus 22 nmol/L PGE1 – as suppressor of intracellular free calcium levels for abating the nonspecific effect of the ADP binding to P2Y1 receptors – is sensitive to thienopyridine treatment and its results are expressed as P2Y12 reaction units (PRU) [68, 105, 106]. VerifyNow system revealed a moderate agreement with LTA, poor with PFA-100 and Plateletworks [107–111]. The definition of cutoff values for the identification of patients not responsive to antiplatelets at high risk of MACE has been exceedingly discussed, and several studies have reported the clinical value of this system [105–113]. In particular, various indexes of high on-treatment platelet reactivity in patients on P2Y12 inhibitors deemed at increased risk of thromboembolic events are considered: cutoff values of 240 PRU [105, 114] or 208/203 PRU [110] were found. On the other hand, in different surgical settings, the assessment of response to thienopyridine by using the VerifyNow system is recently growing for attempting to predict postoperative hemorrhage. So, different cutoff values were considered: results below 60 PRU [114] or 95 PRU [115] and 207 PRU [116] were assumed as suggesting low on-treatment platelet reactivity with an increased risk of bleeding events [117, 118]. Moreover, bleeding and transfusion requests in cardiac surgery were significantly correlated with preoperatively measured PRU values [119], and low PRU values have been reported to have a predictive value of a major rate of platelet transfusions in trauma patients assuming clopidogrel [120].

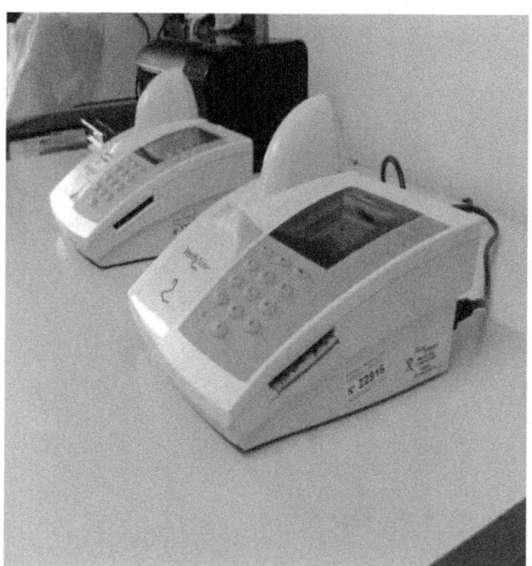

Fig. 3.3 VerifyNow system device

3.3.4 Plateletworks System

The Plateletworks aggregation kits and Ichor full blood counter system is a WB POCT based on the measure of platelet counts before and after aggregation. Plateletworks aggregation kit consists of EDTA tubes (as baseline controls) and citrate tubes filled with platelet agonists, ADP or AA, as aggregation test samples. By using the Ichor blood counter (Helena Laboratories, Beaumont, United States), the Plateletworks method compares the platelet count measured in the control sample (EDTA tube) with that in citrate blood added either ADP or AA or collagen. The decrease of platelet count measured in citrate tubes is related to the extent of aggregation [45]. The main advantages of this method are that no manipulation of blood sample is needed and results are obtained in few minutes. The main disadvantage is the very short interval for performing the test consisting in few minutes after blood sampling. In acute care condition, such as cardiac surgery and cath lab, Plateletworks shows the clinical value of giving information about both platelet count and function [121–124]. Significant correlations between Plateletworks and LTA, VerifyNow system, and Thromboelastography have been found [125–127]. These evidences give a clinical value of useful tool for monitoring antiplatelet treatment to this system. Indeed, in elective surgery patients, this POC system test has been used preoperatively for monitoring reversal of clopidogrel therapy [127]. In addition, in cardiac surgery, preoperative high platelet inhibition measured by Plateletworks either with collagen [128], either that, or with ADP test [129] was associated with increased postoperative blood loss.

3.4 Assays Based on Platelet Adhesion Under Shear Stress

3.4.1 The Platelet Function Analyzer (PFA)-100/Innovance PFA-200

This platelet POCT uses the device Innovance PFA-200 (Siemens, Munich, Germany) [130], formerly called PFA-100 [44] (Fig. 3.4). Based on the capacity of platelets to adhere to collagen under high shear stress conditions and aggregate in response to specific agonists (primary hemostasis), this test has been considered the in vitro standardization of BT [131–134]. Originally, the prototype of this device was the Thrombostat 4000 system that was further settled into the PFA- 100 by Dade-Behring [135, 136].

Primary hemostasis is simulated in WB by using disposable cartridges in which citrated WB (0.8 ml) is moved at high shear rates (5000–6000/s) through a capillary that at its top presents a collagen-coated membrane with a microscopic aperture (147 μm). Based on different reagents beyond the collagen, three assays are available: (1) test cartridge containing the membrane coated with collagen (C) plus ADP (CADP cartridge) sensible to platelet dysfunctions [132, 133], (2) that with collagen plus epinephrine (EPI) (CEPI cartridge) also sensible to aspirin therapy [108,

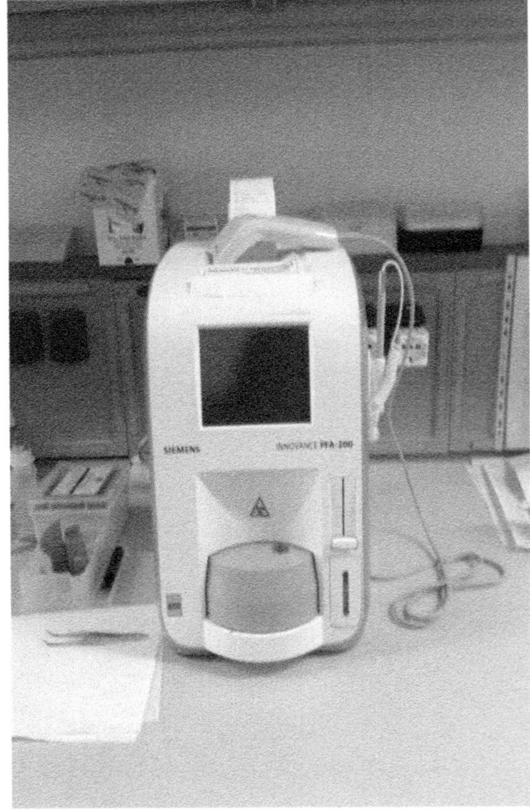

Fig. 3.4 Platelet function analyzer – 200 (Innovance PFA-200)

137], and (3) the Innovance PFA P2Y assay with a membrane coated with ADP, prostaglandin E1, and calcium designed for monitoring the treatment with P2Y12 inhibitors [130, 138]. The presence of different agonists in association with the high shear rates provoked by the system induces platelet activation and aggregation leading to an occlusion of the hole by the forming platelet plug. The time taken by platelets for occluding the aperture and stopping the WB flow is defined as closure time (CT) and it is expressed in seconds (s). The extent of CT is inversely correlated to overall platelet-related hemostasis [134]. The test requires a lead time of 5–8 min (maximum CT is 300 s) and must be performed within 4 h of citrated blood withdrawal. The method is automated – with the exception of dispensing the WB to the cartridge – and non-skilled personnel is requested for performing it.

The contemporary application of two cartridge tests – CEPI and CADP – allows to discriminate inherited platelet defects (prolonged times obtained with CADP test alone or plus CEPI test) such as VW defects or Bernard-Soulier syndrome or Glanzmann thrombasthenia from those due to antiplatelet therapy with ASA (prolonged time of CEPI test) [132, 134, 137, 139]. Karger and associates (2007) [140] reported that this methodology screens primary hemostasis with a sensitivity and specificity of 82.5 and 66.9 % for the CEPI test and 88.7 and 85.5 % for the COL/ADP. In comparison to BT, this assay has shown to be more sensitive [141] especially for diagnosis of VWD and platelet function defects [134]. But, it is not so sensitive for all platelet disorders as it could give false-negative results in patients with the storage pool disease or mild type I VWD [139]. A short/normal CEPI CT reflects a high residual platelet reactivity on aspirin therapy, and this test was reported to be able in predicting the risk of thromboembolic events [108, 139, 142–145]. In addition, a CT more than 106 s by using the new Innovance P2Y1cartridge was indicated as a cutoff value for the identification of patient responsive to clopidogrel [138]. Notwithstanding the scarcity of information, two studies reported its clinical value for detecting P2Y12 antagonist effect [146, 147].

Different variables can influence this test in prolonging or shorting its results. CTs may be prolonged by low platelet count (<150,000 plt/μL) and hematocrit (<35 %), conditions often associated to thrombocytopathies. Thus, the clinicians should consider these limitations. Conversely, high levels of fibrinogen or VWF, or an increased count of erythrocytes, have been reported to shorten CEPI CT [148–150]. In particular, Harrison and associates 2005 [151] reported that high levels of VW in ACS patients might really mask a reduced response to ASA therapy evidenced with this system.

By using the PFA system, the evaluation of platelet function of patients undergoing different types of surgical procedure device may offer useful information for the postoperative blood transfusion management [152]. Indeed, it was a useful tool for identifying platelet dysfunction before surgery [153, 154]. In particular, this system showed a high sensitivity and specificity in revealing preoperative platelet dysfunction in patients with bleeding history [153]. In cardiac surgery, PFA methodology showed a high predictive value of platelet function for management of intra- and postoperative blood loss [154–158], but contradictory results are reported regarding its predictive potential of postoperative hemorrhage. Certain findings provide positive predictive values: in a small study, Raman and associates [155], firstly, found that the prolonged CT by CADP cartridge was able to identify with high sensitivity (94 %) and specificity (85 %) those bleeding patients responsive or not to platelet concentrates. The prolonged value of CADP CT in association with a reduced angle alpha measured with thromboelastography was predictive of significant postoperative hemorrhage in cardiac surgery [154] . Furthermore, Davidson and associates [158] found that prolonged CTs obtained before cardiac surgery were predictive of postoperative bleeding (more than 200 mL/h during the first four postoperative hours). In aortic valve replacement, the maximally prolonged CT by both CEPI and CADP tests were found associated to an increased probability (up to 80–90 %) of intraoperative RBC transfusions [156]. On the other hand, other authors did not report this capacity due to its poor positive predictive value. It was stated that platelet POCT is not helpful for routine use after cardiac surgery, and thus, it is not helpful in transfusion algorithms [159–161]. Indeed, Slaughter and associates [162] determined the potential for the PFA-100 to predict postoperative bleeding reporting a poor positive predictive value (18 %) and a high negative (96 %) predictive value useful only in identifying patients who are unlikely to need platelet transfusion to reduce bleeding.

Recently, PFA system, used as screening test also in different clinical settings, was found significantly associated with an increased mortality in trauma patients [163]; it was correlated with increased postoperative drain output in orthopedic surgery [164], and it was considered an independent risk factor for postpartum hemorrhage (PPH) severity and significantly related to menorrhagia [165, 166]. Moreover, in neurosurgical patients with preoperative prolonged CTs, the correction with desmopressin allowed to maintain a similar amount of transfusions to those provided to patients with normal presurgical CTs [167].

3.4.2 IMPACT: Analyzer

Impact: Cone And Plate(Let) Analyzer (Image Analysis Monitoring Platelet Adhesion Cone and Plate Technology-CPA) (DiaMed, Cressier sur Morat, Switzerland) – or the recent released research version of the instrument called the Impact-R – is a platelet POC test based on in vitro platelet activation, adhesion, and aggregation upon a polystyrene plate or a plate coated with collagen or extracellular matrix (ECM) under high shear conditions of 1800 s−1 [53, 168]. The shear stress force activates the sample platelets by the spinning of a cone coaxial to the plate. Primary hemostasis with this fully automated methodology is assessed by an automatic and computerized system. Indeed, the instrument contains a microscope, the reaction device – cone and plate – an automatic staining device, and an image analysis software that measures and records the platelets that have adhered and aggregated on the plate. The software, computes a number of parameters, including the percentage of the well surface covered by platelet aggregates, representing platelet adhesion; the average size of the aggregates (per μm2), representing platelet aggregation; and the distribution histogram of adhered platelets [169].

Initial data suggest that this assay could be a consistent system for the diagnosis of platelet defects. Glanzmann thrombasthenia, afibrinogenemia, and von Willebrand disease (VWD) were demonstrated by using Impact test that revealed the complete lack of adhesion to the polystyrene surface [170, 171]. On the other hand, Impact test has been able to see an excessive platelet adhesion induced by plasma from thrombotic thrombocytopenic purpura (TTP) patients or by plasma of patients with erythrocytosis and thrombocytosis [170, 171]. In addition, the use of platelet agonists AA and ADP in the system has allowed to monitor the efficacy of dual antiplatelet therapy [170–177].

Preoperatively, this methodology has been shown to be helpful in the evaluation of platelet function in thrombocytopenic patients and in predicting the risk of bleeding among these patients [169]. During cardiac surgery, platelet dysfunction, ascertained by Impact test, was found significantly correlated with postoperative bleeding [178–180]. To date, only Solomon and associates [181] found that preoperative platelet function evaluation with this methodology did not correlate with postoperative bleeding. So, this methodology appears to be a poor useful tool to determine perioperative platelet function and to help in prediction of postoperative bleeding. These open preliminary data might suggest that the use of Impact test might be an interesting tool for the evaluation of platelet function in surgical care. However, this method still needs an experienced use, and additional studies should be tried for assessing its feasible role in the management of bleeding in surgical care.

3.4.3 The Global Thrombosis Test

The Global Thrombosis Test (GTT) (Montrose Diagnostics Ltd, London, UK) monitors platelet function in native non-anticoagulated WB, without the use of agonists in an environment similar to physiological conditions [42, 46, 182, 183]. The principle of the method is based on the in vitro platelet activation triggered by high shear stress, likewise that existing in the stenosis of coronary artery. The device consists of a conical tube in which two ceramic balls are placed. A flat segment present along the inner wall of the tube prevents its full occlusion due to the inserted beads. When the native WB flows under the effect of gravity through the four narrow gaps on the level of first ball, a high shear stress activates platelets to aggregate. The low shear and turbulent flow produced below the first bead promote a platelet plug that closes the gaps of the second ball. In this first phase of the test, the closure of the tube system is expressed as the occlusion time (OT) in seconds. The WB withdraws more and more slowly in the form of drops, and the time of interval (*d*) between two consecutive drops is recorded until an arbitrary endpoint ($d \geq 15$ s) is reached. The second phase concerns the restart of blood flow at the bottom of the tube due to the lysis of plug expressed as lysis time (LT) in seconds [42, 182].

This POC test, whose purpose is supplying results on the patient's thrombotic status, is used both in acute critical settings and for general screening [183–186]. Studies about the clinical value of GTT as a diagnostic tool in association with clinical outcomes are still in progress. The ability of this global assay in investigating the full process of hemostasis could play a role in clinical practice [182, 187].

3.5 Assays in Combination with Viscoelastic Methodologies

Thromboelastography and thromboelastometry are systems that globally assay the hemostatic process (see Chap. 2). These assays investigate the full occurrence of clot formation analyzing the modifications of viscoelastic forces of WB during the clotting formation [187]. The means of this methodology is related to its capacity to study the extent of platelet count and function and the clotting and fibrinolytic activation [188]. In these tests, platelets play all their functional roles in hemostasis: thrombin generation, clot formation, clot retraction, and lysis.

3.5.1 TEG Platelet Mapping System

The Thromboelastography® Platelet Mapping™ test (Haemoscope Corp, Niles, Ill) is a modification of the original Thrombelastograph (TEG) assay that provides a quantitative analysis of platelet function [55, 189].

It has been developed for monitoring the effect of antiplatelet drugs specially in cardiological, neurological, and perioperative settings. The test is performed in a whole-blood sample, which is a more physiological approach according to the cellular model of hemostasis [190]. Monitoring antiplatelet therapy is relevant in order to prevent perioperative bleeding complications when an inappropriate timing of discontinuance has not been guaranteed, but also in order to prevent thromboembolic complications specially in patients with coronary or cerebral stents and ventricular assist devices.

The examination consists in establishing the degree of inhibition of platelet function adding the agonist of a specific platelet receptor to a blood sample in order to activate platelets that are not inhibited by antiplatelet drugs. First, a kaolin-activated test is performed to evaluate the maximal hemostatic activity as kaolin causes a thrombin burst, and thrombin is the most potent platelet activator known. It represents the 100 % of platelet aggregation potential or the maximum uninhibited platelet function of the specific subject. The following measurements are performed with heparin to eliminate thrombin activity. Second, a test in the presence of heparin and a special activator containing reptilase and Factor XIIIa (activator F) is performed to produce a cross-linked fibrin weak clot that isolates the only fibrin contribution to the clot strength [55, 189, 191]. This represents the lower limit of the range of platelet aggregation (0 %) for this specific patient. Then, the addition of adenosine diphosphate (ADP) or arachidonic acid (AA) stimulates differentially the platelet ADP or thromboxane A2 (TXA2) receptors leading to platelet aggregation in case the receptor is not occupied by the antiplatelet drug or antagonist. So, the contribution of P2Y12 and cyclooxygenase pathways to platelet aggregation is tested by the addition of respective agonist, ADP or AA [192]. The effect of therapy with aspirin (AA addition) or thienopyridines (ADP addition) is evaluated by comparing the TEG kaolin-activated test trace with the AA- or ADP-triggered trace. The maximum amplitude (MA) is the key analyzed parameter. In original TEG, the MA represents the maximum strength and stability of the clot. MA depends on the contribution of both platelets and fibrin. TEG MA parameter measures the percent change in clot strength after the addition of platelet agonist to the cuvette with reptilase and FXIIIa [55]. The platelet inhibition provided by the antiplatelet drug is calculated according to the formula (100 % – % aggregation). The percentage of aggregation is [(MA ADP – MA Fibrin)/(MA thrombin – MA Fibrin)] × 100.

The method has been shown to be reliable with low analytical variation [193] that could reflect the use of whole-blood samples, obviating pre-analytical and analytical factors such as platelet count and size, preparation of platelet-rich plasma, including centrifugation steps [191].

The TEG Platelet Mapping assay enables relating the percent platelet inhibition to the individual's maximum uninhibited platelet function. Therefore, the individual response to antiplatelet therapy is related to their own maximum uninhibited platelet function with potential therapeutic consequences [192] regarding both bleeding and thrombotic matters [194, 195].

TEG platelet mapping correlates well with optical platelet aggregation that still represents the gold standard for platelet function evaluation [55].

Postoperative bleeding remains one of the major complications after cardiac surgery needing cardiopulmonary bypass. Re-exploration and transfusions are associated with a significant increase of perioperative mortality and morbidity such as sepsis, renal failure, acute respiratory distress syndrome, and prolonged mechanical ventilation [196]. In this context, some authors have demonstrated a correlation between the transfusion of platelet concentrate and MA ADP in patients undergoing coronary artery surgery who presented postoperative bleeding tendency [194]. Despite the role of standard TEG in predicting postoperative bleeding is controversial; some authors have speculated the usefulness of platelet mapping to predict postoperative bleeding in patient assuming thienopyridines. The parameter MA ADP presents a significant ability to predict bleeding tendency in patients treated with clopidogrel requiring coronary surgery. MA ADP of <42.5 mm could predict bleeding tendency with a sensitivity of 78 % and specificity of 84 % [194].

According to some authors, agonist resistance is defined as >50 % agonist activation [197].

Nevertheless, the cutoff points to define effectiveness or resistance to antiplatelet drugs have still been insufficiently investigated. Regarding noncardiac surgery populations, the cutoff values indicating adequate normal inhibition levels are different depending on the drug, the cross-over inhibition, the time from suspension of medications, type of surgery, expected complication rate, and acceptable blood losses [198].

Nowadays, further large prospective studies should be performed in order to define the possible role of Thromboelastography® Platelet Mapping™ in monitoring antiplatelet therapy and to establish validated cutoff points.

3.5.2 ROTEM Platelet System

Thromboelastometry, formerly called rotational thromboelastography, is currently performed on a new device, the most recent in technology, the ROTEM *delta* (TEM Int., Germany) [56]. Recently, the ROTEM Platelet System has been added to the machine as an integrated module. The operating principle of the Rotem Platelet System is based on platelet impedance aggregometry in WB, similarly to MEA system. This allows the contemporary analysis of platelet function and clotting activation in a single instrument so that the ROTEM platelet equipment can simultaneously run in conjunction with the ROTEM *delta* system. Because there is a single software of data analysis for this double system, the platelet function analysis is visualized simultaneously with the thromboelastometric measurements on the same screen. Some characteristics of the ROTEM platelet are similar to those of MEA such as disposable cuvettes, measured platelet indexes, and agonists used. The assay is just available, but only a few data have been published regarding its laboratory and clinical value [199].

Conclusions

Platelet function assays have been up to now employed either for screening or diagnosing idiopathic or acquired pathological platelet conditions that lead to hemorrhagic and/or prothrombotic status [15–18]. Recently, these methodologies have been also utilized for monitoring antiplatelet therapies in order to identify those patients at risk of thromboembolic adverse events [19–22]. Traditional tests are not so complex to perform, but are time consuming, expensive, and affected by a great number of different methodological aspects requiring an adequate degree of expertise and experience. These numerous different aspects have produced an intra- and/or interlaboratory variability of results and have delayed a clear standardized procedure [73–76]. This fact has mostly restricted their wide clinic use, notwithstanding the effort in the amelioration of ongoing standardization and the use of flow charts for the correction of platelet defects. Actually, these assays are still performed only in specialized clinical laboratories dedicated to the studies of hemostasis and thrombosis, often in close nearness to the associated clinics.

As the assessment of platelet (dys)function play a crucial role in the management of severe hemorrhage, a skillful competence to perform platelet function assays in a timely and efficient manner is indispensable. During the last year, the introduction of simpler assays utilized as POCT or within nonspecialized laboratories has allowed to investigate platelet function [15, 23–29]. So, platelet function POCT, that shows a standardized operating procedure and consists of easy-to-use devices, has overwhelmed the important drawbacks of traditional tests. Moreover, these methodologies, by using WB as milieu, may evaluate in vitro platelet adhesion and aggregation in which also other blood cells play a role. Fianally, platelet POC can achieve either the study of global platelet function (Innovance PFA-200, IMPACT, GTT) or the evaluation of particular aspects of platelet activation (MEA, VerifyNow, TEG Platelet Mapping, Plateletworks) (Tables 3.1 and 3.2).

Now, platelet function POCT seems to be able in predicting bleeding (e.g., peri- or postoperatively) and/or thrombosis in high-risk surgical patients.

A peri-postoperative coagulopathy might occur (e.g., cardiopulmonary bypass), and this defective status might also be complicated by the use of pharmacological thromboprophylaxis [200]. So, the use of a platelet function assay that rapidly can give information about platelet function status could be advantageous. In this contest, the question is: Are platelet function and global hemostatic assays able to predict either bleeding or thrombosis in surgical patients? Preoperative and perioperative breakdowns of platelet function are principally due to unobserved (acquired or inherited) bleeding defects and to surgical procedures that may cause platelet defects and coagulopathies resulting in massive hemorrhage [201]. Although platelet POCT has demonstrated to be able to identify platelet function defects, its helpfulness in perioperative setting is still debated [23–28, 202, 203].

In 2013, guidelines about the management of severe perioperative bleeding were delivered by The European Society of Anaesthesiology (ESA) [204]. This release has recommended the preoperative use of platelet function analysis only when a positive bleeding anamnesis there was, or in presence of a platelet function affected by antiplatelet therapy or medical conditions. In this issue, platelet POCT has had the task of identifying preoperatively potential bleeding patients and those at high risk of thrombosis for the rapid diagnosis of emerging platelet defects and coagulopathies. The consequent management of hemorrhage during surgical procedures by using de facto platelet function POCT does consist in providing proper transfusions or specific targeted hemostatic treatments in the meantime of surgery, reducing unnecessary transfusions and their consequent related risks [201].

In addition, platelet POCT has demonstrated to be a useful tool in monitoring antiplatelet therapy, in guiding its titration, and in orienteering the possible choice of a different drug. Thus, it may be a control for minimizing the risk of either thrombosis or bleeding.

Recently, guidelines, released by the Society of Thoracic Surgeons (STS) [205], have recommended that the timing of cardiac and noncardiac surgery in patients on antiplatelet drugs should be objectively decided on the basis of test results rather than arbitrarily defined delays. Thus, the preoperative assessment of platelet function might be useful for identifying those patients with or without high residual platelet reactivity, that may undergo surgery reducing the bleeding risk. In addition, perioperative use of platelet function POCT has been described as a useful tool in regulating blood transfusions.

In the light of this, novel non-POC platelet adhesion methods such as microfluidic devices or platelet spreading tests, using fluorescence microscopy or scanning electron microscopy, are under evaluation [206, 207]. Different test such as immunological assay, HPLC, fluorescence microscopy, or flow cytometry that investigate the expression or the release of several compounds as ATP, ADP, 5-HT, CXCL12, CD34, P-selectine, or thromboxanes are by now available. As previously reported, many platelet tests like platelet aggregometry in PRP or different prototypes gave rise to the current available platelet function POCT. Given the plethora of the novel tests in studio, it seems to be reasonable to expect that other new platelet POCT similarly are quickly available. In the future, it would be desirable that specific, standardized, more rapid, and easy tests – whose clinical value has been well defined – are available.

The effort in translating the traditional platelet function tests in platelet function POC assays able to predict bleeding disorders or high on treatment platelet reactivity is over in progress, and the interest on this issue is constantly increasing. An ideal assay should be rapid, reliable, maximally standardized, possibly inexpensive, and should offer a global evaluation of hemostasis such as viscoelastic systems. Indeed, by using these methodologies, algorithms for the correct use of blood components and proper pharmacological treatment in surgical patients at high risk have been developed. With these tools, the number of transfusions has been reduced and postoperative hemorrhage decreased [208, 209]. Along viscoelastic method, also platelet POCT has been progressively used in cardiovascular intensive care, trauma coagulopathy, liver transplantation, and obstetric care for the prediction of bleeding [25, 194, 210]. However, the "ideal" and widely acknowledged platelet POCT is still not available. Due to the intrinsic peculiarities, each assay has its own strengths and drawbacks [211]. Nevertheless, the correct identification of pros and cons of each platelet POC assay might guide the clinicians for the correct use of transfusions and for the rapid identification of bleeding risk directly in perioperative care [25, 153, 204, 209, 210]. This underlines the need for an evidence-based critical assessment of further studies supplying clinically relevant results on platelet POCT.

References

1. George JN (2000) Platelets. Lancet 355:1531–1539
2. Broos K, Feys HB, De Meyer SF, Vanhoorelbeke K, Deckmyn H (2011) Platelets at work in primary hemostasis. Blood Rev 25:155–167
3. Katz JN, Kolappa KP, Becker RC (2011) Beyond thrombosis: the versatile platelet in critical illness. Chest 139:658–668
4. Caudrillier A, Kessenbrock K, Gilliss BM et al (2012) Platelets induce neutrophil extracellular traps in transfusion-related acute lung injury. J Clin Invest 122:2661–2671
5. Lievens D, von Hundelshausen P (2011) Platelets in atherosclerosis. Thromb Haemost 106:827–838
6. Linden MD, Jackson DE (2010) Platelets: pleiotropic roles in atherogenesis and atherothrombosis. Int J Biochem Cell Biol 42:1762–1766
7. Pakala R, Waksman R (2011) Currently available methods for platelet function analysis: advantages and disadvantages. Cardiovasc Revasc Med 12:312–322
8. Harrison P (2009) Assessment of platelet function in the laboratory. Hamostaseologie 29:25–31
9. The British Society for Haematology (BCSH) Haemostasis and Thrombosis Task Force (2003) Guidelines on platelet function testing. J Clin Pathol 41:1322–1330
10. Michelson AD (2003) How platelets work: platelet function and dysfunction. J Thromb Thrombolysis 16:7–12
11. Ruggeri ZM (2002) Platelets in atherothrombosis. Nat Med 8:1227–1234

12. Ruggeri ZM, Mendolicchio GL (2007) Adhesion mechanisms in platelet function. Circ Res 100:1673–1685
13. de Groot PG, Urbanus RT, Roest M (2012) Platelet interaction with the vessel wall. Handb Exp Pharmacol 210:87–110
14. Badimon L, Vilahur G (2014) Thrombosis formation on atherosclerotic lesions and plaque rupture. J Intern Med 276:618–632
15. Rand ML, Leung R, Packham MA (2003) Platelet function assays. Transfus Apher Sci 28:307–317
16. Hayward CP, Rao AK, Cattaneo M (2006) Congenital platelet disorders: overview of their mechanisms, diagnostic evaluation and treatment. Haemophilia 12:128–136
17. Podda G, Femia EA, Pugliano M, Cattaneo M (2012) Congenital defects of platelets function. Platelets 23:552–563
18. Harrison P, Lordkipanidzé M (2013) Testing platelet function. Hematol Oncol Clin North Am 27:411–441
19. Collet JP, Montalescot G (2009) Platelet function testing and implications for clinical practice. J Cardiovasc Pharmacol Ther 14:157–169
20. Mylotte D, Foley D, Kenny D (2011) Platelet function testing: methods of assessment and clinical utility. Cardiovasc Hematol Agents Med Chem 9:14–24
21. Bonello L, Tantry US, Marcucci R et al (2010) Consensus and future directions on the definition of high on-treatment platelet reactivity to adenosine diphosphate. J Am Coll Cardiol 56:919–933
22. Buonamici P, Marcucci R, Migliorini A et al (2007) Impact of platelet reactivity after clopidogrel administration on drug-eluting stent thrombosis. J Am Coll Cardiol 49:2312–2317
23. Harle CC (2007) Point-of-care platelet function testing. Semin Cardiothorac Vasc Anesth 11:247–251
24. Dickinson KJ, Troxler M, Homer-Vanniasinkam S (2008) The surgical application of point-of-care haemostasis and platelet function testing. Br J Surg 5:1317–1330
25. Enriquez LJ, Shore-Lesserson L (2009) Point-of-care coagulation testing and transfusion algorithms. Br J Anaesth 103(suppl 1):i14–i22
26. Gibbs NM (2009) Point-of-care assessment of antiplatelet agents in the perioperative period: a review. Anaesth Intensive Care 37:354–369
27. Darling CE, Sala Mercado JA, Quiroga-Castro W et al (2014) Point-of-care assessment of platelet reactivity in the emergency department may facilitate rapid rule-out of acute coronary syndromes: a prospective cohort pilot feasibility study. BMJ Open 4, e003883
28. Kehrel BE, Brodde MF (2013) State of the art in platelet function testing. Transfus Med Hemother 40:73–86
29. Cardigan R, Turner C, Harrison P (2005) Current methods of assessing platelet function: relevance to transfusion medicine. Vox Sang 88:153–163
30. Duke WW (1985) The relation of blood platelets to hemorrhagic disease. JAMA 55:1185–1192
31. Rodgers RP, Levin J (1990) A critical reappraisal of the bleeding time. Semin Thromb Hemost 16:1–20
32. Born GV (1962) Aggregation of blood platelets by adenosine diphosphate and its reversal. Nature 194:927–929
33. Zhou L, Schmaier AH (2005) Platelet aggregation testing in platelet-rich plasma: description of procedures with the aim to develop standards in the field. Am J Clin Pathol 123:172–183
34. Hayward CP, Pai M, Liu Y, Moffat KA et al (2009) Diagnostic utility of light transmission platelet aggregometry: results from a prospective study of individuals referred for bleeding disorder assessments. J Thromb Haemost 7:676–684
35. Wu KK, Hoak JC (1974) A new method for the quantitative detection of platelet aggregates in patients with arterial insufficiency. Lancet 2:924–926
36. Grotemeyer KH (1991) The platelet reactivity test: A useful "by-product" of the blood-sampling procedure? Thromb Res 61:423–431
37. Koscielny J, Aslan T, Meyer O et al (2005) Use of the platelet reactivity index by Grotemeyer, platelet function analyzer, and retention test Homburg to monitor therapy with antiplatelet drugs. Semin Thromb Hemost 31:464–469
38. Hellem AJ (1960) The adhesiveness of human blood platelets in vitro. Scand J Clin Lab Invest 12(suppl):1–117
39. O'Brien JR, Etherington MD (1998) Antiglycoprotein Ib causes platelet aggregation: Different effects of blocking glycoprotein Ib and glycoprotein IIb/IIIa in the high shear filterometer. Blood Coagul Fibrinolysis 9:453–461
40. Krischek B, Morgenstern E, Mestres P et al (2005) Adhesion, spreading, and aggregation of platelets in flowing blood and the reliability of the retention test Homburg. Semin Thromb Hemost 31:449–457
41. Nowak G, Wiesenburg A, Schumann A, Bucha E (2005) Platelet adhesion assay: a new quantitative whole blood test to measure platelet function. Semin Thromb Hemost 31:470–475
42. Gorog DA, Kovacs IB (1995) Thrombotic status analyser. Measurement of platelet-rich thrombus formation and lysis in native blood. Thromb Haemost 73:514–520
43. Li CK, Hoffmann TJ, Hsieh PY, Malik S, Watson WC (1998) The xylum clot signature analyzer: a dynamic flow system that simulates vascular injury. Thromb Res 92:S67–S77
44. Kundu SK, Heilmann EJ, Sio R, Garcia C, Davidson RM, Ostgaard RA (1995) Description of an in vitro platelet function analyzer – PFA-100. Semin Thromb Hemost 21:S106–S112
45. Campbell J, Ridgway H, Carville D (2008) Plateletworks: a novel point of care platelet function screen. Mol Diagn Ther 12:253–258
46. Yamamoto J, Yamashita T, Ikarugi H et al (2003) Gorog thrombosis test: A global in-vitro test of

platelet function and thrombolysis. Blood Coagul Fibrinolysis 14:31–39
47. Cardinal DC, Flower RJ (1980) The electronic aggregometer: a novel device for assessing platelet behavior in blood. J Pharmacol Methods 3:135–158
48. Michelson AD (2006) Evaluation of platelet function by flow cytometry. Pathophysiol Haemost Thromb 35:67–82
49. Holmsen H, Holmsen I, Bernhardsen A (1966) Microdetermination of adenosine diphosphate and adenosine triphosphate in plasma with the firefly luciferase system. Anal Biochem 17:456–473
50. Tóth O, Calatzis A, Penz S, Losonczy H, Siess W (2006) Multiple electrode aggregometry: a new device to measure platelet aggregation in whole blood. Thromb Haemost 96:781–788
51. Smith JW, Steinhubl SR, Lincoff AM et al (1999) Rapid platelet-function assay: an automated and quantitative cartridge-based method. Circulation 99:620–625
52. Koessler J, Ehrenschwender M, Kobsar A, Brunner K (2012) Evaluation of the new INNOVANCE® PFA P2Ycartridge in patients with impaired primary haemostasis. Platelets 23:571–578
53. Varon D, Dardik R, Shenkman B et al (1997) A new method for quantitative analysis of whole blood platelet interaction with extracellular matrix under flow conditions. Thromb Res 85:283–294
54. Afshari A, Wikkelsø A, Brok J, Møller AM, Wetterslev J (2011) Thrombelastography (TEG) or thromboelastometry (ROTEM) to monitor haemotherapy versus usual care in patients with massive transfusion. Cochrane Database Syst Rev 16:CD007871
55. Craft RM, Chavez JJ, Bresee SJ et al (2004) A novel modification of the Thromboelastograph assay, isolating platelet function, correlates with optical platelet aggregation. J Lab Clin Med 143:301–309
56. http://www.rotem.de/en/methodology/impedance-aggregometry/
57. O'Brien JM (1962) Platelet aggregation. II some results from a new method of study. J Clin Pathol 15:452–458
58. Frontroth JP (2013) Light transmission aggregometry. In: Monagle P (ed) Haemostasis: methods and protocols, methods in molecular biology. Springer Science+Business Media, New York, pp 227–240
59. Dawood BB, Lowe GC, Lordkipanidzé M et al (2012) Evaluation of participants with suspected heritable platelet function disorders including recommendation and validation of a streamlined agonist panel. Blood 120:5041–5049
60. Kottke-Marchant K, Corcoran G (2002) The laboratory diagnosis of platelet disorders. Arch Pathol Lab Med 126:133–146
61. Hayward CP (2008) Diagnostic approach to platelet function disorders. Transfus Apher Sci 38:65–76
62. Israels SJ (2015) Laboratory testing for platelet function disorders. Int J Lab Hematol 37(Suppl 1):18–24
63. Gadisseur A, Hermans C, Berneman Z, Schroyens W, Deckmyn H, Michiels JJ (2009) Laboratory diagnosis and molecular classification of von Willebrand disease. Acta Haematol 121:71–84
64. Lev EI (2009) Aspirin resistance transient laboratory finding or important clinical entity? J Am Coll Cardiol 53:678–680
65. Harper AR, Price MJ (2013) Platelet function monitoring and clopidogrel. Curr Cardiol Rep 15:321
66. Leé S, Vargová K, Hizoh I et al (2014) High on clopidogrel treatment platelet reactivity is frequent in acute and rare in elective stenting and can be functionally overcome by switch of therapy. Thromb Res 133:257–264
67. Tantry US, Bonello L, Aradi D et al (2013) Consensus and update on the definition of on-treatment platelet reactivity to adenosine diphosphate associated with ischemia and bleeding. J Am Coll Cardiol 62:2261–2273
68. Breet NJ, van Werkum JW, Bouman HJ et al (2010) Comparison of platelet function tests in predicting clinical outcome in patients undergoing coronary stent implantation. JAMA 303:754–762
69. Bouman HJ, van Werkum JW, Breet NJ, ten Cate H, Hackeng CM, ten Berg JM (2011) A case–control study on platelet reactivity in patients with coronary stent thrombosis. J Thromb Haemost 9:909–916
70. Wisman PP, Roest M, Asselbergs FW et al (2014) Platelet-reactivity tests identify patients at risk of secondary cardiovascular events: a systematic review and meta-analysis. J Thromb Haemost 12:736–747
71. Paniccia R, Antonucci E, Maggini N et al (2011) Light transmittance aggregometry induced by different concentrations of adenosine diphosphate to monitor clopidogrel therapy: a methodological study. Ther Drug Monit 33:94–98
72. Femia EA, Pugliano M, Podda G, Cattaneo M (2012) Comparison of different procedures to prepare platelet-rich plasma for studies of platelet aggregation by light transmission aggregometry. Platelets 23:7–10
73. Christie DJ, Avari T, Carrington LR et al (2008) Platelet function testing by aggregometry; approved guideline, Clinical and Laboratory Standards Institute, vol 38; No. 31. CLSI document H58-A, Wayne. Available on-line at www.clsi.org
74. Hayward CP, Moffat KA, Raby A et al (2010) Development of North American consensus guidelines for medical laboratories that perform and interpret platelet function testing using light transmission aggregometry. Am J Clin Pathol 134:955–963
75. Harrison P, Mackie I, Mumford A et al (2011) British Committee for Standards in Haematology. Guidelines for the laboratory investigation of heritable disorders of platelet function. Br J Haematol 155:30–44
76. Cattaneo M, Cerletti C, Harrison P et al (2013) Recommendations for the standardization of light transmission aggregometry: A consensus of the

Working Party from the platelet physiology subcommittee of SSC/ISTH. J Thromb Haemost 11:1183–1189
77. Seyfert UT, Haubelt H, Vogt A, Hellstern P (2007) Variables influencing Multiplate whole blood impedance platelet aggregometry and turbidimetric platelet aggregation in healthy individuals. Platelets 18:199–206
78. Stissing T, Dridi NP, Ostrowski SR, Bochsen L, Johansson PI (2011) The influence of low platelet count on whole blood aggregometry. Clin Appl Thromb Hemost 17:E211–E217
79. Hanke AA, Roberg K, Monaca E et al (2010) Impact of platelet count on results obtained from multiple electroce platelet aggregometry (Multiplate). Eur J Med Res 15:214–219
80. Paniccia R, Antonucci E, Maggini N et al (2010) Comparison of methods for monitoring residual platelet reactivity after clopidogrel by point-of-care tests on whole blood in high-risk patients. Thromb Haemost 104:287–292
81. Paniccia R, Antonucci E, Maggini N et al (2009) Assessment of platelet function on whole blood by multiple electrode aggregometry in high-risk patients with coronary artery disease receiving antiplatelet therapy. Am J Clin Pathol 131:834–842
82. Sibbing D, Braun S, Jawansky S et al (2008) Assessment of ADP-induced platelet aggregation with light transmission aggregometry and multiple electrode platelet aggregometry before and after clopidogrel treatment. Thromb Haemost 99:121–126
83. Sibbing D, Schulz S, Braun S et al (2010) Antiplatelet effects of clopidogrel and bleeding in patients undergoing coronary stent placement. J Thromb Haemost 8:250–256
84. Christ G, Siller-Matula JM, Francesconi M, Dechant C, Grohs K, Podczeck-Schweighofer A (2014) Individualising dual antiplatelet therapy after percutaneous coronary intervention: the IDEAL-PCI registry. BMJ Open 4, e005781
85. Di Dedda U, Ranucci M, Baryshnikova E, Castelvecchio S, Surgical and Clinical Outcome Research Group (2014) Thienopyridines resistance and recovery of platelet function after discontinuation of thienopyridines in cardiac surgery patients. Eur J Cardiothorac Surg 45:165–170
86. Sibbing D, Braun S, Morath T et al (2009) Platelet reactivity after clopidogrel treatment assessed with point-of-care analysis and early drug-eluting stent thrombosis. J Am Coll Cardiol 53:849–856
87. Sibbing D, Morath T, Braun S et al (2010) Clopidogrel response status assessed with Multiplate point-of-care analysis and the incidence and timing of stent thrombosis over six months following coronary stenting. Thromb Haemost 103:151–159
88. Petricevic M, Biocina B, Milicic D et al (2013) Bleeding risk assessment using multiple electrode aggregometry in patients following coronary artery bypass surgery. J Thromb Thrombolysis 35:31–40
89. Ranucci M, Baryshnikova E, Soro G, Ballotta A, De Benedetti D, Conti D, Surgical and Clinical Outcome Research (SCORE) Group (2010) Multiple electrode whole-blood aggregometry and bleeding in cardiac surgery patients receiving thienopyridines. Ann Thorac Surg 91:123–129
90. Ranucci M, Colella D, Baryshnikova E, Di Dedda U, Surgical and Clinical Outcome Research (SCORE) Group (2014) Effect of preoperative P2Y12 and thrombin platelet receptor inhibition on bleeding after cardiac surgery. Br J Anaesth 113:970–976
91. Mengistu AM, Wolf MW, Boldt J, Röhm KD, Lang J, Piper SN (2008) Evaluation of a new platelet function analyzer in cardiac surgery: a comparison of modified thromboelastography and whole-blood aggregometry. J Cardiothorac Vasc Anesth 22:40–46
92. Rahe-Meyer N, Winterhalter M, Boden A et al (2009) Platelet concentrates transfusion in cardiac surgery and platelet function assessment by multiple electrode aggregometry. Acta Anaesthesiol Scand 53:168–175
93. Schimmer C, Hamouda K, Sommer SP, Özkur M, Hain J, Leyh R (2013) The predictive value of multiple electrode platelet aggregometry (multiplate) in adult cardiac surgery. Thorac Cardiovasc Surg 61:733–743
94. Solomon C, Traintinger S, Ziegler B et al (2011) Platelet function following trauma. A multiple electrode aggregometry study. Thromb Haemost 106:322–330
95. Kutcher ME, Redick BJ, McCreery RC et al (2012) Characterization of platelet dysfunction after trauma. J Trauma Acute Care Surg 73:13–19
96. Davies GR, Mills GM, Lawrence M et al (2014) The role of whole blood impedance aggregometry and its utilisation in the diagnosis and prognosis of patients with systemic inflammatory response syndrome and sepsis in acute critical illness. PLoS One 9, e108589
97. Morel-Kopp MC, Aboud M, Tan CW, Kulathilake C, Ward C (2011) Heparin-induced thrombocytopenia: evaluation of IgG and IgGAM ELISA assays. Int J Lab Hematol 33:245–250
98. Bolliger D, Dell-Kuster S, Seeberger MD et al (2012) Impact of loss of high-molecular-weight von Willebrand factor multimers on blood loss after aortic valve replacement. Br J Anaesth 108:754–762
99. Valarche V, Desconclois C, Boutekedjiret T, Dreyfus M, Proulle V (2011) Multiplate whole blood impedance aggregometry: a new tool for von Willebrand disease. J Thromb Haemost 9:1645–1647
100. Małek ŁA, Kłopotowski M, Śpiewak M et al (2014) Platelet reactivity and intramyocardial hemorrhage in patients with ST-segment elevation myocardial infarction. Clin Appl Thromb Hemost 20:553–558
101. Wheeler GL, Braden GA, Steinhubl SR et al (2002) The ultegra rapid platelet function assay: comparison to standard platelet function assays in patients undergoing percutaneous coronary intervention with abciximab therapy. Am Heart J 143:602–611

102. Steinhubl SR, Talley JD, Braden GA et al (2001) Point-of-care measured platelet inhibition correlates with a reduced risk of an adverse cardiac event after percutaneous coronary intervention: results of the GOLD (AU-Assessing Ultegra) multicenter study. Circulation 103:2572–2578
103. Kereiakes DJ, Mueller M, Howard W et al (1999) Efficacy of abciximab induced platelet blockade using arapid point of care assay. J Thromb Thrombolysis 7:265–276
104. Malinin A, Spergling M, Muhlestein B, Steinhubl S, Serebruany V (2004) Assessing aspirin responsiveness in subjects with multiple risk factors for vascular disease with a rapid platelet function analyzer. Blood Coagul Fibrinolysis 15:295–301
105. Marcucci R, Gori AM, Paniccia R et al (2009) Cardiovascular death and nonfatal myocardial infarction in acute coronary syndrome patients receiving coronary stenting are predicted by residual platelet reactivity to ADP detected by a point-of-care assay: a 12-month follow-up. Circulation 119:237–242
106. Jin HY, Yang TH, Kim DI et al (2012) High post-clopidogrel platelet reactivity assessed by a point-of-care assay predicts long-term clinical outcomes in patients with ST-segment elevation myocardial infarction who underwent primary coronary stenting. Int J Cardiol 167:1877–1881
107. Harrison P, Segal H, Blasbery K, Furtado C, Silver L, Rothwell PM (2005) Screening for aspirin responsiveness after transient ischemic attack and stroke: comparison of 2 point-of-care platelet function tests with optical aggregometry. Stroke 36:1001–1005
108. Paniccia R, Antonucci E, Gori AM et al (2007) Comparison of different methods to evaluate the effect of aspirin on platelet function in high-risk patients with ischemic heart disease receiving dual antiplatelet treatment. Am J Clin Pathol 128:143–149
109. Paniccia R, Antonucci E, Gori AM et al (2007) Different methodologies for evaluating the effect of clopidogrel on platelet function in high-risk coronary artery disease patients. J Thromb Haemost 5:1839–1847
110. Price MJ, Endemann S, Gollapudi RR et al (2008) Prognostic significance of post-clopidogrel platelet reactivity assessed by a point-of-care assay on thrombotic events after drug-eluting stent implantation. Eur Heart J 29:992–1000
111. Collet JP, Cuisset T, Rangé G et al; Investigators ARCTIC (2012) Bedside monitoring to adjust antiplatelet therapy for coronary stenting. N Engl J Med 367:2100–2109
112. Jeong YH, Bliden KP, Antonino MJ, Park KS, Tantry US, Gurbel PA (2012) Usefulness of the VerifyNow P2Y12 assay to evaluate the antiplatelet effects of ticagrelor and clopidogrel therapies. Am Heart J 164:35–42
113. Angiolillo DJ, Curzen N, Gurbel P et al (2014) Pharmacodynamic evaluation of switching from ticagrelor to prasugrel in patients with stable coronary artery disease: results of the SWAP-2 Study (Switching Anti Platelet-2). J Am Coll Cardiol 63:1500–1509
114. Delgado Almandoz JE, Kadkhodayan Y, Crandall BM, Scholz JM, Fease JL, Tubman DE (2014) Variability in initial response to standard clopidogrel therapy, delayed conversion to clopidogrel hyper-response, and associated thromboembolic and hemorrhagic complications in patients undergoing endovascular treatment of unruptured cerebral aneurysms. J Neurointerv Surg 6:767–773
115. Aradi D, Kirtane A, Bonello L et al (2015) Bleeding and stent thrombosis on P2Y12-inhibitors: collaborative analysis on the role of platelet reactivity for risk stratification after percutaneous coronary intervention. Eur Heart J 36:1762–1771
116. Reed GW, Kumar A, Guo J et al (2015) Point-of-care platelet function testing predicts bleeding in patients exposed to clopidogrel undergoing coronary artery bypass grafting: verify pre-op TIMI 45--a pilot study. Clin Cardiol 38:92–98
117. Rosengart TK, Romeiser JL, White LJ et al (2013) Platelet activity measured by a rapid turnaround assay identifies coronary artery bypass grafting patients at increased risk for bleeding and transfusion complications after clopidogrel administration. J Thorac Cardiovasc Surg 146:1259–1266
118. Yu PJ, Cassiere HA, Dellis SL, Manetta F, Stein J, Hartman AR (2014) P2Y12 platelet function assay for assessment of bleeding risk in coronary artery bypass grafting. J Card Surg 29:312–316
119. Alström U, Granath F, Oldgren J, Ståhle E, Tydén H, Siegbahn A (2009) Platelet inhibition assessed with VerifyNow, flow cytometry and PlateletMapping in patients undergoing heart surgery. Thromb Res 124:572–577
120. Short S, Kram B, Taylor S, Cheng J, Ali K, Vasquez D (2013) Effect of platelet inhibition on bleeding complications in trauma patients on preinjury clopidogrel. J Trauma Acute Care Surg 74:1419–1424
121. Lakkis NM, George S, Thomas E, Ali M, Guyer K, Carville D (2001) Use of ICHOR/Plateletworks to assess platelet function in patients treated with GP IIb/IIIa inhibitors. Catheter Cardiovasc Interv 53:346–351
122. Lennon MJ, Gibbs NM, Weightman WM, McGuire D, Michalopoulos N (2004) A comparison of Plateletworks and platelet aggregometry for the assessment of aspirin-related platelet dysfunction in cardiac surgical patients. J Cardiothorac Vasc Anesth 18:136–140
123. Mobley JE, Bresee SJ, Wortham DC, Craft RM, Snider CC, Carroll RC (2004) Frequency of nonresponse antiplatelet activity of clopidogrel during pretreatment for cardiac catheterization. Am J Cardiol 93:456–458
124. Holm M, Dalén M, Tornvall P, van der Linden J (2014) Point-of-care testing of clopidogrel-mediated platelet inhibition and risk for cardiovascular events after coronary angiography with or without percutaneous coronary intervention. Blood Coagul Fibrinolysis 25:577–584

125. van Werkum JW, Kleibeuker M, Postma S et al (2010) A comparison between the Plateletworks™-assay and light transmittance aggregometry for monitoring the inhibitory effects of clopidogrel. Int J Cardiol 140:123–126
126. White MM, Krishnan R, Kueter TJ, Jacoski MV, Jennings LK (2004) The use of the point of care Helena ICHOR/Plateletworks and the Accumetrics Ultegra RPFA for assessment of platelet function with GPIIB-IIIa antagonists. J Thromb Thrombolysis 18:163–169
127. Craft RM, Chavez JJ, Snider CC, Muenchen RA, Carroll RC (2005) Comparison of modified Thrombelastograph and Plateletworks whole blood assays to optical platelet aggregation for monitoring reversal of clopidogrel inhibition in elective surgery patients. J Lab Clin Med 145:309–315
128. Ostrowsky J, Foes J, Warchol M, Tsarovsky G, Blay J (2004) Plateletworks platelet function test compared to the thromboelastograph for prediction of postoperative outcomes. J Extra Corpor Technol 36:149–152
129. Dalén M, van der Linden J, Lindvall G, Ivert T (2012) Correlation between point-of-care platelet unction testing and bleeding after coronary artery surgery. Scand Cardiovasc J 46:32–38
130. Koessler J, Kobsar AL, Rajkovic M et al (2011) The new INNOVANCE® PFA P2Y cartridge is sensitive to the detection of the $P2Y_{12}$ receptor inhibition. Platelets 22:20–27
131. Francis J, Francis D, Larson L, Helms E, Garcia M (1999) Can the Platelet Function Analyzer (PFA)-100 test substitute for the template bleeding time in routine clinical practice? Platelets 10:132–136
132. Favaloro EJ (2002) Clinical application of the PFA-100. Curr Opin Hematol 9:407–415
133. Harrison P (2005) The role of PFA-100 testing in the investigation and management of haemostatic defects in children and adults. Br J Haematol 130:3–10
134. Hayward CP, Harrison P, Cattaneo M, Ortel TL, Rao AK (2006) Platelet function analyzer (PFA)-100 closure time in the evaluation of platelet disorders and platelet function. J Thromb Haemost 4:312–331
135. Alshameeri RS, Mammen EF (1995) Performance characteristics and clinical evaluation of an in vitro bleeding time device -- Thrombostat 4000. Thromb Res 79:275–287
136. Mammen EF, Comp PC, Gosselin R et al (1998) PFA-100 system: a new method for assessment of platelet dysfunction. Semin Thromb Hemost 24:195–202
137. Homoncik M, Jilma B, Hergovich N, Stohlawetz P, Panzer S, Speiser W (2000) Monitoring of aspirin (ASA) pharmacodynamics with the platelet function analyzer PFA-100. Thromb Haemost 83:316–321
138. Edwards A, Jakubowski JA, Rechner AR, Sugidachi A, Harrison P (2012) Evaluation of the INNOVANCE PFA P2Y test cartridge: sensitivity to P2Y(12) blockade and influence of anticoagulant. Platelets 23:106–115
139. Favaloro EJ (2001) Utility of the PFA-100 for assessing bleeding disorders and monitoring therapy: a review of analytical variables, benefits and limitations. Haemophilia 7:170–179
140. Karger R, Donner-Banzhoff N, Müller HH, Kretschmer V, Hunink M (2007) Diagnostic performance of the platelet function analyzer (PFA-100) for the detection of disorders of primary haemostasis in patients with a bleeding history-a systematic review and meta-analysis. Platelets 18:249–260
141. Michelson AD, Frelinger AL 3rd, Furman MI (2006) Current options in platelet function testing. Am J Cardiol 98:4N–10N
142. Marcucci R, Paniccia R, Antonucci E et al (2006) Usefulness of aspirin resistance after percutaneous coronary intervention for acute myocardial infarction in predicting one-year major adverse coronary events. Am J Cardiol 98:1156–1159
143. Bevilacqua S, Alkodami AA, Volpi E et al (2009) Risk stratification after coronary artery bypass surgery by a point-of-care test of platelet function. Ann Thorac Surg 87:496–502
144. Hovens MM, Snoep JD, Eikenboom JC, van der Bom JG, Mertens BJ, Huisman MV (2007) Prevalence of persistent platelet reactivity despite use of aspirin: a systematic review. Am Heart J 153:175–181
145. Crescente M, Di Castelnuovo A, Iacoviello L, Vermylen J, Cerletti C, de Gaetano G (2008) Response variability to aspirin as assessed by the platelet function analyzer (PFA)-100. A systematic review. Thromb Haemost 99:14–26
146. Linnemann B, Schwonberg J, Rechner AR, Mani H, Lindhoff-Last E (2010) Assessment of clopidogrel non-response by the PFA-100 system using the new test cartridge INNOVANCE PFA P2Y. Ann Hematol 89:597–605
147. Tsantes A, Ikonomidis I, Papadakis I et al (2012) Evaluation of the role of the new INNOVANCE PFA P2Y test cartridge in detection of clopidogrel resistance. Platelets 23:481–489
148. Chakroun T, Gerotziafas G, Robert F et al (2004) In vitro aspirin resistance detected by PFA-100 closure time: pivotal role of plasma von Willebrand factor. Br J Haematol 124:80–85
149. Wannhoff A, Müller OJ, Friedrich K et al (2014) Effects of increased von Willebrand factor levels on primary hemostasis in thrombocytopenic patients with liver cirrhosis. PLoS One 9:e112583
150. Mannini L, Marcucci R, Paniccia R et al (2006) Erythrocyte deformability and white blood cell count are associated with aspirin resistance in high-risk vascular patients. Clin Hemorheol Microcirc 35:175–181
151. Harrison P, Mackie I, Mathur A et al (2005) Platelet hyper-function in acute coronary syndromes. Blood Coagul Fibrinolysis 16:557–562
152. Rechner AR (2011) Platelet function testing in clinical diagnostics. Hamostaseologie 31:79–87
153. Koscielny J, von Tempelhoff GF, Ziemer S et al (2004) A practical concept for preoperative manage-

ment of patients with impaired primary hemostasis. Clin Appl Thromb Hemost 10:155–166
154. Cammerer U, Dietrich W, Rampf T, Braun SL, Richter JA (2003) The predictive value of modified computerized thromboelastography and platelet function analysis for postoperative blood loss in routine cardiac surgery. Anesth Analg 96:51–57
155. Raman S, Silverman NA (2001) Clinical utility of the platelet function analyzer (PFA-100) in cardiothoracic procedures involving extracorporeal circulation. J Thorac Cardiovasc Surg 122:190–191
156. Sucker C, Litmathe J, Feindt P, Zotz R (2011) Platelet function analyzer (PFA-100) as a useful tool for the prediction of transfusion requirements during aortic valve replacement. Thorac Cardiovasc Surg 59:233–236
157. Steinlechner B, Zeidler P, Base E et al (2011) Patients with severe aortic valve stenosis and impaired platelet function benefit from preoperative desmopressin infusion. Ann Thorac Surg 91:1420–1426
158. Davidson SJ, McGrowder D, Roughton M, Kelleher AA (2008) Can ROTEM thromboelastometry predict postoperative bleeding after cardiac surgery? J Cardiothorac Vasc Anesth 22:655–661
159. Wahba A, Sander S, Birnbaum DE (1998) Are in-vitro platelet function tests useful in predicting blood loss following open heart surgery? Thorac Cardiovasc Surg 46:228–231
160. Fattorutto M, Pradier O, Schmartz D, Ickx B, Barvais L (2003) Does the platelet function analyser (PFA-100) predict blood loss after cardiopulmonary bypass? Br J Anaesth 90:692–693
161. Forestier F, Coiffic A, Mouton C, Ekouevi D, Chêne G, Janvier G (2002) Platelet function point-of-care tests in post-bypass cardiac surgery: are they relevant? Br J Anaesth 89:715–721
162. Slaughter TF, Sreeram G, Sharma AD, El-Moalem H, East CJ, Greenberg CS (2001) Reversible shear-mediated platelet dysfunction during cardiac surgery as assessed by the PFA-100 platelet function analyzer. Blood Coagul Fibrinolysis 12:85–93
163. Jacoby RC, Owings JT, Holmes J, Battistella FD, Gosselin RC, Paglieroni TG (2001) Platelet activation and function after trauma. J Trauma 51:639–647
164. Ng KF, Lawmin JC, Tsang SF, Tang WM, Chiu KY (2009) Value of a single preoperative PFA-100 measurement in assessing the risk of bleeding in patients taking cyclooxygenase inhibitors and undergoing total knee replacement. Br J Anaesth 102:779–784
165. Chauleur C, Cochery-Nouvellon E, Mercier E et al (2008) Some hemostasis variables at the end of the population distributions are risk factors for severe postpartum hemorrhages. J Thromb Haemost 6:2067–2074
166. Philipp CS, Miller CH, Faiz A et al (2005) Screening women with menorrhagia for underlying bleeding disorders: the utility of the platelet function analyser and bleeding time. Haemophilia 11:497–503
167. Karger R, Reuter K, Rohlfs J, Nimsky C, Sure U, Kretschmer V (2012) The Platelet Function Analyzer (PFA-100) as a screening tool in neurosurgery. ISRN Hematol 2012:839242
168. Spectre G, Brill A, Gural A et al (2005) A new point of- care method for monitoring anti-platelet therapy: application of the cone and plate(let) analyzer. Platelets 16:293–299
169. Kenet G, Lubetsky A, Shenkman B et al (1998) Cone and platelet analyser (CPA): a new test for the prediction of bleeding among thrombocytopenic patients. Br J Haematol 101:255–259
170. Shenkman B, Savion N, Dardik R, Tamarin I, Varon D (2000) Testing of platelet deposition on polystyrene surface under flow conditions by the cone and plate(let) analyzer: role of platelet activation, fibrinogen and von Willebrand factor. Thromb Res 99:353–361
171. Dardik R, Varon D, Eskaraev R, Tamarin I, Inbal A (2000) Recombinant fragment of von Willebrand factor AR545C inhibits platelets binding to thrombin and platelet adhesion of thrombin-treated endothelial cells. Br J Haematol 109:512–518
172. Shenkman B, Inbal A, Tamarin I, Lubetsky A, Savion N, Varon D (2003) Diagnosis of thrombotic thrombocytopenic purpura based on modulation by patient plasma of normal platelet adhesion under flow condition. Br J Haematol 120:597–604
173. Peerschke EI, Silver RT, Weksler BB, Yin W, Bernhardt B, Varon D (2007) Examination of platelet function in whole blood under dynamic flow conditions with the cone and plate(let) analyzer: effect of erythrocytosis and thrombocytosis. Am J Clin Pathol 127:422–428
174. Varon D, Lashevski I, Brenner B et al (1998) Cone and plate(let) analyzer: monitoring glycoprotein IIb/IIIa antagonists and von willebrand disease replacement therapy by testing platelet deposition under fl ow conditions. Am Heart J 135:S187–S193
175. Matetzky S, Shenkman B, Guetta V et al (2004) Clopidogrel resistance is associated with increased risk of recurrent atherothrombotic events in patients with acute myocardial infarction. Circulation 109:3171–3175
176. Shenkman B, Einav Y, Salomon O, Varon D, Savion N (2008) Testing agonist-induced platelet aggregation by the Impact-R [Cone and plate(let) analyzer (CPA)]. Platelets 19:440–446
177. Shenkman B, Matetzky S, Fefer P et al (2008) Variable responsiveness to clopidogrel and aspirin among patients with acute coronary syndrome as assessed by platelet function tests. Thromb Res 122:336–345
178. Gerrah R, Snir E, Brill A, Varon D (2004) Platelet function changes as monitored by cone and plate(let) analyzer during beating heart surgery. Heart Surg Forum 7:E191–E195
179. Gerrah R, Brill A, Tshori S, Lubetsky A, Merin G, Varon D (2006) Using cone and plate(let) analyzer to

predict bleeding in cardiac surgery. Asian Cardiovasc Thorac Ann 14:310–315
180. Gerrah R, Brill A, Varon D (2007) Platelet function changes in different cardiac surgery subgroups as evaluated with an innovative technology. Innovations (Phila) 2:176–183
181. Solomon C, Hartmann J, Osthaus A et al (2010) Platelet concentrates transfusion in cardiac surgery in relation to preoperative point-of-care assessment of platelet adhesion and aggregation. Platelets 21:221–228
182. Yamamoto J, Inoue N, Otsui K, Ishii H, Gorog DA (2014) Global Thrombosis Test (GTT) can detect major determinants of haemostasis including platelet reactivity, endogenous fibrinolytic and thrombin generating potential. Thromb Res 133:919–926
183. Saraf S, Christopoulos C, Salha IB, Stott DJ, Gorog DA (2010) Impaired endogenous thrombolysis in acute coronary syndrome patients predicts cardiovascular death and nonfatal myocardial infarction. J Am Coll Cardiol 55:2107–2115
184. Saraf S, Wellsted D, Sharma S, Gorog DA (2009) Shear-induced global thrombosis test of native blood: pivotal role of ADP allows monitoring of P2Y12 antagonist therapy. Thromb Res 124:447–451
185. Gorog DA, Fuster V (2013) Platelet function tests in clinical cardiology: unfulfilled expectations. J Am Coll Cardiol 61:2115–2229
186. Rosser G, Tricoci P, Morrow D et al (2014) PAR-1 antagonist vorapaxar favorably improves global thrombotic status in patients with coronary disease. J Thromb Thrombolysis 38:423–429
187. Ganter MT, Hofer CK (2008) Coagulation monitoring: current techniques and clinical use of viscoelastic point-of-care coagulation devices. Anesth Analg 106:1366–1375
188. Bischof D, Dalbert S, Zollinger A, Ganter MT, Hofer CK (2010) Thrombelastography in the surgical patient. Minerva Anestesiol 76:131–137
189. Price MJ (2009) Bedside evaluation of thienopyridine antiplatelet therapy. Circulation 119:2625–2632
190. Hoffman M, Monroe DM (2001) A cell-based model of hemostasis. Thromb Haemost 85:958–965
191. Bochsen L, Wiinberg B, Kjelgaard-Hansen M, Steinbrüchel DA, Johansson PI (2007) Evaluation of TEG® platelet mapping™ assay in blood donors. Thromb J 5:3
192. Preisman S, Kogan A, Itzkovsky K, Leikin G, Raanani E (2010) Modified thromboelastography evaluation of platelet dysfunction in patients undergoing coronary artery surgery. Eur J Cardiothorac Surg 37:1367–1374
193. Paniccia R, Priora R, Alessandrello Liotta A, Abbate R (2015) Platelet function test: a comparative review. Vasc Health Risk Manag 11:133–148
194. Chen L, Bracey AW, Radovancevic R et al (2004) Clopidogrel and bleeding in patients undergoing elective coronary artery bypass grafting. J Thorac Cardiovasc Surg 128:425–431
195. Bliden KP, DiChiara J, Tantry US, Bassi AK, Chaganti SK, Gurbel PA (2007) Increased risk in patients with high platelet aggregation receiving chronic clopidogrel therapy undergoing percutaneous coronary intervention: is the current antiplatelet therapy adequate? J Am Coll Cardiol 49:657–666
196. Moulton MJ, Creswell LL, Mackey ME, Cox JL, Rosenbloom M (1996) Reexploration for bleeding is a risk factor for adverse outcomes after cardiac operations. J Thorac Cardiovasc Surg 111:1036–1046
197. Tantry US, Bliden KP, Gurbel PA (2005) Overestimation of platelet aspirin resistance detection by thromboelastograph platelet mapping and validation by conventional aggregometry using arachidonic acid stimulation. J Am Coll Cardiol 46:1705–1709
198. Cattano D, Altamirano AV, Kaynak HE et al (2013) Perioperative assessment of platelet function by Thromboelastograph Platelet Mapping in cardiovascular patients undergoing non-cardiac surgery. J Thromb Thrombolysis 35:23–30
199. Lang T, Tollnick M, Rieke M (2014) Evaluation of the new device ROTEM® platelet. In: Poster presented at: 58th annual meeting of society of thrombosis and haemostasis research (GTH2014); 12–15 Feb, Wien
200. Paparella D, Brister SJ, Buchanan MR (2004) Coagulation disorders of cardiopulmonary bypass: a review. Intensive Care Med 30:1873–1881
201. Koh MB, Hunt BJ (2003) The management of perioperative bleeding. Blood Rev 17:179–185
202. Avidan MS, Alcock EL, Da Fonseca J et al (2004) Comparison of structured use of routine laboratory tests or near-patient assessment with clinical judgment in the management of bleeding after cardiac surgery. Br J Anaesth 92:178–186
203. Poston R, Gu J, Manchio J et al (2005) Platelet function tests predict bleeding and thrombotic events after off-pump coronary bypass grafting. Eur J Cardiothorac Surg 27:584–591
204. Kozek-Langenecker SA, Afshari A, Albaladejo P et al (2013) Management of severe perioperative bleeding: guidelines from the European Society of Anaesthesiology. Eur J Anaesthesiol 30:270–282
205. Ferraris VA, Saha SP, Oestreich JH et al (2012) 2012 update to the Society of Thoracic Surgeons guideline on use of antiplatelet drugs in patients having cardiac and noncardiac operations. Ann Thorac Surg 94:1761–1781
206. Van Kruchten R, Cosemans JM, Heemskerk JW (2012) Measurement of whole blood thrombus formation using parallel-plate flow chambers – a practical guide. Platelets 23:229–242
207. Aslan JE, Itakura A, Gertz JM, McCarty OJ (2012) Platelet shape change and spreading. Methods Mol Biol 788:91–100

208. Petricevic M, Kopjar T, Biocina B et al (2015) The predictive value of platelet function point-of-care tests for postoperative blood loss and transfusion in routine cardiac surgery: a systematic review. Thorac Cardiovasc Surg 63:2–20
209. Pearse BL, Smith I, Faulke D et al (2015) Protocol guided bleeding management improves cardiac surgery patient outcomes. Vox Sang. doi:10.1111/vox.12279
210. Mishra PK, Thekkudan J, Sahajanandan R et al (2015) The role of point-of-care assessment of platelet function in predicting postoperative bleeding and transfusion requirements after coronary artery bypass grafting. Ann Card Anaesth 18:45–51
211. Berger PB, Kirchner HL, Wagner ES et al (2015) Does preoperative platelet function predict bleeding in patients undergoing off pump coronary artery bypass surgery? J Interv Cardiol 28:223–232

4 Other Coagulation Point-of-Care Tests

Ekaterina Baryshnikova

4.1 Introduction

A point-of-care (POC) device is a kind of diagnostic testing placed and performed at or in proximity of the site where the patient is receiving medical care. The ideal POC assay should be rapid with results readily available to the healthcare personnel and applicable to the clinical setting, poorly influenced by environmental factors, simple to perform and understand, and convenient and cost efficient if compared to the traditional laboratory technologies. This kind of device is normally positioned outside the laboratory, generally in intensive care units, clinical wards, or operating rooms. Multiple attempts have been made in order to achieve these characteristics in the field of coagulation monitoring, both for hemostasis and for anticoagulation purposes. Some of the devices gained success and acknowledgment and are now widely used in the hospitals, many more have been proposed in the past, and others are just at the beginning of their development and recognition route. The present chapter will address coagulation POC devices not treated in Chaps. 2 and 3.

4.2 Viscosity-Based Devices

The viscosity of a fluid is a measure of its resistance to gradual deformation by shear stress. Under flow conditions, a forming thrombus presents the properties of both a fluid (viscosity) and a solid (elasticity). The combination of the viscoelastic properties of blood has been extensively applied to the coagulation monitoring in devices such as TEG® and ROTEM®. These devices however are not directly assessing viscosity but only a transition from a viscoelastic fluid to a viscoelastic solid detected as a resistance of the sample to a rotation strain. Moreover, in the abovementioned devices, the shear rate is settled at a very low rate (approximately 0.5 s^{-1}), not present in any area of the physiological circulation, and the applied shear rate is not constant. Concerns about the sensitivity, repeatability, and lack of standardization of these devices have been raised with conflicting findings reported so far [1–4].

Blood viscosity and its correlation with different blood components have been studied since the early twentieth century. The importance of changes in blood viscosity in many pathological conditions has been elucidated, and instruments allowing this kind of analysis were developed and refined – from homemade capillary viscosimeters to complex modern semi-automized devices with specifically dedicated software. Most of the applications to the coagulation monitoring proposed so far do not totally fulfill the POC requirements but show promising potentiality for a wider clinical use and deserve a mention.

E. Baryshnikova, PhD
Department of Cardiothoracic-Vascular Anesthesia and ICU, IRCCS Policlinico San Donato, San Donato Milanese, MI, Italy
e-mail: ekaterina.baryshnikova@gmail.com

M. Ranucci, P. Simioni (eds.), *Point-of-Care Tests for Severe Hemorrhage: A Manual for Diagnosis and Treatment*, DOI 10.1007/978-3-319-24795-3_4

4.2.1 Cone-on-Plate Viscosimetry

Historically, blood viscosity was assessed in anticoagulated blood and is normally 3–4 centipoise (cP). However, dynamic measurement of blood and plasma viscosity during coagulation is feasible. Whole blood is a non-Newtonian fluid, for which viscosity decreases for increasing shear rates in a nonlinear manner and is mainly dependent on hematocrit and temperature. A cone-on-plate rheometer is able to generate a range of shear rates that reproduce flow conditions in different areas of the circulatory system. Shear rate is a fundamental parameter affecting the dynamics of coagulation and blood viscosity [5], influencing platelet adhesion and activation, as well as thrombin generation [6–8]. After a liquid phase with a duration depending on the efficacy of the thrombin generation by the coagulation cascade, there is a transition from the liquid to the gel phase of the blood, and this turning point can be identified as the gel point (GP). Time-to-gel point (TGP) is prolonged when thrombin generation is impaired, for example, in presence of anticoagulation drugs and in case of congenital or acquired deficiency of coagulation factors (due to consumption, loss, or hemodilution). The viscosity of the growing clot increases until the maximum clot viscosity (MCF) is reached; a clot lysis could be detected as well [9]. MCF represents the overall clot strength and is influenced by platelet count, fibrinogen concentration, and factor XIII.

The direct measurement of the viscosity of blood coagulation is very sensitive and presents the undeniable advantages of applying a constant shear rate throughout the whole coagulation process and the possibility to change shear rate to conform to different physiology of circulation districts, as well as measuring the process in standard instead of arbitrary units. The cone-on-plate viscosimeter is still to be conformed to the POC requirements but already presents significant potential to overcome the limitations of the existing viscoelastic POC devices, besides offering the basis for the development of more sophisticated instrumentation.

4.2.2 Free Oscillation Rheometry (FOR) and ReoRox®

The application of the free oscillation rheometry concept to body fluids viscosity assessment was first described and patented in 1994 [10], and assays for the measurement of coagulation factors activity in whole blood were developed afterwards [11, 12].

In the ReoRox® (Medirox AB, Sweden) device blood is added to a cup that is set in free oscillation by a torsion wire with a cylinder submerged into the blood sample. The cup is initially rotated around its longitudinal axis and then released. At release, the torsion wire sets the cup into free oscillation, and the movement is recorded by an optical detector. FOR allows the detection of a wide range of elasticity changes. No external force is applied during measurement with no mechanical interference with the damping and frequency change in oscillating movement.

ReoRox® shows elasticity and viscosity in separate curves as compared to TEG® and ROTEM® that only presents the overall viscoelastic data. The detected variables include COT1 (clot onset time 1, determined from the viscosity curve) which represents the start of clot formation, COT2 (determined from the frequency/elasticity curve) which represents the time to a fully formed clot and equals the ROTEM variable CT, and G′ max (maximum elasticity which equals ROTEM MCF and elastic modulus). Common ReoRox® analyses include Fibscreen1 (thromboplastin activation, Fib1) and Fibscreen2 (thromboplastin activation and platelet inhibition with abciximab); Fib 1 and Fib2 correspond to EXTEM and FIBTEM in ROTEM.

ReoRox® works both on whole blood and plasma. The assay is usually performed on citrate-anticoagulated blood then recalcified with $CaCl_2$ with no artificial activators or inhibitors.

Changes in clot properties have been explored in supposed hypercoagulation (pregnancy) and hypocoagulation (thrombocytopenia) conditions [13]. It was found that pregnant women presented with shorter clotting times and higher clot elasticity than matched nonpregnant female donors with elasticity values higher in the late pregnancy. The thrombocytopenic patients presented low elasticity values that were readily increased by platelet transfusion with no change in corresponding clotting time.

There are two studies comparing fibrin-based clot elasticity parameters as measured by ReoRox® versus thromboelastometry (ROTEM®). Both methods were performed under platelet inhibition. Sølbeck and associates performed an in vitro comparison of ReoRox® and ROTEM® in trauma patients upon hospital admission [14]. Clot parameters were found to correlate between the two devices, including clot strength parameters. Solomon and associates applied FIBTEM test and Fibscreen2 test to native and hemodiluted whole blood samples from healthy volunteers, concluding that ReoRox® Fibscreen2 test has a higher than expected coefficient of variation and that both tests reflected elasticity impairment due to hemodilution [15].

In vitro-induced fibrinolysis is also detectable using a specifically designed ReoLyse test [16]. Spiking whole blood samples from healthy volunteers with different amounts of tissue plasminogen activator (t-PA), it was assessed that neither ReoRox® nor ROTEM® could detect low degrees of fibrinolysis. The authors concluded that ReoRox® could be a valuable alternative to ROTEM® to study high degrees of fibrinolysis and should be evaluated in clinical situations with increased fibrinolysis.

A study evaluating the contribution of various blood components to the viscous and elastic properties of the clot as measured by free oscillation rheometry reported that increasing the number of platelets and fibrinogen concentration resulted in higher elasticity while increasing hematocrit gave lower elasticity. In spiking samples with receptor GPIIb/IIIa inhibitor, the clot elasticity was severely impaired. The use of citrate-anticoagulated blood versus non-anticoagulated blood samples did not have significant differences in the clot properties [17].

ReoRox® is sensitive to the effect of the antiplatelet agents, like the receptor P2Y12 inhibitors [18]. ADP-receptor inhibition prolonged the clotting time for whole blood activated with collagen-related peptide, but it did not affect the properties of the subsequently formed clot.

ReoRox® device begins to be employed to produce research in the setting of cardiac pathologies [19]. Incubating blood samples from patients with a history of myocardial infarction complicated by ventricular fibrillation versus patients without ventricular fibrillation with lipopolysaccharide (LPS), a coagulation activator, and measuring the relative clotting times, Kälsch and associates concluded that the first group showed an enhanced coagulation activation which may be at least partially due to an enhanced platelet activation.

FOR technology presents significant qualities, but a few concerns regarding its reproducibility and precision need to be solved through appropriate investigations. Clinical applications of the ReoRox® device and its addition to the bleeding management decision helping charts should be further explored by specifically designed clinical studies.

4.3 Cone-and-Plate(let) Analyzer (CPA)

The CPA platelet function analyzer is based upon a method in which platelets from a whole blood sample aggregate on an extracellular matrix (ECM) when subjected to high shear stress. The surface coverage (SC) and the average size (AS) of the surface-bound particles (platelet aggregates) can be evaluated after staining the samples with a histologic stain by an inverted light microscope connected to an image analysis system [20]. Under shear stress, platelets adhere to ECM, and, following a release reaction, then other platelets aggregate on the first layer of adhered platelets. In these conditions, SC and AS are positively correlated with both platelet count and hematocrit. Blood samples from patients with von Willebrand disease showed reduced SC and AS, whereas those with Glanzmann thrombasthenia presented an almost normal SC but an AS close to that of single platelet. Previous data also showed a good correlation between the aggregate size and the bleeding tendency among patients undergoing pulmonary bypass [21]. In a modified CPA without ECM, treatment of blood samples with arachidonic acid or ADP significantly decreased the surface coverage, partially reversed by preincubation of the sample with aspirin and AMP, respectively [22]. The CPA technology presents the advantage of platelet aggregation taking place on an ECM-covered surface and under shear stress conditions, closely resembling physiological setting. However, this method still has steps requiring specialized personnel, and more data in prospective monitoring of coagulation and hemostasis should be collected.

4.4 Optical TEG (oTEG) and Laser Speckle Rheology (LSR)

Laser speckle rheology is an optical technology potentially capable of providing a noncontact rapid mechanical assessment of tissue properties [23]. Laser speckles represent a pattern of random intensity spots caused by the interference of coherent light scattered from tissue. This pattern is sensitive to the passive Brownian motion of intrinsic light-scattering particles. The analysis of laser speckle patterns has already been investigated for a number of biomedical applications, especially for the measurement of blood flow and tissue perfusion. In a viscoelastic medium such as blood, the Brownian motion of light-scattering centers is directly related to the viscoelastic properties of the medium. Consequently, during the coagulation process, the increasing stiffness of the blood clot caused by the formation of a fibrin-platelet network limits scatter displacements, eliciting a slower rate of speckle intensity fluctuations compared to un-clotted blood. Because scatter motion causes a modulation of the laser speckle pattern, the measurement of the time scale of speckle intensity fluctuations with a high-speed camera should provide information about the viscoelastic properties of clotting blood.

Applicability to the blood properties assessment was first presented in 2012 [24], employing heparinized blood from a swine animal model and then specifically designed for real-time coagulation testing with results compared to the conventional coagulation tests [25]. For each patient, the LSR clotting time (CT_{LSR}) and maximum clot stiffness (τ_{Max}) were calculated. Coagulation of citrate-anticoagulated samples was kaolin activated. Blood samples with normal activated partial thromboplastin time (aPTT) and prothrombin time (PT) showed shorter clotting times CT_{LSR} than samples with prolonged aPTT and PT values. Blood samples with increased fibrinogen concentration presented higher τ_{Max}.

The development of a point-of-care handheld LSR technology will certainly boost the assessment of blood and coagulation properties in various clinical settings. Until then, a wider application of LSR to bleeding management remains a potential.

4.5 Resonant Acoustic Spectroscopy with Optical Vibrometry (RASOV)

RASOV is a micro-elastometry via acoustic spectroscopy that measures the elastic modulus of the clot (CEM). Vibration produced by a magnetic force applied to the sample surface causes the clot to react with a specific resonant frequency. CEM is then computed and expressed in kPa. This method is not capable of assessing coagulation dynamics but offers a major sensitivity in assessing CEM and the ability to rapidly repeat measurements on a single sample. The first exploratory study was able to confirm that CEM is strongly influenced by fibrinogen concentration and is sensitive to a wide range of fibrinogen content variation [26].

4.6 Global Thrombosis Test (GTT)

The Global Thrombosis Test or Görög Thrombosis Test is a global coagulation test which allows the assessment of the overall coagulation process, from thrombosis to thrombolysis [27]. Native blood is placed in a test tube and flows through two consecutive series of narrow gaps, exposing platelets to high shear stress and consequently activating them. Activated platelets aggregate and thrombin is generated, and the gaps are finally occluded by the formed clot. Blood flow reduction and arrest is detected as the time interval between two consecutive blood drops falling from the tube increases and the occlusion time (OT) is registered. The displacement of the thrombi is indicative of occurred thrombolysis.

Platelets play a major role in the obstruction flow. Monoclonal antibodies against platelet GPIIb/IIIa receptor completely prevented occlusion [27]. GTT is capable of detecting the effect of antiplatelet (clopidogrel) and anticoagulation (heparin, dabigatran, and argatroban) drugs that significantly prolonged OT [28, 29]. The occlusion time was inversely correlated with von Willebrand factor, ristocetin cofactor activity, and von Willebrand factor antigen, as well as with hemoglobin and hematocrit, whereas platelet count showed no correlation with OT [30].

GTT was applied in studies on large series of smokers [31], patients with metabolic syndrome [32], and patients with cerebral infarction [33], but bleeding and cardiovascular setting have not been explored yet.

4.7 Microfluidics-Based Devices

Recent technological advances allowed miniaturization and development of new application of already acquired methodologies to the monitoring of blood coagulation. Sophisticated constructions could be potentially downscaled and optimized to fulfill point-of-care requirements into a lab-on-a-chip devices. The advantages of these technologies are small size and need for small volumes of blood and reagents with consequent lower waste and costs, faster analysis and response times due to short diffusion distances, faster sample conditioning and high surface to volume ratio, high level of automation with no or limited need for sample manipulation, and no specialized personnel demand. Most of the published methodologies are still prototype devices, but the proposed ideas and results seem promising for future application in POC setting.

Microfluidics could be combined with other technologies in order to perform dynamic analysis of blood coagulation. In one of the recently developed prototypes, Rayleigh surface-acoustic waves (SAW) have been implemented into a miniaturized device for observation of ongoing thrombogenesis [34]. Rayleigh waves are a type of surface-acoustic wave traveling near the surface of solids. When a SAW encounters a solid/liquid interface, it is transferred into a sound wave that generate a pressure gradient and a flow in the liquid (acoustic steaming). Consequently, SAW could be used for instantly mixing and recalcifying a drop of citrated whole blood and induce coagulation. A small amount of fluorescent microspheres is added to blood, then the sample is placed within the reaction chamber, calcium chloride is added, and mixing is immediately started by inducing the SAW. Before coagulation is started, the fluorescent beads could freely move within the sample, but when coagulation is initiated, their degree of freedom is more and more reduced until the majority of the microspheres are trapped in the formed clot and the movement cease. The fluorescence displacement is registered by a fluorescence microscope and analyzed digitally through an image processing technique. Specific software measures the correlation between two successive images, with images becoming increasingly identical as the clot is forming. These coefficients are finally normalized between 0 % (no correlation) and 100 % (identical pictures), and the time corresponding to 50 % of maximal response is referred to as SAW-clotting time (CT).

In untreated blood of healthy volunteers, SAW-CT was approximately 200 s. Treatment with unfractioned heparin, argatroban, dabigatran, rivaroxaban, and GPIIb/IIIa inhibitor abciximab significantly prolonged SAW-CT, whereas acetylsalicylic acid together with clopidogrel had no influence on coagulation measured with this device.

In another kind of microdevice, fluorescently labeled fibrinogen combined with microstructured lateral flow platforms is able to detect the clot formation. The incorporation of the labeled molecules into the growing thrombus induces changes in fluorescence intensity and distribution easily detectable with appropriate instrumentation. This assay was shown to be specifically sensitive to heparin [35].

Microfluidic chips could be also used for studying the electrical impedance spectrum of whole blood [36]. Applying a frequency of about 1000 Hz to a whole blood sample placed into a micro-well, it is possible to observe the magnitude of the electrical impedance growing from approximately 10^4 Ω of the fluid phase to 10^6–10^7 Ω of the solid clot with a distinct point at which blood coagulation begins. Electrical impedance of blood is sensitive to hematocrit and temperature variations. It was shown that native blood clotting time was increasingly prolonged lowering the temperature, from approximately 1600 s at 37 °C to more than 4000 s at 18 °C. Blood coagulation time was linearly associated to hematocrit with higher values for increasing hematocrit. This technology is at its very beginning with no data in clinical settings available.

References

1. Evans PA, Hawkins RH, Morris N et al (2010) Gel point and fractal microstructure of incipient blood clots are significant new markers of hemostasis for healthy and anticoagulated blood. Blood 116:3341–3346
2. Ågren A, Wikman AT, Holmström M, Östlund A, Edgren G (2013) Thromboelastography (TEG®) compared to conventional coagulation tests in surgical patients – a laboratory evaluation. Scand J Clin Lab Invest 73:214–220
3. Theusinger OM, Schröder CM, Eismon J et al (2013) The influence of laboratory coagulation tests and clotting factor levels on Rotation Thromboelastometry (ROTEM®) during major surgery with hemorrhage. Anesth Analg 117:314–321
4. Haas T, Spielmann N, Mauch J et al (2012) Comparison of thromboelastometry (ROTEM®) with standard plasmatic coagulation testing in paediatric surgery. Br J Anaesth 108:36–41
5. Ranucci M, Laddomada T, Ranucci M, Baryshnikova E (2014) Blood viscosity during coagulation at different shear rates. Physiol Rep 2:e12065
6. Chen H, Angerer JI, Napoleone M et al (2013) Hematocrit and flow rate regulate the adhesion of platelets to von Willebrand factor. Biomicrofluidics 7:64113
7. Li M, Hotaling NA, Ku DN, Forest CR (2014) Microfluidic thrombosis under multiple shear rates and antiplatelet therapy doses. PLoS One 9:e82493
8. Haynes LM, Dubief YC, Orfeo T, Mann KG (2011) Dilutional control of prothrombin activation at physiologically relevant shear rates. Biophys J 100:765–773
9. Ranucci M, Ranucci M, Laddomada T, Baryshnikova E, Nano G, Trimarchi S (2014) Plasma viscosity, functional fibrinogen, and platelet reactivity in vascular surgery patients. Clin Hemorheol Microcirc. http://content.iospress.com/articles/clinical-hemorheology-and-microcirculation/ch1866?resultNumber=0&totalResults=5&start=0&q=baryshnikova&resultsPageSize=10&rows=10
10. Method of measuring rheological properties and rheometer for carrying out the method, patent WO 1994008222 A1
11. Ungerstedt JS, Kallner A, Blombäck M (2002) Measurement of blood and plasma coagulation time using free oscillating rheometry. Scand J Clin Lab Invest 62:135–140
12. Rånby M, Ramström S, Svensson PO, Lindahl TL (2003) Clotting time by free oscillation rheometry and visual inspection and a viscoelastic description of the clotting phenomenon. Scand J Clin Lab Invest 63:397–406
13. Tynngärd N, Lidanhl TL, Ramström S, Räf T, Rugarn O, Berlin G (2008) Free oscillation rheometry detects changes in clot properties in pregnancy and thrombocytopenia. Platelets 19:373–378
14. Sølbeck S, Vindeløv NA, Bæek NH, Nielasen JD, Ostrowski SR, Johansson PI (2012) In-vitro comparison of free oscillation rheometry (ReoRox) and rotational thromboelastometry (ROTEM) in trauma patients upon hospital admission. Blood Coagul Fibrinolysis 23:688–692
15. Solomon C, Schöchl H, Ranucci M, Schött U, Schlimp CJ (2015) Comparison of fibrin-based clot elasticity parameters measured by free oscillation rheometry (ReoRox®) versus thromboelastometry (ROTEM®). Scand J Clin Lab Invest 75:239–246
16. Nilsson CU, Tynngård N, Reinstrup P, Engström M (2013) Monitoring fibrinolysis in whole blood by viscoelastic instruments: a comparison of ROTEM and ReoRox. Scand J Clin Lab Invest 73:457–465
17. Tynngård N, Lindahl T, Ramström S, Berlin G (2006) Effects of different blood components on clot retraction analysed by measuring elasticity with a free oscillating rheometer. Platelets 17:545–554
18. Rämstrom S, Rånby M, Lindahl TL (2003) Effects of inhibition of P2Y(1) and P2Y(12) on whole blood clotting, coagulum elasticity and fibrinolysis resistance studied with free oscillation rheometry. Thromb Res 109:315–322
19. Kälsch T, Elmas E, Nguyen DX et al (2005) Enhanced coagulation activation by in vitro lipopolysaccharide challenge in patients with ventricular fibrillation complicating acute myocardial infarction. J Cardiovasc Electrophysiol 16:858–863

20. Varon D, Dardik R, Shenkman B et al (1997) A new method for quantitative analysis of whole blood platelet interaction with extracellular matrix under flow conditions. Thromb Res 85:283–294
21. Golan M, Modan M, Lavee J et al (1990) Transfusion of fresh whole blood stored (4 °C) for short period fails to improve platelet aggregation on extracellular matrix and clinical hemostasis after cardiopulmonary bypass. J Thorac Cardiovasc Surg 99:354–360
22. Spectre G, Brill A, Gural A et al (2005) A new point-of-care method for monitoring anti-platelet therapy: application of the cone and plate(let) analyzer. Platelets 16:293–299
23. Hajjarian Z, Tripathi MM, Nadkarni SK (2015) Optical thromboelastography to evaluate whole blood coagulation. J Biophotonics 8:372–381
24. Hajjarian Z, Nadkarni SN (2012) Evaluating the viscoelastic properties of tissue from laser speckle fluctuations. Sci Rep 2:316
25. Tripathi MM, Hajjarian Z, Van Cott EM, Nadkarni SK (2014) Assessing blood coagulation status with laser speckle rheology. Biomed Opt Express 5:817–831
26. Wu G, Krebs CR, Lin FC, Wolberg AS, Oldenburg AL (2013) High sensitivity micro-elastometry: applications in blood coagulopathy. Ann Biomed Eng 41:2120–2129
27. Yamamoto J, Yamashita T, Ikarugi H et al (2003) Görög Thrombosis Test: a global in-vitro test of platelet function and thrombolysis. Blood Coagul Fibrinolysis 14:31–39
28. Saraf S, Wellsted D, Sharma S, Gorog DA (2009) Shear-induced global thrombosis test of native blood: pivotal role of ADP allows monitoring of P2Y12 antagonist therapy. Thromb Res 124:447–451
29. Yamamoto J, Inoue N, Otsui K, Ishii H, Gorog DA (2014) Global Thrombosis Test (GTT) can detect major determinants of haemostasis including platelet reactivity, endogenous fibrinolytic and thrombin generating potential. Thromb Res 133:919–926
30. Nishida H, Murata M, Miyaki K, Omae K, Watanabe K, Ikeda Y (2006) Gorog Thrombosis Test: analysis of factors influencing occlusive thrombus formation. Blood Coagul Fibrinolysis 17:203–207
31. Suehiro A, Wakabayashi I, Yamashita T, Yamamoto J (2014) Attenuation of spontaneous thrombolytic activity measured by the global thrombosis test in male habitual smokers. J Thromb Thrombolysis 34:414–418
32. Suehiro A, Wakabayashi I, Uchida K, Yamashita T, Yamamoto J (2012) Impaired spontaneous thrombolytic activity measured by global thrombosis test in males with metabolic syndrome. Thromb Res 129:499–501
33. Taomoto K, Ohnishi H, Kuga Y et al (2010) Platelet function and spontaneous thrombolytic activity of patients with cerebral infarction assessed by the global thrombosis test. Pathopysiol Haemost Thromb 37:43–48
34. Meyer dos Santos S, Zorn A, Guttenberg Z et al (2013) A novel μ-fluidic whole blood coagulation assay based on Rayleigh surface-acoustic waves as a point-of-care method to detect anticoagulants. Biomicrofluidics 7:56502
35. Dudek MM, Kent NJ, Gu P, Fan ZH, Killard AJ (2011) Development of a fluorescent method for detecting the onset of coagulation in human plasma on microstructured lateral flow platforms. Analyst 136:1816–1825
36. Lei KF, Chen KH, Tsui PH, Tsang NM (2013) Real-time electrical impedimetric monitoring of blood coagulation process under temperature and hematocrit variations conducted in a microfluidic chip. PLoS One 8:e76243

Coagulation and Point of Care in Clinical Practice: History

5

Luca Spiezia and Paolo Simioni

This was the historical and cultural context that framed the work and studies of a young German physiologist, Dr. Hellmut Hartert (1918 Tübingen – 1993 Kaiserslautern). He started his research from the two main limitations of PT and aPTT: (a) these tests evaluated only the initiation of the clotting process; (b) the information obtained was limited to plasma.

Dr. Hartert conceived the first thromboelastograph in Germany, in 1948 [6]. He started from the concept that blood clot has both viscous and elastic properties. Based on these premises, he developed an apparatus able to measure the elastic shear modulus or storage modulus of clotting blood. The method provided that an aliquot of whole blood be placed in the sample cup. A pin suspended by a calibrated torsion wire was lowered into the sample. To measure the elastic shear modulus of the sample, the cup was oscillated through an angle of 4° 45″ over a 10s interval, including 1s rest periods at the end of the rotation in each direction to prevent viscosity errors. The torque of the cup is transmitted to the pin through the sample in the cup. The width of the tracing is proportional to the magnitude of elastic shear modulus of the sample that is affected by platelet count and fibrinogen levels in whole blood [7]. Thromboelastographic information was obtained from an uninterrupted recorded tracing called the thromboelastogram. At the very beginning, only reusable steel sets of cups and pins were available and whole blood (350 uL) containing no anticoagulants would be placed directly in the instrument immediately after being drawn with the sample being recalcified to start the procedure. In 1974, Caprini [8] and colleagues introduced a modified technique called celite-activated TEG, consisting of comparing two simultaneously performed thromboelastograms: one was a native whole-blood thromboelastogram and the other was performed in native whole-blood activated with celite.

Since the initial four parameters introduced by Hartert on each thromboelastogram tracing, namely: the reaction time *R*; the coagulation time K o k; the angle α; and the maximum amplitude, MA [7] (see subsequent paragraphs for further details), several new parameters, ratios, indexes, and even mathematical equations have been proposed.

Originally, the thromboelastography (TEG) assay was considered interesting from a theoretical standpoint, but the clinical applicability was not well understood. Therefore, TEG was seen as being a bit too esoteric and too shock sensitive for routine clinical use. Performing the test was also technically challenging and the results of the TEG analysis were scarcely reproducible. In the subsequent years, several European researchers

L. Spiezia, MD (✉)
Department of Medicine, University of Padua Medical School, Padua, Italy
e-mail: luca.spiezia@unipd.it

P. Simioni, MD, PhD
Department of Medicine, Hemorrhagic and Thrombotic Diseases Unit, University of Padua Medical School, Padua, Italy

M. Ranucci, P. Simioni (eds.), *Point-of-Care Tests for Severe Hemorrhage: A Manual for Diagnosis and Treatment*, DOI 10.1007/978-3-319-24795-3_5

between the 1950s and the 1970s developed the possible clinical applicability of this new apparatus. The American use of TEG began with von Kaulla and Caprini in the 1960s but minimal growth occurred until the 1980s.

While the TEG assay experienced growth in clinical interest as new surgical procedures evolved and perioperative bleeding became more of a serious complication, it remained mainly outside the scope of conventional diagnostic application in clinical practice. Even the TEG technology itself had not significantly evolved from its original design and continued to be performed only by an astute few. Nonetheless, the TEG maintained a level of interest because it provided a unique, comprehensive way to assess hemostasis in a whole-blood sample, in vitro, which more closely mirrored the physiologic conditions in vivo. Through the work of the dedicated scientific and medical community, realization of its diagnostic advantages and its clinical application began to spread.

In the early 1990s, a modified thromboelastography system was developed in Munich, Germany. Calatzis et al. reported the development of an improved method of viscoelastic testing called "rotational thromboelastography" or RoTEG [9]. This new method minimized many of the interferences that plagued classic thromboelastography. Later termed "rotational thromboelastometry" or "RoTEM," the test was made simpler by automating much of the analytical process, e.g., by using an automated pipette. The sensitivity to agitation was also minimized, which allowed the device to be used in a broader range of clinical settings. The testing could now be performed more easily by clinicians outside of the laboratory setting and could deliver more reliable and reproducible results.

References

1. Die MP, der Blutgerinnung C (1905) Die chemie der blutgerinnung. Ergeb Physiol 4:307–422
2. Quick AJ, Stanley-Brown M, Bancroft FW (1935) A study of the coagulation defect in hemophilia and in jaundice. Am J Med Sci 190:501–511
3. Langdell RD, Wagner RH, Brinkhous KM (1935) Effect of antihemophilic factor on one-stage clotting tests; a presumptive test for hemophilia and a single one-stage antihemophilic factor assay procedure. J Lab Clin Med 41:637–647
4. Davie EW, Ratnoff OD (1964) Waterfall sequence for intrinsic blood clotting. Science 145:1310–1312
5. MacFarlane RG (1964) An enzyme cascade in the blood clotting mechanism, and its function as a biochemical amplifier. Nature 202:498–499
6. Hartert H (1948) Blutgerinnungsstudien mit der Thrombelastographie, einem neuen Untersuchungsverfahren. Klin Wochenschr 26:577–583
7. Hartert H, Schaeder JA (1962) The physical and biological constants of thromboelastography. Biorheology 1:31–39
8. Caprini JA, Eckenhoff JB, Ramstack JM, Zuckerman L, Mockros LF (1974) Contact activation of heparinized plasma. Thromb Res 5:379–400
9. Calatzis A, Hipp R, Mössmer G, Stemberger A (1996) The roTEG coagulation analyser: a new thrombelastographic system for whole blood coagulation analysis. Int Congr Clin Chem abstract B610

6 Blood Products, Derivates, and Prohemostatic Drugs

Vanessa Agostini, Peter Santer, Guido Di Gregorio, and Vincenzo Tarzia

6.1 Fresh Frozen Plasma

Fresh frozen plasma is human donor plasma either obtained from a single whole-blood donation or collected by apheresis (jumbo plasma in the USA), frozen within a specific time period after collection, and stored at a defined temperature, typically −30 °C.

Plasma frozen within 6–8 h after the collection is called fresh frozen plasma (FFP) [1].

FFP contains approximately 1 IU per ml of each clotting factor, and for the quality control not less than 70 IU factor VIII per 100 mL and at least similar quantities of the other labile coagulation factors are required. This quality control is required by UK and EU guidelines [2], but not by the American Association of Blood Banks (AABB) standards [3]. This level needs to be met for a proportion of units (typically 75 %).

V. Agostini, MD (✉)
Transfusion Medicine Cesena/Forlì and Blood Establishment, Clinical Pathology Department-Cesena Azienda U.S.L Romagna, Romagna, Italy
e-mail: vani.agostini@gmail.com

P. Santer, MD
Clinical Pathology Laboratory, Brunico Hospital, Brunico, Italy

G. Di Gregorio, MD
Anesthesia and Intensive Care Unit, Department of Medicine, Padua University Hospital, Padua, Italy

V. Tarzia, MD
Division of Cardiac Surgery, Department of Cardiac, Thoracic and Vascular Sciences, University of Padua, Padua, Italy

Plasma frozen at slightly longer intervals (up to 24 h) after collection is referred as frozen plasma (FP, known as F24 in the USA). Levels of labile coagulation factors V and VIII may be lower in FP in comparison with FFP [1]. Both components are largely considered clinically equivalent by physicians and are both termed FFP.

After thawing, if plasma is not transfused within 24 h, it can be relabeled as thawed plasma and can be used within 5 days [3–5].

Different forms of industrial plasma are available in Europe. These components are prepared from pools of 300 to 5000 plasma donation and are pathogen inactivated in order to guarantee additional safety against transfusion-transmitted infections [4].

The main methods used for the pathogen-inactivation are solvent/detergent (S/D plasma) treatment in which pooled plasma is exposed to a solvent and detergent; methylene blue treatment in which a single donor unit of plasma is treated with an aniline dye (methylene blue) and light with the generation of reactive oxygen species able to inactivate enveloped and some non-enveloped viruses [4]; and amotosalen treatment in which psoralens are added to plasma prior to exposure to UVA light. Psoralens have virus- and bacteria-killing properties.

Due to biological variations in coagulation factor levels among plasma donors, an inter-unit variability exists in plasma preparations. Such variation seems to be less marked for industrial pathogen inactivated plasma together with a reduc-

M. Ranucci, P. Simioni (eds.), *Point-of-Care Tests for Severe Hemorrhage: A Manual for Diagnosis and Treatment*, DOI 10.1007/978-3-319-24795-3_6

tion in the levels of cytokines such as IL-8 and IL-10 responsible for immune-modulatory adverse events associated with plasma transfusion [6].

6.1.1 Indications

The clinical use of FFP has grown steadily in the last two decades in many countries, and there is also evidence of variation in usage among countries.

It is well known the widespread inappropriate utilization despite the available national and professional guidelines. This is true both for adult and children as documented in a recent international scenario-based survey on plasma transfusion practice in critically ill children [7].

Plasma for transfusion is given primarily for two indications: therapeutically to stop bleeding or as prophylaxis to prevent bleeding in patients with coagulation defects determined by the measurement of the prothrombin time (PT) or international normalized ratio (INR) and the activated partial thromboplastin time (aPTT).

Several worldwide guidelines recommend plasma transfusions when PT/INR and/or aPTT is greater than 1.5 times normal [8–12] in a bleeding patient.

However, a consensus on laboratory value triggers for plasma transfusion has not been reached. Recently the American Society of Anesthesiologists [13] proposed an INR grater the 2, in the absence of heparin, as a plasma transfusion trigger for the correction of excessive microvascular bleeding.

A recent systematic review [14] of 80 randomized controlled trials (RCTs) failed to demonstrate a significant benefit for both prophylactic and therapeutic plasma transfusion across a wide range of intervention.

Kozek-Langenecker and coworkers [15] analyzed outcome data (blood loss, allogeneic blood transfusion requirement, length of stay and survival) from 70 studies on FFP and 21 studies on fibrinogen concentrate and concluded against the evidence for the efficacy of FFP on all assessed outcomes.

Other classical indications for plasma transfusion are: replacement of a single factor deficiency for which no coagulation factor concentrate is available, disseminated intravascular coagulation (DIC) [16–19], liver failure [20, 21], massive transfusion [22–24], and plasma exchange and/or transfusion for thrombotic thrombocytopenic purpura.

6.1.2 Monitoring the Effects of FFP

The efficacy of plasma transfusion is generally assessed by measuring PT/INR and aPTT after the transfusion. Nevertheless it is well documented the inability of FFP to correct mild coagulation abnormalities [25, 26].

Holland and associates [26] have calculated the volume of FFP likely to achieve a target INR. To correct a mild prolonged INR, large volume of FFP is required, and the potential benefits of plasma transfusion, in terms of normalization of coagulation test results, are minimal in patients with a INR of less than 1.7. Similar conclusions derived from a small prospective cohort study [27] demonstrating a correction of coagulation tests and a rise in the concentration of coagulation factors only with a high volume of FFP (33. 5 ml/kg).

Using viscoelastic test performed on whole blood, a shortening in EXTEM CT (ROTEM) or R (TEG) and an increase in EXTEM MCF (ROTEM) or MA (TEG) after the transfusion of a therapeutic dose of fresh frozen plasma are expected.

6.1.3 Adverse Events

A comprehensive review of adverse plasma transfusion reactions is beyond the scope of this chapter.

However, plasma transfusion is associated with several infectious and noninfectious adverse events (www.shotuk.org). Transfusion-transmitted diseases include HIV, hepatitis B virus, and hepatitis C virus infections, which are to date rare events. Noninfectious complications include: transfusion-associated cardiac overload (TACO) [28], transfusion-related lung injury (TRALI) [29], and allergic reactions.

6.2 Platelets

Platelets can be obtained by two different methods: from donor whole blood or from apheresis. Platelet concentrates from whole blood are prepared from platelet-rich plasma [30], and this kind of product is named whole-blood random donor platelets (WB-RDP) or from buffy coat [31]. Four to 6 buffy coats are pooled in a larger bag to obtain a single unit.

Apheresis platelets are collected by cell separators through processing 4–5 l of donor blood. The major advantage of apheresis platelet transfusion is the reduction in donor exposure and consequently a lower risk of transfusion-transmitted infection and alloimmunization.

Platelet products are stored at 20–24 °C with continuous gentle agitation for up to 5 days.

Quality controls are required for the institution that prepares platelet concentrates in order to detect problems in the collection, processing, or storage of these products. These quality control include serological tests for transfusion-transmitted infection, platelet content (minimum of 2×10^{11} per unit), residual leukocyte counting ($<1 \times 10^{6}$ per unit), and pH measurement (>6.4) at the end of the shelf half-life.

6.2.1 Indications

Platelets transfusions are typically used for prophylaxis or treatment of bleeding episodes in patients with thrombocytopenia or congenital and acquired platelet dysfunction. Prophylactic transfusions are recommended in patients with hypoproliferative thrombocytopenia after chemotherapy or hematopoietic progenitor cell transplantation to reduce the risk of for spontaneous bleeding when the platelet count is below or equal to 10×10^{9}/L [32–36].

For patients having elective central venous placement, prophylactic platelet transfusions are indicated when platelet count is below or equal to 20×10^{9}/L [32, 37], while a trigger of 50×10^{9}/L is used for patients undergoing major non-neuraxial surgery [32, 38, 13] and 100×10^{9}/L for neurosurgical interventions [39].

In case of active bleeding and in patients undergoing massive transfusion, there is consensus for using a higher trigger [39, 40].

For patients on antiplatelet drugs who have spontaneous or traumatic hemorrhage, there is no consensus on platelet transfusion trigger [32, 41].

6.2.2 Monitoring the Effects of Platelet Concentrates

The efficacy of platelet transfusion is generally assessed by measuring immediate and late platelet count increments. The immediate effects of the transfusion of platelet concentrates on coagulation may be also evaluated in whole blood by viscoelastic tests (ROTEM, TEG).

A shortening in EXTEM CFT (ROTEM) or K (TEG) may be observed, but the most specific change is an increase in EXTEM MCF (ROTEM) or MA (TEG) after the transfusion of a therapeutic dose of platelet concentrate (Fig. 6.1).

6.2.3 Adverse Events

A comprehensive review of adverse plasma transfusion reactions is beyond the scope of this chapter. Basically, the most frequent adverse events are febrile and allergic reactions, bacterial sepsis, and TRALI [29].

6.3 Cryoprecipitate

Cryoprecipitate, originally known as cryoprecipitated antihemophilic factor, was developed for the treatment of congenital hemophilia A, von Willebrand disease, and hypofibrinogenemia.

It is a concentrate of high-molecular-weight plasma proteins that precipitate when plasma is slowly thawed at 1–6 °C and the supernatant (cryosupernatant or cryoprecipitate poor plasma) is removed. The product is refrozen and contains factor VIII, von Willebrand factor, factor XIII, fibronectin, and small amounts of other plasma proteins.

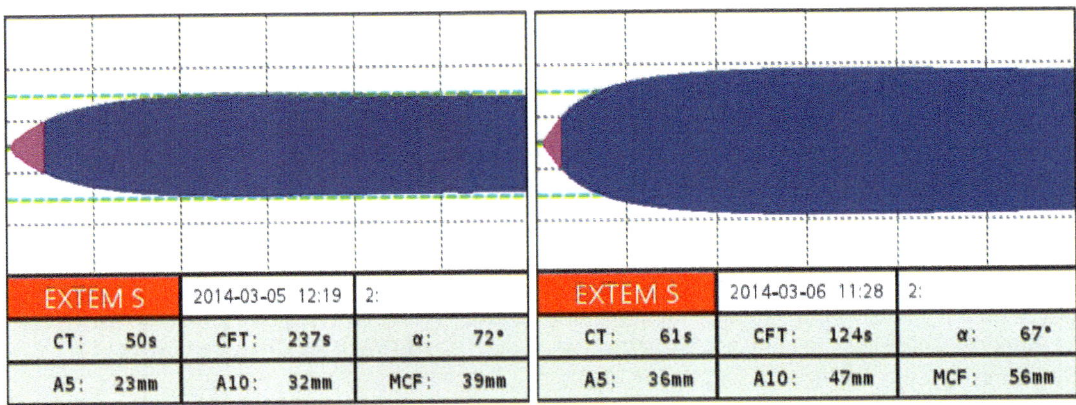

Fig. 6.1 EXTEM ROTEM trace of low platelet count in a patient with cirrhosis pre and post platelet transfusion

One unit of cryoprecipitate is manufactured from one unit of fresh frozen plasma and generally has a volume of 10–15 mL despite a great variability in the volume as described in literature [2, 3, 42, 43].

Despite it is believed that cryoprecipitate contains the majority of fibrinogen present in plasma, in fact it contains about one-third. Nevertheless, because of its small volume, the final fibrinogen concentration is higher than in plasma. Actually, the fibrinogen concentration derives from donors, so there is a wide variation (3.5–30 g/L) in the final content of each unit [44].

Cryoprecipitate can be infused as single unit or as a pool of 5–10 single donor units. Pooling of cryoprecipitate can be prepared before freezing or after thawing [45].

The cryoprecipitate specification requires that 75 % of units contain at least 140 mg of fibrinogen and 70 UI/ml of factor VIII [9].

6.3.1 Indications

Cryoprecipitate was historically used for the treatment of congenital factor VIII deficiency and von Willebrand disease, but now, more safe, purified, and virus-inactivated products or recombinant drugs are available, making it contraindicated for this indication in the developed world.

The most common indication for cryoprecipitate is to increase fibrinogen levels in acquired hypofibrinogenemia seen in trauma setting, in obstetric patients with postpartum hemorrhage, and in disseminated intravascular coagulopathy (DIC).

To date, it is recognized that patients with major trauma (ISS > 15) will develop, early, a relative hypofibrinogenemia, defined as a fibrinogen level <1.5 g/L [46, 47].

The use of cryoprecipitate in this setting was investigated by Morrison and associates in the MATTERs II study [48]. Over a 5-year period, 1332 patients, requiring at least 1 unit of red blood cell concentrate, were identified from the UK and US Joint Theater Trauma registries. Eleven percent of the cohort received tranexamic acid only, 12.6 % received cryoprecipitate only, 19.4 % received both tranexamic and cryoprecipitate, and 56.9 % received no treatment. Mortality was the highest in the non-treatment group (23.6 %) and the lowest in tranexamic acid/cryoprecipitate group (11.6 %). The benefit of tranexamic acid and cryoprecipitate was similar: in fact both were associated with an odds ratio for mortality of 0.61 and 95 % confidence interval of 0.42–0.89 and 0.40–0.94, respectively.

In the civilian setting, Rourke and associates [46] investigated cryoprecipitate in coagulophatic trauma patients demonstrating that the standard UK dose of 2 pool of cryoprecipitate maintained basal fibrinogen level during transfusion of red blood cells without significantly increasing the level compared with patients who had not received cryoprecipitate.

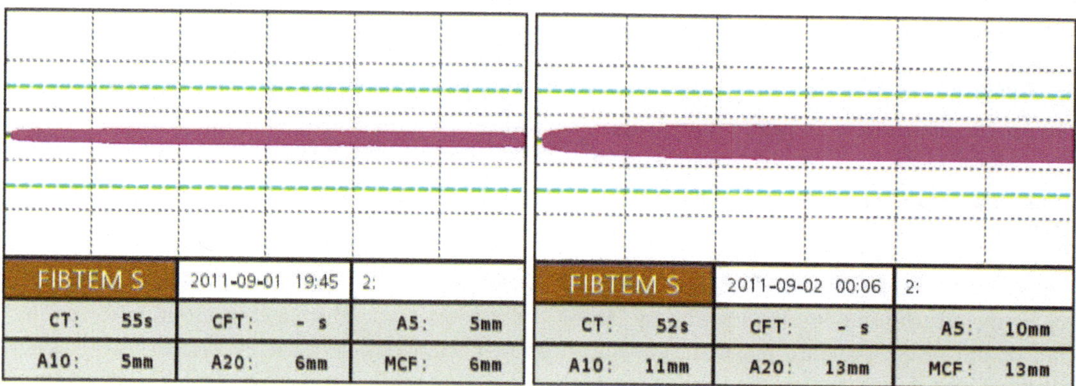

Fig. 6.2 FIBTEM ROTEM trace in a severely injured patient pre and after administration of 10 single units of cryoprecipitate

In 2007 the European guidelines [49] on the management of bleeding after major trauma recommended treatment of acquired hypofibrinogenemia if significant bleeding is accompanied by a plasma fibrinogen level <1 g/L. This trigger was increased to 1.5–2 g/L in the update to the guidelines in 2013 [50], and cryoprecipitate is a therapeutic option.

In obstetric bleeding patients, UK guidelines for the management of postpartum hemorrhage published in 2009 and updated in 2011 [40] recommend fibrinogen supplementation with cryoprecipitate if fibrinogen levels are <1 g/L. The European guidelines on the management of severe perioperative bleeding suggest a higher trigger (2 g/L) due to the physiologically elevated fibrinogen concentration in pregnancy [51].

6.3.2 Monitoring the Efficacy of Cryoprecipitate

It is possible to monitor the efficacy of cryoprecipitate as hemostatic therapy measuring fibrinogen plasma concentration by Clauss method or by viscoelastic tests such as rotational thromboelastometry (ROTEM) or thromboelastography (TEG). Cryoprecipitate transfusion significantly improves clot firmness measured by EXTEM test and FIBTEM test (Fig. 6.2). Similar changes are observed for the MA at standard TEG and functional fibrinogen test.

In a recent study Lee and associates [52] investigated the efficacy of cryoprecipitate in increasing plasma fibrinogen concentration (fibrinogen recovery) and quality of the fibrin-based clot in patients with bleeding during aortic surgery.

FIBTEM A10 was the test chosen to monitor the replacement therapy and the value of 6 mm as trigger for the administration of 10 units of cryoprecipitate.

The authors demonstrated that cryoprecipitate is able to increase clot firmness in FIBTEM A 10 and that the dose required to increase FIBTEM A10 by 1 mm was 13.2 mg fibrinogen/kg body weight or approximately 0.5 units per 10 kg body weight.

6.3.3 Adverse Events

A comprehensive review of adverse plasma transfusion reactions is beyond the scope of this chapter. However, typical adverse events include allergic reactions, transfusion-transmitted disease, TACO [28], and TRALI [29].

6.4 Antifibrinolytic Agents

Antifibrinolytic agents are commonly used to reduce blood loss and allogeneic blood transfusion during major surgery at high risk of bleeding such as cardiac, orthopedic, gynecological, urological, and neurosurgery.

The main antifibrinolytic agents are aprotinin, tranexamic acid, and e-aminocaproic acid.

6.4.1 Aprotinin

Aprotinin is a nonspecific serine protease inhibitor extracted from bovine lung acting by inhibition of the serine protease plasmin. The site of action is the active center of serine proteases. Aprotinin also inhibit trypsin, kallikrein, elastase, and thrombin and can interfere with the contact factor of coagulation (FXII).

Aprotinin was introduced for the first time in 1950 for the treatment of hyperfibrinolysis but became routinely used around 1990s in patients undergoing complex cardiac surgery [53].

The use of aprotinin came to the end after the publication of the BART (Blood conservation using Antifibrinolytic in a Randomized Trial) trial [54] conducted on 2331 patients at high risk of bleeding during cardiac surgery and randomized to receive aprotinin, e-aminocaproic acid, and tranexamic acid. The study was early interrupted because of an increased 30-day mortality rate in the aprotinin arm compared with the other two antifibrinolytic drugs (RR 1.53, 95 % CI, 1.06–2.22).

After these results, aprotinin was withdrawn from the market in 2008, but in 2011 the Canadian Health authorities [55] reviewed the BART trial results and authorized aprotinin in coronary bypass graft surgery. In 2012 the European Medicines Agency [56] removed the suspension after having reevaluated the risk profile of aprotinin.

Between 2011 and 2013, a number of meta-analyses and trials [57–60] in adult and pediatric populations have been published documenting that the aprotinin debate is still unresolved.

6.4.2 Tranexamic Acid

Tranexamic acid is a synthetic lysine amino acid derivative that exerts antifibrinolytic activity reversibly binding to plasminogen and preventing its interaction with fibrin. Tranexamic acid also blocks the binding of alfa2-antiplasmin to plasma and its inactivation of plasmin and inhibits trypsin and weakly thrombin [61].

Tranexamic acid can be used intravenously, orally, or topically, and the ideal dosage for each route of administration is not well defined. In vivo and in vitro data demonstrated that the effective therapeutic plasma concentration for inhibiting fibrinolysis has been reported to be 5–10 mg/L or 10–15 mg/L, respectively [62, 63]. Intravenous administration of 1 g dose achieves plasma concentration >10 mg/l for up to 5–6 h; after oral and intramuscular administration, the maximum plasma concentration is reached at 2–3 h and 0.5 h, respectively [64]. The absorption of oral tranexamic acid is not markedly affected by food; therefore, it can be administered without regard to meals.

Tranexamic acid crosses the placenta and the blood-brain barrier, penetrates eyes, and rapidly diffuses into joint fluid and sundial membranes. It requires adjustment in case of renal impairment while there is no need in case of hepatic impairment.

Few pharmacokinetic data are available for pediatric patients. Recently the first pharmacokinetic study in children undergoing craniofacial surgery was published demonstrating that a loading dose of 10 mg/kg over 15 min followed by continuous infusion of 5 mg/kg/h is optimal to reach the minimal therapeutic plasma level of 16 μg/mL during this kind of surgery [65].

Renewed interest in tranexamic acid stems from the CRASH-2 (Clinical Randomization of an Antifibrinolytic in Significant Hemorrhage-2) trial [66] assessing the effects of early administration of tranexamic acid in trauma patients with or at risk of substantial bleeding. 20,211 trauma patients from 40 countries were randomized within 8 h of injury to receive either tranexamic acid (1 g loading dose then 1 g over 8 h) or placebo.

The study demonstrated that all-cause mortality was significantly lower in the tranexamic acid group compared to placebo (14.5 % vs 16 %;

relative risk 0.91; 95 % CI 0.85–0.97, $P=0.0035$). Also death due to bleeding was reduced from 5.7 to 4.9 % ($p=0.0077$).

After the publication of CRASH-2 study, a number of systematic reviews, meta-analysis, and randomized clinical trials have been published in the setting of trauma [67] and surgical bleeding [68], in pediatric noncardiac surgery [69], and in orthopedic surgery [70, 71].

The topical application of tranexamic acid reduces the blood loss by 29 % (pooled ratio 0.71, 95 % CI 0.69–0.72; $p<0.0001$) versus placebo as recently documented in a Cochrane systematic review [72].

6.4.3 Monitoring the Efficacy of Antifibrinolytic Drugs

Whole-blood viscoelastic tests are established methods for the detection of fibrinolysis. Fibrinolysis is usually determined by detecting more than 15 % breakdown in clot strength as compared to MCF within 1 h after clotting time (maximum lysis, ML >15 %) in INTEM, EXTEM, and FIBTEM. After the administration of antifibrinolytic drugs, INTEM, EXTEM, and FIBTEM reveal stable clot trace (Fig. 6.3). Similar response is observed at TEG tests, where the clot lysis is expressed in terms of % changes in the MA.

6.4.4 Adverse Events

The most frequently reported side effects are gastrointestinal symptoms such as nausea and vomiting. Concerns have been raised regarding the prothrombotic potential and the increased risk of vascular events related to antifibrinolytic drugs. No increase in the rate of myocardial infarction, stroke, deep vein thrombosis, or pulmonary embolism has been described in recent meta-analysis and CRASH-2 trial.

6.5 Fibrinogen

Fibrinogen (factor I) is a plasma-soluble protein synthetized in the liver. It is the first clotting factor to decrease to critically low levels during hemorrhage, because the hepatic synthesis remains inadequate to compensate for the deficit in case of massive blood loss [73].

Fibrinogen plays an essential role in coagulation and is a central element of hemostasis [74]. It has a dual role as it enhances platelet aggregation and it is converted into fibrin to form an insoluble clot. During primary hemostasis, platelets become activated, resulting in an activation of platelet GPIIb/IIIa receptors that become the docking station for fibrinogen, linking platelets to platelets and thereby stabilizing the platelet plug. Activated platelets present highly efficacious surfaces for plasma coagulation, resulting

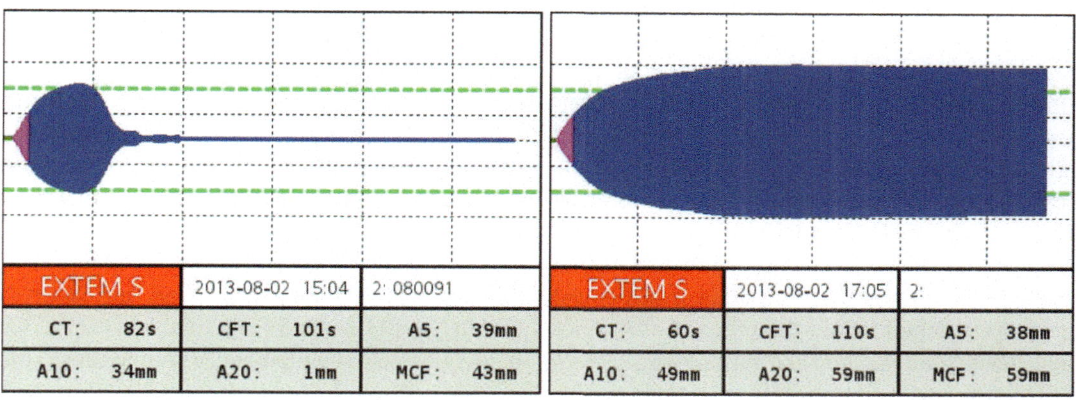

Fig. 6.3 ROTEM trace of fulminant hyperfibrinolysis in a severely injured patient pre and post administration of 2g of tranexamic acid

in the thrombin burst. As a result, fibrinogen is converted to fibrin and factor XIII (FXIII) is activated. The activated FXIII cross-link the soluble fibrin into solid fibrin strands [75, 76].

Low preoperative fibrinogen levels have been associated with increased perioperative bleeding and the need for transfusion of blood products [50, 77–82].

Thus, fibrinogen supplementation to restore plasma levels is an important component for normalizing clot formation in bleeding patients with low fibrinogen levels.

Fibrinogen concentrate is a plasma-derived, pasteurized, and lyophilized human fibrinogen, manufactured from pooled plasma donations that undergo purification, viral inactivation, and removal processes. The risk of immunological and allergic reactions is greatly reduced by viral inactivation and removal processes [83]. Fibrinogen concentrate is available for almost immediate use as no screening for blood type is needed and can be stored at room temperature (2–25 °C); thus, relatively high doses can be administered in a short time.

In addition to the advantages mentioned above, fibrinogen concentrate can be used to deliver a standardized dose, with a concentration of 0.9–1.3 g/vial (final concentration of 20 g/L), unlike fresh frozen plasma and cryoprecipitate, which contain variable amounts of fibrinogen.

Haemocomplettan/RiaSTAP (CSL Behring) is the only fibrinogen concentrate globally available and is licensed in a number of countries for multiple indications including treating acute bleeding episodes with hypofibrinogenemia. Other fibrinogen concentrate products with more limited availability are licensed in specific countries such as China, Japan, and France (Clottagen/Clottafact, Fibrinogen HT, FibroRAAS) [84].

Fibrinogen concentrate is widely used to correct hypofibrinogenemia with the goal of reducing coagulopathy, bleeding, and transfusion requirements. In particular, a number of clinical trials have demonstrated the efficacy of fibrinogen concentrate in aortic and cardiac surgery [85, 86]. Furthermore fibrinogen concentrate administration has been described as effective and safe in trauma patients and patients with postpartum hemorrhage by retrospective analyses and several systematic reviews [18, 87–94].

Recently, the European Society of Anaesthesiology (ESA) published guidelines for the management of perioperative bleeding which recommends substitution therapy with fibrinogen concentrate if significant bleeding is accompanied by at least suspected hypofibrinogenemia (Grade 1C: Strong recommendation, but with low quality of evidence) and suggests including fibrinogen concentrate in goal-directed treatment algorithms [51].

6.5.1 Monitoring the Efficacy of Fibrinogen Supplementation

Fibrinogen concentrate dosing should depend upon bleeding status and laboratory or point-of-care test results. The maximum clot firmness (MCF) in the FIBTEM test on the ROTEM device (or the equivalent parameter maximum amplitude, MA, in the functional fibrinogen assay on the TEG device) has been used extensively to determine fibrinogen levels [77, 85, 95, 96]. The fibrinogen dose can be calculated as follows:

$$\text{Fibrinogen concentrate dose}(\text{g}) = \begin{pmatrix} \text{target FIBTEM MCF}[\text{mm}] \\ -\text{actual FIBTEM MCF}[\text{mm}] \end{pmatrix} \times (\text{bodyweight}[\text{kg}]/70) \times 0.5\,\text{g}/\text{mm}$$

Normal MCF values are 9–25 mm, and they should correlate with a normal fibrinogen levels [77]; however, a target MCF of 22 mm has been used in aortic surgery patients (achieved using mean fibrinogen doses of 5.7 g) [97]. In the algorithm by Weber, 25 mg/kg fibrinogen concentrate is recommended if EXTEM A10 and FIBTEM A10 are below 40 mm and 8 mm, respectively. If FIBTEM A10 is <6 mm and EXTEM A10 is <40 mm, the recommended dose increases to 50 mg/kg [98]. According to the recent ESA guidelines, the recommended initial dose for adults is 25–50 mg/kg (children: 30–50 mg/kg) in the perioperative management [51] or 3–4 g in trauma management [50] (Fig. 6.4).

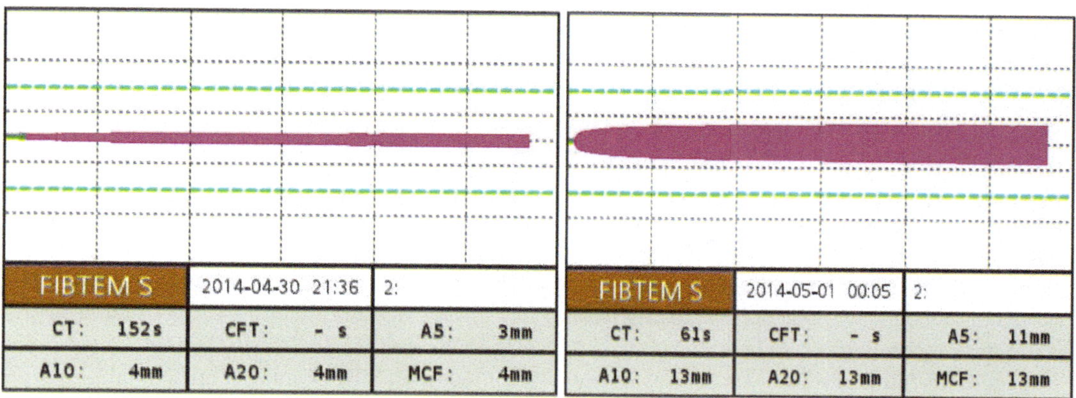

Fig. 6.4 FIBTEM ROTEM trace in a severely injured patient pre and post administration of 4 g of fibrinogen concentrate

However, the critical threshold for fibrinogen substitution and the target level to achieve are still a matter of debate, and the value of 22 mm at FIBTEM should be considered arbitrary.

6.5.2 Adverse Events

When administering a prohemostatic factor such as fibrinogen concentrate, the risk of thromboembolic complication should be considered. However, in a recent published descriptive analysis of over 27 years of pharmacovigilance, data indicates that the rate of adverse drug reactions reported following the administration of Haemocomplettan P/RiaSTAP across diverse clinical settings is low. In this analysis the authors identified approximately 4.3 thromboembolic events (TEE) per 105 treatment episodes (calculated from 28 cases reporting a possible TEE, corresponding to one case for every 23,300 standard doses of 4 g each) including all reported TEEs, regardless of their relationship to fibrinogen concentrate. Moreover, no allergic reactions or virus transmission events were identified during this literature review [99].

6.5.3 Desmopressin

Desmopressin (DDAVP, 1-deamino-8-D-arginine vasopressin) is a synthetic vasopressin derivate that increases plasma concentration of factor VIII (FVIII), von Willebrand factor (vWF), and tissue plasminogen activator (t-PA). It also has a vasodilatory action via activation of endothelial nitric oxide synthase.

Its effect on vWF and t-PA is likely explained by a direct action on the endothelium. It is postulated that activation of endothelial V2 receptors results in c-AMP-mediated exocytosis of vWF and t-PA from Weibel-Palade bodies where both are stored [100]. As a result of the increase in vWF, there is an increase in the number of FVIII binding sites; FVIII is therefore better protected against proteolytic breakdown. Desmopressin also induces the release and membrane presentation of P-selectin, which mediates platelet rolling on endothelial cells under high shear conditions [101]. A recent study demonstrated that desmopressin increases endothelial adhesiveness for platelets and platelet adhesion to collagen by releasing a proadhesive factor, likely vWF, from endothelial cells [102].

6.5.4 Indications

DDAVP has a proven hemostatic efficacy in mild hemophilia A, in von Willebrand disease (VWD), in uremia and liver cirrhosis as well as in congenital and acquired, drug-induced platelet dysfunction [103].

Desmopressin has been used as a hemostatic agent in patients without preexisting coagulation disorders undergoing high blood loss surgeries such as cardiac, spinal, and orthopedic procedures. A meta-analysis of 38 randomized, placebo-controlled trials indicated that desmopressin (usually at a dose of 0.3 μg/kg) had a statistically significant (albeit clinically modest) effect on reducing perioperative bleeding and transfusion of blood components without significant increased risk of thromboembolic complications [104].

In patients undergoing liver resection, desmopressin does not reduce transfusion requirement [105].

Although there is no evidence for DDAVP routine use after cardiac surgery, desmopressin may be considered whenever bleeding is suspected to stem from GPIIb/IIIa inhibitors and other antiplatelet agents [106] and in the setting of acquired von Willebrand disease (aortic stenosis patients) [107].

However, there is no convincing evidence that desmopressin minimizes perioperative bleeding or perioperative allogeneic blood transfusion in patients without a congenital bleeding disorder [51].

A decreased biological response has been observed after DDAVP doses repeated over short time intervals (tachyphylaxis), due likely to a V2 receptors desensitization or a slow vWf stores replenished [100].

6.5.5 Adverse Events

Adverse effects of DDAVP include mild facial flushing, headache, palpitations, and hypotension. Desmopressin should be used with caution in cases of severe congestive heart failure because of its potent antidiuretic effect. An increased risk of thrombotic events (i.e., myocardial infarction, stroke, arterial thrombosis, venous thromboembolism) has been reported [108, 109]. DDAVP should, therefore, be used with caution in patients with coronary artery disease.

6.6 Prothrombin Complex Concentrates

Prothrombin complex concentrates (PCCs) represent a highly purified concentrate of coagulation factors prepared from pooled normal plasma and contain a heterogeneous combination of coagulation factors and counterbalancing inhibitor components.

On market three-factor PCCs (containing factor II, IX and X) and four-factor PCCs (containing factor II, VII, IX and X) are available..

Initially PCCs were developed for the treatment of hemophilia B as a source of factor IX, and, to date, they are standardized on the basis of factor IX content. Concentrations of the other coagulation factors differ between batches.

6.6.1 Indications

1. *Reversal of vitamin K antagonists in major, life-threatening bleeding or for urgent surgery*

   PCCs replenish the coagulation factors suppressed by vitamin K antagonists (warfarin, acenocoumarol, or phenprocoumon) together with the administration of vitamin K i.v. [110–113]. The recommended dosages are related to the patient body weight and the INR value. Generally PCCs 25–50 IU/kg plus 10 mg of vitamin K are administered [114] with the goal to lower the INR below 1.5 as early as possible [113, 115]. This is particularly true in cases of intracranial hemorrhage which represent a serious anticoagulant-related bleeding complication, even though there is no solid evidence from literature of an improvement in prognosis [116, 117]. A close monitoring of INR is required in order to adjust quickly dosages in cases of unsatisfactory reversal.

   There is a well-known inverse no linear relationship between factor VII levels and INR, and for INR values over 4, the level of factor VII is under 5–10 %. It is reasonably believed that the non-complete reversal of higher INR values by 3 factors PCCs is due to the low content of factor VII [118].

Although randomized control trials do not exist to compare directly the efficacy and safety of 4-factor PCCs versus 3-factor PCCs, recent guidelines suggest the use of 4-factor PCCs because of the presence of anticoagulant factor proteins C and S. These more balanced drugs achieve a rapid reversal of anticoagulation at a higher rate [114, 115, 117, 119–121].

2. *Reversal of direct oral anticoagulants (direct thrombin inhibitors, direct factor Xa inhibitors)*

   Direct oral anticoagulants do not have specific antidotes, although this is an area of intense research. Treatment approach for the reversal of their effects derives mainly from studies on animals or in vitro studies or on healthy volunteers [122, 123].

   It has been suggest to administer 4-factor PCCs as first-line therapy at the dosages of 30–50 UI/kg [124–126].

3. *Major bleeding without vitamin K antagonists*

   In the past few years, several reports have been published on the efficacy of PCCs in the management of major bleeding in patients not on oral anticoagulation.

   Schols and associates [127, 128] demonstrated an increased risk of postoperative bleeding in patients with a low thrombin generation, while in vitro studies showed the possibility to restore thrombin generation through the infusion of fibrinogen concentrate and PCCs [129–131]. Based on these studies, recent guidelines [50, 51] suggest to administer PCCs at the dosages of 20–30 U/kg in bleeding patients with abnormal coagulation results (INR >1.5 or EXTEM clotting time >80 s).

4. *Treatment and prophylaxis of bleeding in congenital vitamin K-dependent factors deficiency*

   PCCs are the treatment of choice in congenital bleeding disorders in case the specific factor concentrate is not available.

   In particular PCCs are indicated for the management of bleeding episodes in congenital factor X and factor II (prothrombin) deficiency [132–135].

6.6.2 Monitoring the Efficacy of PCCs Therapy

It is possible to monitor the efficacy of PCCs treatment with POC devices such as ROTEM or TEG. A reduction of vitamin K coagulation factors cause a prolongation of clotting time (EXTEM ROTEM) or (TEG) which return in normal range after the administration of PCCs (Fig. 6.5).

6.6.3 Adverse Events

Potential adverse events related to PCCs infusion are allergic reaction, alloantibody development, chills, pyrexia, disseminated intravascular dissemination, and thromboembolic events [136] (microvascular thrombosis and myocardial infarction).

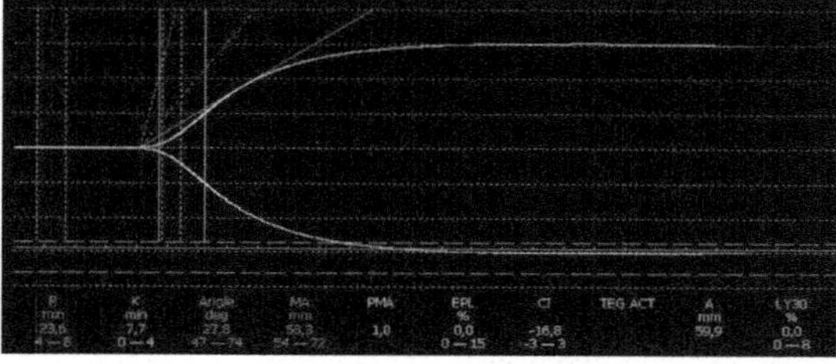

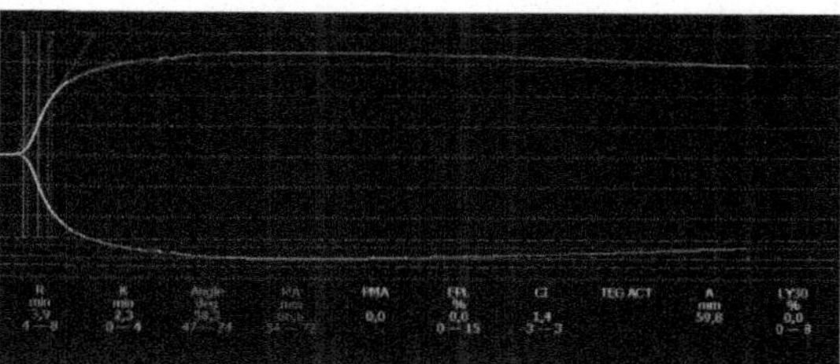

Fig. 6.5 TEG trace in a patient on oral anticoagulant therapy pre and post administration of 30UI/kg of 3-factor PCC

6.7 Bypassing Agents: Activated Prothrombin Complex Concentrates (aPCC) and Recombinant Factor VIIa

Bypassing agents consist of activated prothrombin complex concentrates (aPCC) and recombinant factor VIIa (rVIIa). There is only one manufactured rFVIIa (NovoSeven; Novo Nordisk, Bagsvaerd, Denmark) and one factor eight inhibitor bypassing activity (FEIBA; Baxter Bioscience, Vienna, Austria).

Their bypassing activities induce and facilitate thrombin generation, via pathways that do not require factor VIII and IX, but for which factor X and factor V play critical roles. It should, however, be emphasized that the two drugs are dissimilar even though both lead to thrombin generation and fibrin formation in patients with inhibitors [137, 138].

It is important to underline that neither of these two agents are able to completely restore thrombin generation in contrast to factor VIII and IX administration. Both agents have an overall efficacy rate above 80 % with similar rates of adverse events [139, 140].

FEIBA is a mixture of vitamin K-dependent coagulation factors obtained from a pooled human plasma after removal of cryoprecipitate and include factor II (prothrombin), factor VII, factor IX, and factor X and a small amount of factor IXa, Xa, and thrombin and a larger amount of factor VIIa [141–144]. The protein complex, apart from routine tests for pharmacological products, is subjected to a two-step vapor heat-treatment procedure for inactivation of lipid and non-lipid-enveloped viruses.

Originally it was believed rFVIIa would drive the activation of factor X via TF-FVIIa complex, bypassing the need for FVIII and FIX in hemophiliac patients. Later it was demonstrated that rFVIIa can directly activate FX on a negatively charged phospholipid surface in the absence of TF [145]. Furthermore at high doses [146], it can form the complex TF-VIIa competing with zymogen FVII for binding TF and can activate factor IX directly on the surface of activated platelets independent of FVIIIa or IXa [147–149]. To date, although a TF-dependent mechanism of action is not ruled out, it is believed that the major contributor to the hemostatic effect of rFVIIa is the ability to induce the thrombin burst on the platelet surface.

6.7.1 Indications

The principal indication for FEIBA and rFVIIa is the treatment of bleeding in patients with hemophilia A and B with inhibitors.

The usual dosages for FEIBA are 50–100 U/kg every 6–12 h with a maximum daily dose of 200 U/kg, while rFVIIa is administered at the dose of 90 mcg/kg given every 2–3 h by bolus infusion until hemostasis is achieved. For severe bleeding, the treatment with rFVIIa should continue at 3–6 h intervals to maintain hemostatic plug.

In acquired hemophilia rFVIIa is infused at the dosage of 70–90 mcg/kg repeated every 2–3 h until hemostasis is achieved. For the management of bleeding in congenital factor VII deficiency, dosages of 15–30 mcg/kg every 4–6 h until hemostasis is achieved are recommended.

Recently FEIBA and rFVIIa have been proposed as reversal hemostatic drugs in patients on direct oral anticoagulants who need urgent or emergency surgery or in case of life-threatening hemorrhage (e.g., intracranial or in critical organs) at the dose of 30–50 U/kg [150–152] and 90 mcg/kg, respectively.

rFVIIa has been used also in the treatment of acquired bleeding episodes in patients on oral anticoagulants, in intracranial hemorrhage, in traumatic bleeding, in postpartum hemorrhage, in cardiac surgery [153], and in surgical bleeding as rescue therapy.

Nevertheless the published CONTROL trial [154] failed to demonstrate a mortality benefit in using rFVIIa in blunt and penetrating trauma, and the study was terminated early. In this phase 3 randomized clinical trial, patients were assigned to receive 200 mcg/kg initially and 100 mcg/kg at 1 and 3 h or a placebo. Despite the fact that the rate of allogeneic blood transfusion was reduced in the rFVIIa arm, there wasn't any effect on mortality.

Safety data on 4468 subjects (4119 patients and 349 healthy volunteers) were recently analyzed [155] to determine the frequency of thromboembolic events. A higher rate of arterial thrombosis has been described in patients who received rFVIIa compared to placebo, while the rate of venous thromboembolism was similar in the two arms (rFVIIavs placebo).

6.7.2 Adverse Events

Further safety concerns derived from a Cochrane Systematic Review [156] of 29 randomized clinical trials comparing rFVIIa with a placebo for the prevention or treatment of bleeding in patients without hemophilia. Sixteen trials involved 1361 participants with prophylactic use of rFVIIa and 13 trials involved 2929 patients receiving therapeutic doses. The results indicated a trend toward an increased risk of arterial thromboembolic events in patients receiving rFVIIa (RR 1.14; 95 % CI 0.89–1.47).

Choice of bypassing agents depends on the current clinical situation, efficacy for single patient, and convenience.

6.7.3 Monitoring the Efficacy of Bypassing Agents

Clinical responsiveness to bypassing agents is difficult to predict, and no validated laboratory method is available for monitoring their therapeutic efficacy [157, 142].

Recently the capability of rotational thromboelastometry (ROTEM) and thrombin generation assay (TGA) to monitor the treatment response of bypassing agents has been evaluated in patients with hemophilia and high titer inhibitors [158].

On ROTEM, MaxVel and maximum clot firmness (MCF) increased to levels comparable to that of healthy controls after 15–30 min following infusion of FEIBA and NovoSeven, without substantial differences between the two drugs. The coefficient variation (CV) on healthy controls analysis of ROTEM parameters ranged between 4 and 31 %.

On TGA, lag time (LG) and time to peak shortened to minimum values at 15–30 min after the infusion of both FEIBA and NovoSeven; endogenous thrombin potential (ETP) and peak thrombin increased two- to threefolds 15–30 min after infusion. The individual variation was more evident for aPCC than for rFVIIa.

The CV ranged between 7 and 30 % for TGA parameters.

In conclusion, both methods are promising in monitoring response to bypassing agents although the clinical values need to be further evaluated in future clinical trials.

6.8 Factor XIII

FXIII concentrate is a highly purified, heat-treated plasma derivate, which has been available in Europe as Fibrogammin P (CSL Behring GmbH, Marburg, Germany) since 1993 and was approved by the US Food and Drug Administration (FDA) in 2011 as CorifactTM.

A recombinant FXIII concentrate, catridecacog (NovoThirteen, Novo Nordisk), which contains the A subunit of human factor XIII produced in yeast cells (*Saccharomyces cerevisiae*) and associated in plasma with factor XIII-B subunit to form a stable heterotetramer, has been licensed by the European Medical Agency for prophylaxis in patients with congenital factor XIII deficiency aged>6 years at recommended dose of 35 U/kg once a month (www.ema.europa.eu).

6.8.1 Indications

FXIII concentrate is approved for routine prophylaxis of congenital factor XIII deficiency every 28 days at a loading dose of 40 U/kg adjusted to maintain factor XIII activity between 5 and 20 %.

Acquired factor XIII deficiency may be caused by perioperative hemodilution in cardiac surgery, neurosurgery, and trauma in adults and children [159–161]. In these cases, plasma FXIII levels are usually in the range of 30–70 %.

A randomized clinical trial in surgical cancer patients [162] and other studies [163, 164] suggest maintaining FXIII levels above 50–60 % of normal during perioperative bleeding through the administration of 20 U/kg [165] of factor XIII concentrate or FFP transfusions.

6.8.2 Monitoring the Efficacy of FXIII Treatment

Factor XIII deficiency is not detected by standard coagulation tests (PT/aPTT), and specific factor XIII assay is available only in specialized laboratory. This makes monitoring of factor XIII levels and the response to treatment challenging during perioperative period.

Point-of-care (POC) monitoring of blood coagulation is becoming increasingly used providing real-time results, and the detection of FXIII deficiency with POC devices would be desirable.

References

1. Stanworth SJ (2007) The evidence-based use of FFP and Cryoprecipitate for abnormalities of coagulation tests and clinical coagulopathy. Hematololgy Am Soc Hematol Educ Program 179–186
2. European Committee on Blood Transfusion (2010) Guide to the preparation, use and quality assurance of blood components. 16th ed. European Directorate for the quality of Medicine and HealthCare. website:www.edqm.eu
3. AABB (2013) Circular information for the use of Human Blood and Blood Components. 2013. Available at www.aabb.org/tm/coi/Documents/coi1113.pdf
4. Benjamin RJ, McLauglin LS (2012) Plasma components: properties, differences, and uses. Transfusion 52(Suppl 1):9S–19S
5. Eder AF, Sebok MA (2007) Plasma components: FFP, FP24 and thawed plasma. Immunohematology 23:150–157
6. Theusinger OM, Baulig W, Seifert B et al (2011) Relative concentrations of haemostatic factors and cytokines in solvent/detergent-treated and fresh-frozen plasma. Br J Anaesth 106:505–511
7. Karam O, Tucci M, Lacroix J et al (2014) International Survey on plasma transfusion practices in critically ill children. Transfusion 54:1125–1132
8. Practice guidelines for blood component therapy: a report by the American Society of Anesthesiologists Task Force on Blood Component Therapy (1996) Anesthesiology 84:732–747
9. British Committee for Standards in Hematology, Blood Transfusion Task Force (2004) Guidelines for the use of fresh-frozen plasma, cryoprecipitate and cryosupernatant. Br J Haematol 126:11–28
10. American Red Cross (2002) Practice guidelines for blood transfusion: a compilation from recent peer-review literature, 2002. Available at http://www.redcrossblood.com
11. Ferraris VA, Brown JR, Despotis GJ et al (2011) 2011 Update to the Society of Thoracic Surgeons and Society of Cardiovascular Anesthesiologists blood conservation clinical practice guidelines. Ann Thorac Surg 91:944–982
12. Roback JD, Caldwell S, Carson J et al (2010) Evidence-based practice guidelines for plasma transfusion. Transfusion 50:1227–1239
13. Practice guidelines for perioperative blood management an updated report by the American Society of Anesthesiologists Task Force on Perioperative Blood Management (2015) Anesthesiology 122: 241–275
14. Yang L, Stanworth S, Hopewll S et al (2012) Is fresh-frozen plasma clinically effective? An update of a systematic review of randomized controlled trials. Transfusion 52:1673–1686
15. Kozek-Langenecker S, Sorensen B, Hess JR et al (2011) Clinical effectiveness of fresh frozen plasma compared with fibrinogen concentrate: a systematic review. Crit Care 15:R239
16. Wada H, Tachil M, Di Nisio M et al (2013) Guidance for diagnosis and treatment of disseminated intravascular coagulation from harmonization of the recommendation from three guidelines. Thromb Haemost 11:761–767
17. Levi M, Toh CH, Hoots WK et al (2001) Towards definition, clinical and laboratory criteria, and scoring system for disseminated intravascular coagulation. Thromb Haemost 86:1327–1330
18. Di Nisio M, Baudo F, Cosmi B et al (2012) Diagnosis and treatment of disseminated intravascular coagulation: Guidelines of the Italian Society for Haemostasis and Thrombosis (SISET). Thromb Res 129:e177–e184
19. Kawasugi K, Wada H, Hatada T et al (2011) Prospective evaluation of hemostatic abnormalities in overt DIC due to various underlying diseases. Thromb Res 128:186–190
20. Lisman T, Porte RJ (2010) Rebalanced hemostasis in patients with liver disease: evidence and clinical consequences. Blood 116:878–885
21. Mallett SV, Chowdary P, Burroughs AK (2013) Clinical utility of viscoelastic tests of coagulation in patients with liver disease. Liver Int 33:961–974
22. Borgman M, Spinella P, Perkins M et al (2007) The ratio of blood products transfused affects mortality in patients receiving massive transfusions at a combact support hospital. J Trauma 63:805–813
23. Holcomb JB, Wade CE, Michalek JE et al (2008) Increased plasma and platelet to red blood cell ratios

improves outcome in 466 massively transfused civilian trauma patients. Ann Surg 248:447–458
24. Cohen MJ, Kutcher M, Redick B et al (2013) Clinical and mechanistic drivers of acute traumatic coagulopathy. J Trauma Acute Care Surg 75(1 Suppl 1):S40–S47
25. Abdel-Wahab OI, Healy B, Dzik WH (2006) Effect of fresh-frozen plasma transfusion on prothrombin time and bleeding in patients with mild coagulation abnormalities. Transfusion 46:1279–1285
26. Holland LL, Brooks JP (2006) Toward rational fresh frozen plasma transfusion. The effect of plasma transfusion on coagulation tests results. Am J Clin Pathol 126:133–139
27. Chowdary P, Saayman AG, Paulus U et al (2004) Efficacy of standard dose and 30 ml/kg fresh frozen plasma in correcting laboratory parameters of haemostasis in critically ill patients. Br J Haematol 125:69–73
28. Clifford L, Jia Q, Yadav H et al (2015) Characterizing the epidemiology of perioperative transfusion-associated circulatory overload. Anesthesiology 122:21–28
29. Clifford L, Jia Q, Subramanian A et al (2015) Characterizing the epidemiology of postoperative transfusion-related acute lung injury. Anesthesiology 122:12–20
30. Slichter SJ, Harker LA (1976) Preparation and storage of platelet concentrates. I factors influencing the harvest of viable platelets from whole blood. Br J Haematol 134:395–402
31. Pietersz RNI, Loos JA, Reesink HW (1985) Platelet concentrates stored in plasma for 72 hours at 22oC prepared from buffy coats of citrate-phosphate-dextrose blood collected in a quadruple-bag saline-adenine-glucose-mannitol system. Vox Sang 49:81–85
32. Kaufman RM, Djulbegovic B, Gernsheimer T et al (2015) Platelet transfusion: a clinical practice guidelines from the AABB. Ann Intern Med 162:205–213
33. Nahirniak S, Slichter S, Tanael S et al (2015) Guidance on platelet transfusion for patients with hypoproliferative thrombocytopenia. Transfus Med Rev 29:3–13
34. Stanworth SJ, Estcourt LJ, Powter G et al (2013) A no-prophylaxis platelet transfusion strategy for hematologic cancer. N Engl J Med 368:1771–1780
35. Wandt H, Schaefer-Eckart K, Wendelin K et al (2012) Therapeutic platelet transfusion versus routine prophylactic transfusion in patients with haematological malignancies: an open-label, multicentre, randomized study. Lancet 380:1309–1316
36. Stanworth SJ, Estcourt LJ, Llewelyn CA et al (2014) Impact of prophylactic platelet transfusion on bleeding events in patients with hematologic malignancies: a subgroup analysis of a randomized trial. Transfusion 54:2385–2393
37. Zeidler K, Arn K, Senn O et al (2011) Optimal preprocedural platelet transfusion threshold for central venous catheter insertions in patients with thrombocytopenia. Transfusion 51:2269–2276
38. Practice guidelines for perioperative blood transfusion and adjuvant therapies: an update report by the American Society of Anesthesiologists Task Force on Perioperative Blood transfusion and Adjuvant Therapies (2006) Anestesiology 105:198–208.
39. British Committee for Standards in Haematology and Blood Transfusion Task Force (2003) Guidelines for the use of platelet transfusions. Br J Haematol 122:10–23
40. Royal College of Obstetricians and Gynaecologists (2009) Prevention and management of post-partum haemorrhage. Green-top guideline No 52
41. Morgenstern LB, Hemphill JC, Andreson C et al (2010) Guidelines for the management of spontaneous intracerebral hemorrhage. A guideline for healthcare professionals from the American Heart Association/American Stroke Association. Stroke 41:2108–2129
42. United Kingdom Blood Transfusion Services (2013) Guidelines for the blood transfusion Services in the UK. 8th ed. Available from http://transfusionguidelines.org/red-book
43. Patanowitz L, Kruskall MS, Uhl L (2003) Cryoprecipitate. Patterns of use. Am J Clin Pathol 119:874–881
44. Miller Y, Bachowski G, Benjamin R et al (2007) Practice guidelines for blood transfusion: a compilation from recent peer-reviewed literature. 2nd ed. American Red Cross. Available from http://www.slc.cu/galerias/pdf/anestesiologia/practical_guidelines_blood_transfusion.pdf
45. Alport EC, Callum JL, Nahirniak S et al (2008) Cryoprecipitate use in 25 Canadian hospitals: commonly used outside of the published guidelines. Transfusion 48:2122–2127
46. Rourke C, Curry N, Khan S et al (2012) Fibrinogen level during trauma hemorrhage, response to replacement therapy and association with patient outcomes. J Thromb Haemost 10:1342–1351
47. Schlimp CJ, Voelckel W, Inaba K et al (2013) Estimation of plasma fibrinogen levels based on hemoglobin, base excess and Injury Severity Score upon emergency room admission. Crit Care 17:R137
48. Morrison JJ, Ross JD, Dubose JJ et al (2013) Association of cryoprecipitate and tranexamic acid with improved survival following wartime injury. Findings from the MATTERs II study. JAMA 148:218–225
49. Spahn DR, Cerny V, Coats TJ et al (2007) Management of bleeding following major trauma: a European guideline. Crit Care 11:R17
50. Rossaint R, Bouillon B, Cerny V et al (2013) Management of bleeding following major trauma: an updated European guideline. Crit Care 17:R76
51. Kozek-Langenecker SA, Afshari A, Albaladejo P et al (2013) Management of severe perioperative bleeding: guidelines from the European Society of Anaestesiology. Eur J Anaesthesiol 30:270–382

52. Lee SH, Lee SM, Kim CS et al (2014) Fibrinogen recovery and changes in fibrin-based clot firmness after cryoprecipitate administration in patients undergoing aortic surgery involving deep hypothermic circulatory arrest. Transfusion 54:1379–1387
53. Royston D, Bidstrup BP, Taylor KM et al (1987) Effect of aprotinin on need for blood transfusion after repeat open-heart surgery. Lancet 2:1289–1291
54. Fergusson DA, Hebert PC, Mazer CD et al (2008) A comparison of aprotinin and lysine analogues in high-risk cardiac surgery. N Engl J Med 358:2319–2331
55. Health Canada. Health Canada decision on Trasylol (aprotinin), http://www.hc-sc.ca/ahc-asc/media/advisories-avis/_2011/2011_124-eng.php
56. European Medicines Agency. European Medicines Agency recommends lifting suspension of aprotinin: review finds that benefits of all antifibrinolytic medicines outweigh risk in restricted range of indications. 2012
57. Trzebicki J, Kosieradzki M, Flakiewick E et al (2011) Detrimental effect of aprotinin ban on amount of blood loss during liver transplantation: single-center experience. Transplant Proc 43:1725–1727
58. Walkden GJ, Verheyden V, Goudie R et al (2013) Increased perioperative mortality following apportion withdrawal: a real-world analysis of blood management strategies in adult cardiac surgery. Intensive Care Med 39:1808–1817
59. Martin K, Gertler R, MacGuill M et al (2013) Replacement of aprotinin by e-aminocaproic acid in infants undergoing cardiac surgery: consequences for blood loss and outcomes. Br J Anaesth 110:615–621
60. Meybohm P, Hermann E, Nierhoff J et al (2013) Aprotinin may increase mortality in low and intermediate risk but not in high risk cardiac surgical patients compared to tranexamic acid and e-aminocaproic acid: meta-analysis of randomized and observational trials over 30.000 patients. PLoS One 8:e58009
61. Dunn CJ, Goa KL (1999) Tranexamic acid: a review of its use in surgery and other indications. Drugs 57:1005–1032
62. Benoni G, Bjorkman S, Fredin H (1995) Application of pharmacokinetic data from healthy volunteers for the prediction of plasma concentrations of tranexamic acid in surgical patients. Clin Drug Invest 10:280–287
63. Fiechtner BK, Nuttal GA, Johnson ME et al (2001) Plasma tranexamic acid concentration during cardiopulmonary bypass. Anesth Analg 92:1131–1136
64. Pilbrant A, Schannong M, Vessman J (1981) Pharmacokinetics and bioavailability of tranexamic acid. Eur J Clin Pharmacol 20:65–72
65. Goobie SM, Meier PM, Sethna NF et al (2013) Population pharmacokinetics of tranexamic acid in pediatric patients undergoing craniosynostosis. Clin Pharmacokinet 52:367–376
66. Shakur H, Roberts I, Bautista R et al (2010) Efficacy of tranexamic acid on death, vascular occlusive events, and blood transfusion in trauma patients with significant hemorrhage (CRASH-2): a randomised, placebo-controlled trial. Lancet 376:23–32
67. Roberts I, Shakur H, Afolabi A et al (2012) CRASH-2 Trials Collaborators. Antifibrinolytic drugs for acute traumatic injury. Cochrane Database Syst Rev 12:CD004896
68. Perel P, Ker K, Morales Uribe CH et al (2013) Tranexamic acid for reducing mortality in emergency and urgent injury. Cochrane Syst Rev 1:CD010245
69. Faraoni D, Goobie SM (2014) The efficacy of antifibrinolyitic drugs in children undergoing non cardiac surgery: a systematic review of the literature. Anesth Analg 118:628–636
70. Zuffery P, Marquial F, Laporte S et al (2006) Do antifibrinolytics reduce allogeneic blood transfusion in orthopedic surgey? Anesthesiology 105:1034–1046
71. Kagoma YK, Crowther MA, Douketis J et al (2009) Use of antifibrinolytic therapy to reduce transfusion in patients undergoing orthopedic surgery: a systematic review of randomized. Thromb Res 123:687–696
72. Ker K, Beecher D, Roberts I (2013) Topical application of tranexamic acid for reduction of bleeding. Cochrane Database Syst Rev 7:CD010562
73. Levy JH, Szlam F, Tanaka KA et al (2012) Fibrinogen and hemostasis: a primary hemostatic target for the management of acquired bleeding. Anesth Analg 114:261–274
74. Furie B, Furie BC (2008) Mechanisms of thrombus formation. N Engl J Med 359:938–949
75. Hoffman M, Monroe DM (2001) A cell-based model of hemostasis. Thromb Haemost 85:958–965
76. Spahn DR, Asmis LM (2009) Excessive perioperative bleeding: are fibrin monomers and factor XIII the missing link? Anesthesiology 110:212–213
77. Rahe-Meyer N, Pichlmaier M, Haverich A et al (2009) Bleeding management with fibrinogen concentrate targeting a high-normal plasma fibrinogen level: a pilot study. Br J Anaesth 102:785–792
78. Gorlinger K, Dirkmann D, Hanke AA et al (2011) First-line therapy with coagulation factor concentrates combined with point-of-care coagulation testing is associated with decreased allogeneic blood transfusion in cardiovascular surgery: a retrospective, single-center cohort study. Anesthesiology 115:1179–1191
79. Fenger-Eriksen C, Lindberg-Larsen M, Christensen AQ et al (2008) Fibrinogen concentrate substitution therapy in patients with massive haemorrhage and low plasma fibrinogen concentrations. Br J Anaesth 101:769–773
80. Karlsson M, Ternstrom L, Hyllner M et al (2009) Prophylactic fibrinogen infusion reduces bleeding after coronary artery bypass surgery. A prospective randomized pilot study. Thromb Haemost 102:137–144

81. Karlsson M, Ternstrom L, Hyllner M et al (2008) Plasma fibrinogen level, bleeding, and transfusion after on-pump coronary artery bypass grafting surgery: a prospective observational study. Transfusion 48:2152–2158
82. Ternstrom L, Radulovic V, Karlsson M et al (2010) Plasma activity of individual coagulation factors, hemodilution and blood loss after cardiac surgery: a prospective observational study. Thromb Res 126:e128–e133
83. Levy JH, Welsby I, Goodnough T (2014) Fibrinogen as a therapeutic target for bleeding: a review of critical levels and replacement therapy. Transfusion 54:1389–1405
84. Franchini M, Lippi G (2012) Fibrinogen replacement therapy: a critical review of the literature. Blood Transfus 10:23–27
85. Rahe-Meyer N, Solomon C, Hanke A et al (2013) Effects of fibrinogen concentrate as first-line therapy during major aortic replacement surgery: a randomized, placebo-controlled trial. Anesthesiology 118:40–50
86. Weber CF, Gorlinger K, Meininger D et al (2012) Point-of-care testing: a prospective, randomized clinical trial of efficacy in coagulopathic cardiac surgery patients. Anesthesiology 117:531–547
87. Schochl H, Nienaber U, Hofer G et al (2010) Goal-directed coagulation managementof major trauma patients using thromboelastometry (ROTEM)-guided administrationof fibrinogen concentrate and prothrombin complex concentrate. Crit Care 14:R55
88. Schochl H, Nienaber U, Maegele M et al (2011) Transfusion in trauma: thromboelastometry-guided coagulation factor concentrate-based therapy versus standard fresh frozen plasma-based therapy. Crit Care 15:R83
89. Bell SF, Rayment R, Collins PW et al (2010) The use of fibrinogen concentrate to correct hypofibrinogenaemia rapidly during obstetric haemorrhage. Int J Obstet Anesth 19:218–223
90. Warmuth M, Mad P, Wild C (2012) Systematic review of the efficacy and safety of fibrinogen concentrate substitution in adults. Acta Anaesthesiol Scand 56:539–548
91. Aubron C, Reade MC, Fraser JF et al (2013) Efficacy and safety of fibrinogen concentrate in trauma patients-a systematic review. J Crit Care 29(471):e11–e17
92. Lunde J, Stensballe J, Wikkelsø A et al (2014) Fibrinogen concentrate for bleeding – a systematic review. Acta Anaesthesiol Scand 58:1061–1074
93. Spahn DR (2013) From plasma transfusion to individualized, goal-directed coagulation factor administration. J Cardiothorac Vasc Anesth 27:S16–S19
94. Levy JH, Goodnough LT (2015) How I use fibrinogen replacement therapy in acquired bleeding. Blood 125:1387–1393
95. Solomon C, Pichlmaier U, Schoechl H et al (2010) Recovery of fibrinogen after administration of fibrinogen concentrate to patients with severe bleeding after cardiopulmonary bypass surgery. Br J Anaesth 104:555–562
96. Lang T, Bauters A, Braun SL et al (2005) Multi-centre investigation on reference ranges for ROTEM thromboelastometry. Blood Coagul Fibrinolysis 16:301–310
97. Rahe-Meyer N, Solomon C, Winterhalter M et al (2009) Thromboelastometry-guided administration of fibrinogen concentrate for the treatment of excessive intraoperative bleeding in thoracoabdominal aortic aneurysm surgery. J Thorac Cardiovasc Surg 138:694–702
98. Weber CF, Zacharowski K, Meybohm P et al (2014) Hemotherapy algorithms for coagulopathic cardiac surgery patients. Clin Lab 60:1059–1063
99. Solomon C, Gröner A, Ye J et al (2015) Safety of fibrinogen concentrate: analysis of more than 27 years of pharmacovigilance data. Thromb Haemost 113:759–771
100. Kaufmann JE, Vischer UM (2003) Cellular mechanism of the hemostatic effects of desmopressin (DDAVP). J Thromb Haemost 1:682–689
101. Datta YH, Ewenstein BM (2001) Regulated secretion in endothelial cells: biology and clinical implications. Thromb Haemost 86:1148–1155
102. Calmer S, Ferkau A, Larmann J et al (2014) Desmopressin (DDAVP) improves recruitment of activated platelets to collagen but simultaneously increases platelet endothelial interactions in vitro. Platelets 25:8–15
103. Svensson PJ, Bergqvist PBF, VinterJuul K et al (2014) Desmopressin in treatment of haematological disorders and in prevention of surgical bleeding. Blood Rev 28:95–102
104. Crescenzi G, Landoni G, Biondi-Zoccai G et al (2008) Desmopressin reduces transfusion needs after surgery: a meta-analysis of randomized clinical trials. Anesthesiology 109:1063–1076
105. Wong AY, Irwin MG, Hui TW et al (2003) Desmopressin does not decrease blood loss and transfusion requirements in patients undergoing hepatectomy. Can J Anaesth 50:14–20
106. Reiter RA, Mayr F, Blazicek H et al (2003) Desmopressin antagonizes the in vitro platelet dysfunction induced by GPIIb/IIIa inhibitors and aspirin. Blood 102:4594–4599
107. Steinlechner B, Zeidler P, Base E et al (2011) Patients with severe aortic valve stenosis and impaired platelet function benefit from preoperative desmopressin infusion. Ann Thorac Surg 91:1420–1426
108. Cattaneo M, Mannucci PM (1993) Desmopressin and blood loss after cardiac surgery. Lancet 342:812
109. Levy JH (2004) Hemostatic agents. Transfusion 44(12 Suppl):58S–62S
110. Tazarourte K, Riou B, Tremey B et al (2014) Guideline-concordant administration of PCC and vitamin K is associated with decreased mortality in patients with severe bleeding under vitamin K antagonist treatment (EPAHK study). Crit Care 18:R81

111. Ageno W, Gallus AS, Wittkowsky A et al (2012) Oral anticoagulant therapy: antithrombotic therapy and prevention of thrombosis, 9th American College of Chest Physicians Evidence-Based Clinical Practice Guidelines. Chest 141(2 Suppl):e44S–e88S
112. Pernod G, Godiér A, Gozalo CT et al (2010) French clinical practice guidelines on the management of patients on vitamin K antagonists in at-risk situations (overdose, risk of bleeding, and active bleeding). Thromb Res 126:e167–e174
113. Baker RI, Coughlin PB, Gallus AS et al (2004) Warfarin reversal consensus guidelines, on behalf of the Australasian Society of Thrombosis and Haemostasis. Med J Aust 181:492–497
114. Keeling D, Baglin T, Tait C et al (2011) Guidelines on oral anticoagulation with warfarin-fourth edition. Br J Haematol 154:311–324
115. Voils SA, Baird B (2012) Systematic review: 3-factor versus 4-factor prothrombin complex concentrate for warfarin reversal: does it matter? Thromb Res 130:833–840
116. Selim MH, Molina CA (2012) The role of hemostatic therapy in anticoagulation-associated intracerebral hemorrhage intuition versus evidence. Stroke 43:2539–2540
117. Dowlatshahi D, Butcher KS, Asdaghi N et al (2012) Poor prognosis in warfarin-associated intracranial hemorrhage despite anticoagulation reversal. Stroke 43:1812–1817
118. Makris M, van Veen JJ (2011) Three or four factor prothrombin complex concentrate for emergency anticoagulation reversal? Blood Transfus 9:117–119
119. Holland L, Warkentin TE, Refaai M et al (2009) Suboptimal effect of a three-factor prothrombin complex concentrate (Profilnine-SD) in correcting supratherapeutic international normalized ratio due to warfarin overdose. Transfusion 49:1171–1177
120. Tanaka KA, Kor DJ (2013) Emerging haemostatic agents and patient blood management. Best Pract Res Clin Anaesthesiol 27:141–160
121. Tanaka KA, Esper S, Bolliger D (2013) Perioperative factor concentrate therapy. Br J Anaesth 111(S1):i35–i49
122. Lee FM, Chana AK, Lau KK et al (2014) Reversal of new, factor-specific oral anticoagulants by rFVIIa, prothrombin complex concentrate and activated prothrombin complex concentrate: A review of animal and human studies. Thromb Res 133:705–713
123. Dickneite G, Hoffman M (2014) Reversing the new oral anticoagulants with prothrombin complex concentrates (PCCs): what is the evidence? Thromb Haemost 111:189–198
124. Majeed A, Schulman S (2013) Bleeding and antidotes in new oral anticoagulants. Best Pract Res Clin Haematol 26:191–202
125. Steiner T, Böhm M, Dichgans M et al (2013) Recommendations for the emergency management of complications associated with the new direct oral anticoagulants (DOACs), apixaban, dabigatran and rivaroxaban. Clin Res Cardiol 102:399–412
126. Gonsalves WI, Pruth RK, Patnaik MM (2013) The new oral anticoagulants in clinical practice. Mayo Clin Proc 88:495–511
127. Schols S, Lancé MD, Feijge MA et al (2010) Impaired thrombin generation and fibrin clot formation in patients with dilutional coagulopathy during major surgery. Thromb Haemost 103:318–328
128. Schols S, van der Meijden P, van Oerle R, Curvers J, Heemskerk JW, van Pampus EC (2008) Increased thrombin generation and fibrinogen level after therapeutic plasma transfusion: relation to bleeding. Thromb Haemost 99:64–70
129. Fries D, Haas T, Klingler A et al (2006) Efficacy of fibrinogen and prothrombin complex concentrate used to reverse dilutional coagulopathy a porcine model. Br J Anaesth 97:460–467
130. Mitrophanov AY, Rosendaal FR, Reifman J (2012) Therapeutic correction of thrombin generation in dilution-induced coagulopathy: computational analysis based on a data set of healthy subjects. J Trauma Acute Care Surg 73(2 suppl 1):S95–S102
131. Grottke O, Rossaint R, Henskens Y et al (2013) Thrombin generation capacity of prothrombin complex concentrate in an in vitro dilutional model. PLoS One 8:e64100
132. Lancellotti S, De Cristofaro R (2009) Congenital prothrombin deficiency. Semin Thromb Hemost 35:367–381
133. Lancellotti S, Basso M, De Cristofaro R (2013) Congenital prothrombin deficiency: An update. Semin Thromb Hemost 39:596–606
134. Menegatti M, Peyvandi F (2009) Factor X deficiency. Semin Thromb Hemost 35:407–415
135. Bolton-Maggs PH, Perry DJ, Chalmers EA et al (2004) The rare coagulation disorders – review with guidelines for management from the United Kingdom Haemophilia Centre Doctors' Organisation. Haemophilia 10:593–628
136. Dentali F, Marchesi C, Pierfranceschi MG et al (2011) Safety of prothrombin complex concentrates for rapid anticoagulation reversal of vitamin K antagonists. A meta-analysis. Thromb Haemost 106:429–438
137. Negrier C, Goudemand J, Sultan Y et al (1997) Multicenter retrospective study on the utilization of FEIBA in France in patients with factor VIII and IX inhibitors. Thromb Haemost 77:1113–1119
138. Roberts HR, Monroe DM, White GC (2004) The use of recombinant factor VIIa in the treatment of bleeding disorders. Blood 104:3858–3864
139. Abshire T, Kenet G (2004) Recombinant factor VIIa: review of efficacy, dosing regimens and safety in patients with congenital and acquired factor VIII or IX inhibitors. J Thromb Haemost 2:899–909
140. Ehrlich HJ, Henzi MJ, Gomperts ED (2002) Safety of factor VIII inhibitor bypassing activity (FEIBA):

10-year compilation of thrombotic adverse events. Haemophilia 8:83–90
141. Turececk PL, Varadi K, Gritsch H et al (2004) FEIBA: mode of action. Haemophilia 10(suppl 2):3–9
142. Negrier C, Dargaud Y, Bordet JC (2006) Basic aspects of bypassing agents. Haemophilia 12(suppl 6):48–52
143. Negrier C, Gomperts ED, Oldenurg J (2006) The history of FEIBA: a lifetime of success in the treatment of hemophilia complicated by an inhibitor. Haemophilia 12(suppl 5):4–13
144. Gallistl S, Cvirn G, Leschnik B et al (2002) Respective roles of factor II, VII, IX and X in the procoagulant activity of FEIBA. Blood Coagul Fibrinolysis 13:653–655
145. Bom VJ, Bertina RM (1990) The contribution of Ca2+ phospholipid and tissue-factor apoprotein to the activation of human blood-coagulation factor X by activated factor VII. Biochem J 265:327–336
146. Rao LV, Rapaport SI (1996) Cells and the activation of factor VII. Hemostasis 26(Suppl 1):1–5
147. van't Veer C, Golden NJ, Mann KG (2000) Inhibition of thrombin generation by the zymogen factor VII: implication for the treatment of hemophilia A by factor VIIa. Blood 95:1330–1335
148. Hofmann M, Moore DM (2010) Platelet binding and activity of recombinant factor VIIa. Thromb Res 125(suppl 1):S16–S18
149. Shibeko AM, Woodle SA, Lee TK et al (2012) Unifying the mechanism of recombinant FVIIa action: dose dependence is regulated differently by tissue factor and phospholipids. Blood 120:891–899
150. Pernod G, Albaladejo P, Godier A et al (2013) Management of major bleeding complications and emergency surgery in patients on long-term treatment with direct oral anticoagulants, thrombin or factor-Xa inhibitors: proposal of the working group on preoperative hemostasis (GIHP) -March 2013. Arch Cardiovasc Dis 106:382–393
151. Schulman S, Crowther MA (2012) How I treat with anticoagulants in 2012: new and old, and when and how to switch. Blood 119:3016–3023
152. Weitz JL, Quinlan DJ, Eikelboom JW (2012) Periprocedural approach to bleeding in patients taking dabigatran. Circulation 126:2428–2432
153. Alfirevic A, Duncan A, You J et al (2014) Recombinant factor VII is associated with worse survival in complex cardiac surgical patients. Ann Thorac Surg 98:618–624
154. Hauser CJ, Boffard K, Dutton GR et al (2010) Results of the CONTROL trial: efficacy and safety of recombinant activated factor VII in the management of refractory traumatic hemorrhage. J Trauma 69:489–500
155. Levi M, Levy JH, Andersen HF et al (2010) Safety of recombinant activated factor VII in randomized clinical trials. N Engl J Med 363:1791–1800
156. Simpson E, Lin Y, Stanworth S, Birchall J et al (2012) Recombinant factor VIIa for the prevention and treatment of bleeding in patients without haemophilia. Cochrane Database Syst Rev 3:CD005011
157. Varadi K, Turecek PL, Scwarz HP (2004) Thrombin generation assay and other universal tests for monitoring haemophilia therapy. Haemophilia 10(suppl 2):17–21
158. Tran HT, Sorensen B, Bjornsen S et al (2015) Moniotring bypassing agent therapy-a prospective crossover study comparing thromboelastometry and yhrombin generation assay. Haemophilia 21:275–283
159. Gerlach R, Tolle F, Raabe A et al (2002) Increased risk for postoperative hemorrhage after intracranial surgery in patients with decreased factor XIII activity: implications of a prospective study. Stroke 33:1618–1623
160. Korte W (2006) Fibrin monomer and factor XIII: a new concept for unexplained intraoperative coagulopathy. Hamostaseologie 26(3 Suppl 1):S30–S35
161. Haas T, Korte W, Spielmann N et al (2012) Perioperative course of FXIII in children undergoing major surgery. Paediatr Anaesth 22(7):641–646
162. Korte WC, Szadkowski C, Gahler A et al (2009) Factor XIII substitution in surgical cancer patients at high risk for intraoperative bleeding. Anesthesiology 110:239–245
163. Wettstein P, Haeberli A, Stutz M et al (2004) Decreased factor XIII availibility for thrombin and early loss of clot firmness in patients with unexplained intraoperative bleeding. Anesth Analg 99:1564–1569
164. Godje O, Gallmeier U, Schelian M et al (2006) Coagulation factor XIII reduces postoperative bleeding after coronary surgery with extracorporeal circulation. Thorac Cardiovasc Surg 54:26–33
165. Korte W (2010) Factor XIII in perioperative coagulation management. Best Pract Res Clin Anaesthesiol 24:85–93

7 Clinical Management of Severe Bleeding in Trauma Patients

Giuseppe Nardi, Vanessa Agostini, Alberto Grassetto, Emiliano Cingolani, and Concetta Pellegrini

7.1 Trauma-Induced Coagulopathy (TIC)

Trauma is the leading cause of death between the ages of 1 year and 44 years, and uncontrolled bleeding is the primary cause of these deaths [1]. Coagulopathy is a frequent complication of hemorrhage and may occur in up to 25 % of patients, even before hospital admission [2]. While traditionally believed to be a result of iatrogenic causes such as dilution, hypothermia, and acidosis, trauma-induced coagulopathy (TIC) is now interpreted as a multifactorial global failure of the coagulation system to sustain adequate hemostasis after major trauma. Derangements in coagulation may occur soon after a severe trauma, thus supporting the hypothesis of an early endogenous process. This acute coagulopathy, which occurs before and independently from iatrogenic reasons, is driven by the combination of tissue trauma and systemic hypoperfusion and characterized by global anticoagulation and hyperfibrinolysis [3]. Cohen addressed this early onset coagulopathy as endogenous acute coagulopathy (EAC) to distinguish it from the iatrogenic dilutional coagulopathy (systemic acute coagulopathy, SAC). Patients presenting with EAC have a mortality approaching 50 %, a greater need for transfusion of blood products, and significantly higher morbidity. With the term of TIC, we tend to identify all the severe derangements in coagulation response as a consequence of major injuries. The pathophysiology of TIC is not yet [4] fully understood. Early coagulopathy (EC) occurring before hospital admission is caused mainly by tissue hypoperfusion and severe tissue injury. EC might have different causes than coagulopathy associated with hemodilution, acidosis, and hypothermia. Patients with tissue hypoperfusion and severe tissue damage have a strong activation of the protein C pathway. Protein C (PC) is activated as a consequence of tissue damage leading to thrombomodulin expression on endothelial cells. Thrombin-thrombomodulin complex then activates protein C, bringing to a depletion in PC levels and protein C stores. This brings to increased levels of plasminogen activator inhibitor-1 (PAI-1), favoring fibrinolysis. The diversion of thrombin from cleaving fibrinogen to binding to thrombomodulin also reduces activation of thrombin-activatable fibrinolysis inhibitor (TAFI), which further leads to hyperfibrinolysis

G. Nardi, MD (✉) • E. Cingolani, MD
Shock and Trauma Center, S. Camillo-Forlanini Hospital, Roma, Italy
e-mail: giuseppe.nardi54@gmail.com; 4doctornardi@gmail.com

V. Agostini, MD
Transfusion Medicine Cesena/Forlì and Blood Establishment, Clinical Pathology Department-Cesena Azienda U.S.L Romagna, Romagna, Italy

A. Grassetto, MD
UOC Anestesia e Rianimazione, Dipartimento Emergenza Urgenza, Ospedale dell'Angelo di Mestre, Venice, Italy

C. Pellegrini, MD
U.O.C. Anesthesia and Intensive Care, M.Rummo Hospital, Benevento, Italy

M. Ranucci, P. Simioni (eds.), *Point-of-Care Tests for Severe Hemorrhage: A Manual for Diagnosis and Treatment*, DOI 10.1007/978-3-319-24795-3_7

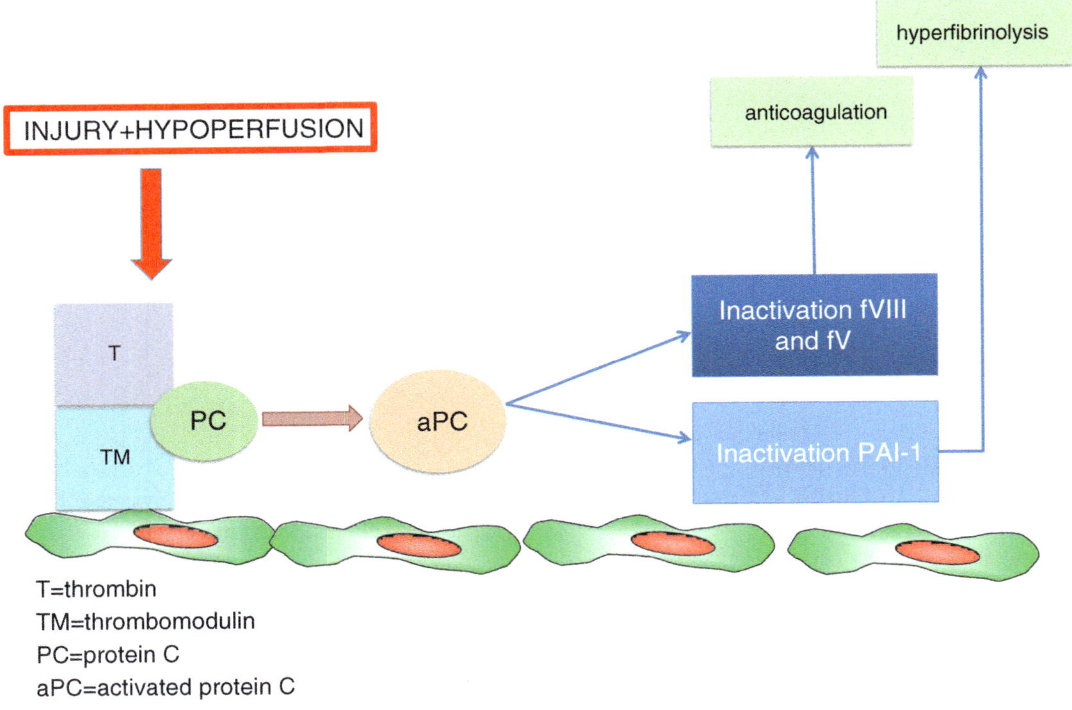

Fig. 7.1 Physiopathology of trauma-induced coagulopathy

[5]. Activated protein C also inactivates factor Va and factor VIIIa [6] bringing to a significant consumption of factor V and VIII. Coagulopathy caused by hypoperfusion is therefore characterized by an acquired deficit in coagulation factor V (and by a less extent, VIII, VII, II, IX, X, and XI [7]) together with a hyperfibrinolytic condition. Acidosis as a consequence of massive hemorrhage has a detrimental effect on the coagulation cascade; a low pH strongly affects the activity of factor VII and to a lesser extent factor X and factor V [8]. Moreover massive bleeding may cause also an acquired deficit of factor XIII which has an important role in clot stabilization and clot firmness. It has been suggested that a decreased factor V activity as well as a deficit in factor XIII concentration might play a role in the pathogenesis of the early onset acute traumatic coagulopathy [9]; however, this hypothesis has not been confirmed by sound clinical data. In addition to EAC and hyperfibrinolysis, further coagulopathy results from infusion of crystalloids, blood products, and severe anemia. Massive hemorrhage leads to anemia, which compromises the marginalization of platelets thus affecting primary hemostasis by impairing platelet adhesion and aggregation. Transfusion of large amount of red blood cells (RBCs) without additional clotting factors or platelets results in further impairment of hemostasis from both hemodilution (dilutional coagulopathy and thrombocytopenia) and metabolic derangement (acidosis and hypocalcaemia). Hypocalcemia develops as a consequence of the administration of relevant amounts of citrate in storage solution and hypothermia from refrigeration. Acidosis and hypocalcaemia are detrimental to normal hemostasis. Furthermore, hypothermia is associated with impairment of both platelet and coagulation factor activity. Although hemodilution and hypothermia are frequently associated, their detrimental effect on coagulation is different: hypothermia impairs coagulation mainly by platelet inhibition, whereas hemodilution principally impairs plasma coagulation. All of these "exogenous" factors contribute to the vicious cycle of pro-

gressive coagulopathy due to the "lethal triad" of refractory coagulopathy, progressive hypothermia, and persistent metabolic acidosis [10]. Trauma patients with uncontrolled bleeding requiring high amount of blood transfusion over a short time (massive transfusion, MT) have a very high mortality. Several definitions of MT exist based on the volume of the blood products transfused and also the time frames over which these transfusions occurred (Fig. 7.1). The three most common definitions of MT in adult patients are:

- Transfusion of ≥10 units of RBCs, which approximates the total blood volume (TBV) of an average adult patient, within 24 h
- Transfusion of at least 4 units of RBCs in 1 h with anticipation of continued need for blood product support
- Replacement of .50 % of the TBV by blood products within 3 h

Patients who undergo massive transfusion have a high mortality rate. A mortality rate ranging between 25 % [11] and 50 % [12–15] has been reported. A recent meta-analysis focused on the association between RBCs transfusion and mortality or other significant outcomes such as multiorgan failure (MOF) and acute respiratory distress syndrome (ARDS) [16]. According to this study, the odds for mortality increases with each additional unit of RBCs transfused as well as the risks of MOF and ARDS. However, these results are based on observational studies only.

7.2 Clinical Management

In recent years, international guidelines [17–19] have been developed aimed at preventing and treating trauma-induced coagulopathy (TIC). The immediate identification of patients who may require transfusion of several units of blood is critical to ensure a timely intervention. Unfortunately clinical criteria as well as predictive scores have a lower than desirable predictive ability for massive transfusion. Predictive models of massive transfusion upon admission have been developed for this purpose. The Trauma-Associated Severe Hemorrhage (TASH) score has been reported to have a high predictive value [20] and is widely used in Germany and other European countries. The TASH score (Table 7.1) is based on a point system taking into consideration clinical and laboratory data as well as the severity of injuries (orthopedic fractures and intra-abdominal fluid). In a multicenter study based on the data of the German Trauma Registry, Borgman [21] divided the population of trauma victims according to their TASH score. A TASH score ≥ 15 was associated with a 40 % risk to receive a massive transfusion. Patients with a TASH score ≥ 15 had a high ISS (42 ± 15.4) and a mortality rate of 39.5 %. Maegele [22] and Brockamp [23] used

Table 7.1 The TASH score

TASH Score (Trauma-Associated Severe Hemorrhage) Predicts the need for massive transfusion based on clinical and laboratory data	
Sex	
Male	+1
Female	0
Hemoglobin	
<7 g/dL	+8
<9 g/dL	+6
<10 g/dL	+4
<11 g/dL	+3
<12 g/dL	+2
≥12 g/dL	0
Base excess	
< −10 mmol/L	+4
< −6 mmol/L	+3
< −2 mmol/L	+1
≥ −2 mmol/L	0
Systolic blood pressure	
<100 mmHg	+4
<120 mmHg	+1
≥120 mmHg	0
Heart rate	
>120 bpm	+2
≤120 bpm	0
Positive FAST for intra-abdominal fluid	
YES	+3
Clinically unstable pelvic fracture	
YES	+6
Open or dislocated femur fracture	
YES	+3

the German Trauma Society database to evaluate the predictive values for MT of six different scoring algorithms. Although the weighted and more complex systems such as the TASH score had the highest overall accuracy, more simple score as the one proposed by Vandromme [24] performed nearly as well. The Vandromme score is based on five parameters four of which immediately available by clinical examination or by the generally available point-of-care devices: blood lactate ≥5 mMol/L, heart rate >105 bpm, INR >1.5, hemoglobin ≤11 g/dL, and systolic blood pressure <110 mmHg. Its predictive value for the need of massive transfusion increases with the number of positive parameters, and the model with ≥3 positive criteria showed a sensitivity of 53 % and a specificity of 98 %. A major limitation of all models is their retrospective nature and the lack of prospective validation. It has been therefore suggested that individual triggers should be considered in order to improve the accuracy of the models [46]. An unpublished analysis of about 1700 major trauma cases from the Italian Trauma Registry (RIT) showed that hypotension (systolic blood pressure, SBP ≤90 mmHg) on hospital admission is associated with a mortality rate as high as 50 % mainly due to uncontrolled hemorrhage. However many hypotensive patients do not meet the MT criteria as they do not survive enough time to receive 10 units of RBCs.

Based on the available data from the literature and the trauma registries, the Italian Trauma Network (TUN) suggests to start an aggressive coagulation support in all the patients presenting with a significant uncontrolled bleeding associated with one or more of the following criteria (Fig. 7.2): SBP <100 mmHg, base excess (BE) < –6, lactate >5 mMol/L, hemoglobin <9 g/dL, or a international normalized ratio (INR) >1.5. The last criterion is thought to be relevant in the case of patients referred from other hospitals with laboratory data showing an impaired coagulation.

Any therapeutic strategy should rapidly tackle acute traumatic coagulopathy through the early replacement of clotting factors. However, due to the heterogeneous availability of hemocomponents and clotting factors in different countries and to the lack of sound data in the literature, there is not a widely agreed clinical strategy yet.

Moreover, because of the aging population in western countries, elderly people with cardiovascular comorbidities and on antiplatelet agents or oral anticoagulants are increasingly represented, thus introducing further complexity in identifying an adequate treatment approach for most of the bleeding patients.

An ideal strategy to prevent and treat the coagulopathy trauma should focus on four key points to be addressed in quick succession:

1. Prevention and treatment of hyperfibrinolysis
2. Identification and reverse of drug-induced coagulopathy

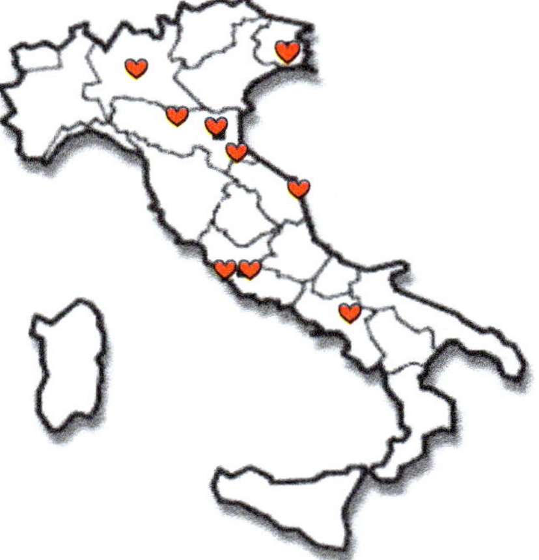

Fig. 7.2 Criteria to start coagulation support by "blind" administration of 2 g of Fibrinogen concentrate according to the ECS protocol

3. Early support to the hemostatic process
4. Goal-directed correction of specific coagulation abnormalities

7.2.1 Prevention and Treatment of Primary Hyperfibrinolysis

Hyperfibrinolysis has been identified in a significant percentage of severely injured patients. Acutely injured patients with severe hyperfibrinolysis (maximum clot lysis >15 % after 30 min) are reported to have mortality rates exceeding 70 % [25, 26]. The CRASH-2 [27] trial demonstrated the potential benefit of empiric antifibrinolytic therapy in injured patients. This study led to a Level 1A recommendation for early administration of antifibrinolytic agents. Based on the results of the CRASH-2 study, administration of tranexamic acid (TA) to all patients with ongoing bleeding or at risk of significant bleeding is now standard care. Although, hyperfibrinolysis may be identified only in a limited number of severely injured patients by viscoelastic tests Raza [28] demonstrated that as many as 57 % of the severely injured patients had fibrinolytic activation measured by plasmin-antiplasmin complex. These data may better explain the results of the CRASH-2 study. Although according to the current recommendations, all the bleeding patients should receive TA soon after injury, TA is probably to be avoided at a later stage. A new analysis of the CRASH-2 study shows that if treatment is not given until 3 h after injury, it is less effective and could even be harmful [29].

Recently, Moore and associates [30] observed three distinct phenotypes of fibrinolysis in response to trauma. Despite having similar demographics and injury patterns, 64 % of their patients presented with a fibrinolysis shutdown, while physiologic fibrinolysis was observed in 18 % of the patients and hyperfibrinolysis in another 18 %. Hyperfibrinolytic patients had a higher mortality rate due to exsanguination occurring early after injury, whereas shutdown patients had an increased delayed mortality more frequently due to organ failure. Modest levels of fibrinolysis seem to be protective. Therefore, according to this data, there might be a U-shaped curve in mortality with the highest peak for patients with acute hyperfibrinolysis and a second peak for patients with a fibrinolysis shutdown. This finding comes from a retrospective study and needs to be considered with caution. However, if they were confirmed, this could lead to reconsider the present indications for a mandatory initial administration of TA.

7.2.2 Identification and Reversal of Drug-Induced Coagulopathy

The number of patients on antiplatelet or anticoagulation therapies is increasing. A retrospective cohort study of trauma centers submitting data to the National Trauma Databank (NTDB) from 2002 to 2007 demonstrated an increase in vitamin K antagonists (VKA) use in the general trauma population from 2.3 % in 2002 to 4 % ($p<0.001$) in 2006. In patients older than 65 years, the use of VKA increased from 7.3 to 12.8 % in the same period ($p<0.001$). Pre-injury VKA use is age related with a sharp increase between the age of 45 and 70 years. Head trauma patients on VKA have an increased risk of intracranial hemorrhage. The younger patients on anticoagulants have a 50 % higher mortality [31]. Recent guidelines recommend emergency anticoagulation reversal with prothrombin complex concentrate (PCC) and vitamin K in trauma patients with major bleeding or cerebral hemorrhage who are on VKA treatment [32–34]. PCCs are classified into three-factor and four-factor products. Three-factor concentrates have therapeutically useful level of FII, FIX, and FX; four-factor PCCs contain FII, FVII, FIX, and FX together with protein C and S. PCC is associated with a non-negligible risk of thrombogenicity and disseminated intravascular coagulation (DIC) [35]. Eight retrospective studies have evaluated the outcomes associated with pre-injury anticoagulation therapy in patients admitted for traumatic head injury. In two of these studies, the mortality was similar between the control and warfarin-treated patients; in the other six studies, there was an increased mortality in the warfarin-treated group compared to the control group [36]. While mortality has been shown to increase in patients with traumatic brain injury on VKAs, data for trauma patients without brain injury are less clear. "Time to correction of the INR" or "extent of correction of the INR" has been used as a surrogate outcome of clinical effectiveness rather than the cessation of clinical bleeding or mortality. Only one retrospective analysis could demonstrate that in trauma patients receiving warfarin, the addition of PCC treatment to fresh frozen plasma (FFP) and vitamin K results in a quicker INR reversal. However, no outcome improvement was observed [37]. Notwithstanding the lack of strong evidence, all international guidelines agree in recommending the use of PCC for the emergency reversal of vitamin K-dependent oral anticoagulation. According to the ECS protocol, patients with significant active bleeding known to be on VKAs should immediately receive 25 UI/kg of PCC even before INR results. PCC treatment will be subsequently adjusted according to INR results [38, 39]. The italian F.C.S.A. recommendations [40] for the management of intracranial hemorrhage have been endorsed to guide treatment once INR is known (Fig. 7.3).

Recently, several new oral anticoagulants (NOACs) have been introduced in the clinical practice, and a few more are under clinical development. These drugs are thought to have a more balanced benefit/risk ratio and several advantages over warfarin: a rapid onset of action, a more predictable anticoagulant effect so that routine laboratory monitoring is not required, and minor food and drugs interactions. Moreover they may carry less hemorrhagic risks, particularly, less intracranial bleeding [41]. NOACs are still relatively known to the practicing community, and there is little or no evidence to guide practical management when patients present with acute bleeding. The use of NOACs as well as the strategies to reverse their effects in case of bleeding is addressed in a separate section of the book (Chap. 12). We will therefore focus on a few simple concepts important to manage trauma patients with critical bleeding. Major and/or life-threatening bleeding should be treated with immediate anticoagulant withdrawal. However, neither FFP nor cryoprecipitate is effective in reversing the anticoagulant effect of the new drugs [42]. A few studies have investigated reversal agents; all of these, except one, have used animal model to evaluate the role of different reversal drugs. The only human study focused on the effect of four-factor PCC on coagulation tests [43]. The use of activated charcoal has been suggested if oral drug assumption is within a couple of hours. High doses of 3-factor or 4-factor PCC are probably effective for the reversal of factor Xa inhibitor such as rivaroxaban, but not for thrombin inhibitor as dabigatran [44]. The Italian Federation of Thrombosis Centers produced a consensus document suggesting the use of hemodialysis as a therapeutic option in case of assumption of dabigatran and the administration of 4-factor PCC for the reversal of rivaroxaban in the one-shot dose of 50 IU/kg [45]. The European Guidelines suggest to start with a similar dose (25–50 IU/kg).

Antiplatelet drugs – mostly aspirin and P2Y12 antagonists (clopidogrel, prasugrel, ticlopidine, and ticagrelor) are prescribed for prophylaxis and treatment in patients with cardiovascular or cerebrovascular diseases. These drugs are associated

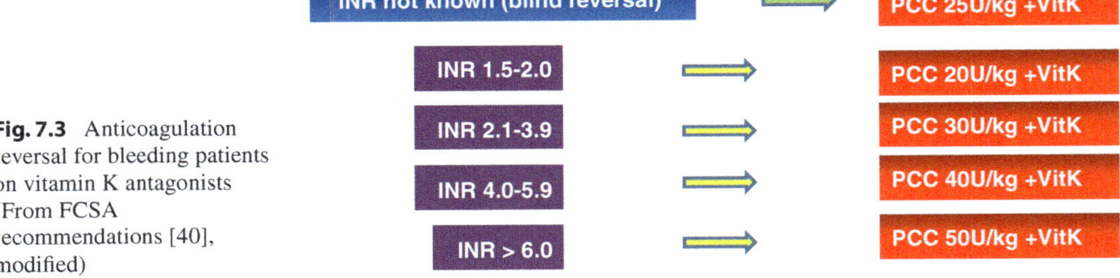

Fig. 7.3 Anticoagulation reversal for bleeding patients on vitamin K antagonists (From FCSA recommendations [40], modified)

with an increased risk of intracranial hemorrhage. Drugs of both classes (with the exception of ticagrelor) irreversibly inhibit platelets function making their short half-lives clinically irrelevant. For each day after the interruption of these medications, the 10–14 % of normal platelet function is restored; so it takes 7–10 days for the entire platelet pool to be refurbished.

There is little evidence to guide platelet transfusion in major trauma patients on antiplatelet medications. A recent meta-analysis of six studies failed to demonstrate any clear benefit of platelet transfusions in patients with either spontaneous or traumatic intracranial hemorrhage [46]. In a retrospective analysis of a cohort of 113 patients with traumatic intracerebral hemorrhage (TICH) on antiplatelet medications, Washington and associates [47] could not find any statistically significant difference in outcome between patients treated with platelets and those who were not transfused. Similar data were reported by Downey in a retrospective study involving two level 1 trauma centers over a 4-year period [48]. Ivascu [49] and Fortuna [50] in two separate studies observed a nonsignificant trend toward higher mortality in patients with traumatic brain injury treated with platelets transfusion, but patients transfused were older and presented a lower Glasgow Coma Scale (GCS) and higher Injury Severity Score (ISS) [35]. All of these studies have some weakness: they are retrospective and relative small, and the indication and timing for platelet transfusion were not standardized. The timing of transfusion might play a key role as the hematoma may set up very early after trauma [51].

Despite the lack of evidence supporting the use of platelets, many institutions have implemented protocols for the reversal of platelet medications in the presence of TICH. According to a multidisciplinary institutional protocol published by Campbell et al. [52], 5 units of platelet concentrate (PLT) should be transfused right on admission to the patients on aspirin who present with a small TICH. Patients on P2Y12 antagonists or with large TICH should receive 10 units of platelets together with 0.3 mcg/kg of desmopressin. As patients with major trauma and critical bleeding often require surgical or intravascular procedures, many authors recommend the use of platelet concentrates even in the absence of brain injury [53].

7.2.3 Early Support to the Hemostatic Process

Hemostasis is critically dependent on fibrinogen as a substrate for clot formation. Fibrinogen is the single factor which is more and earlier affected in case of TIC. Many bleeding trauma patients with TIC present with a depletion of fibrinogen below levels currently recommended for therapeutic supplementation. Recently, Schlimp et al. [54] demonstrated that fibrinogen levels upon admission show strong correlation with rapidly obtainable routine laboratory parameters such as hemoglobin and BE. A level of fibrinogen lower than 150 mg/dL is detected in as many as 73 % of the patients with admission hemoglobin lower than 10 g/dL and in 63 % of those with a BE lower than −6. Moreover Rourke and Brohi [55] found low fibrinogen in 41 % of the patients who were hypotensive on admission. In their study, hypotension, increasing shock severity (as measured by the base deficit), and high degree of injury (ISS ≥25) were all associated with a reduction in fibrinogen levels. Fibrinogen depletion is associated with poor outcomes, and survival improves with the amounts of fibrinogen administered [56]. Fibrinogen is by far the most extensively represented coagulation protein in plasma. One liter of FFP contains on average 2 g of fibrinogen. However, until a few years ago, FFP transfusion was not recommended for the bleeding trauma patients in absence of a prolongation of the prothrombin time (PT) or INR or fibrinogen decrease to less than 1.5 g/L [57]. In the year 2007 retrospective evidences from both military [58] and civilian [59] practice were published suggesting improved outcomes in patients with massive bleeding, after the adoption of a massive transfusion protocol (MTP), including the early administration of high-dose FFP therapy. According to these first reports, a 1:1 FFP/RBCs ratio was associated with a sharp decrease in mortality. Because of these findings, significant changes in the treatment strategy of patients with critical bleeding were introduced, bringing to anticipate coagulation support by administering FFP with a high FFP/RBCs ratio. Several studies focused on this strategy trying to determine if standard doses of FFP and platelets in a fix ratio RBCs were able to improve survival. Notwithstanding a large number of studies, there are still conflicting evidences regarding the use of high ratios. Although many authors suggested that early and aggressive FFP transfusion may reduce mortality [60], the optimal FFP/RBC and PLT/RBCs ratio is controversial because of the possible survival bias flawing most studies [61, 62]. Survival bias is the bias resulting from the fact that surviving patients are more likely to receive more FFP and platelets compared with non-survivors, because they lived long enough to receive those blood products. This issue is still under debate: a multicenter prospective study on a large population of patients undergoing MT showed that high FFP/RBCs and PLT/RBCs ratios are associated with a survival benefit also when time dependency is accounted for [63], but more recently other authors came to opposite conclusion [64]. In their study, Khan and Brohi [65] observed that there was no consistent correction of any measure of clot function nor any large increases in the procoagulant factor level, when FFP was delivered during the acute phase of ongoing bleeding. Furthermore, FFP/RBCs ratios above 1:2 were not associated with any major hemostatic benefit.

Despite the widespread use of blood components to treat TIC, their effects on the coagulation profile when administered during damage control resuscitation remain therefore largely unknown. To define which is the best FFP/RBC and PTL/RBC ratio, a large multicenter randomized study has been designed: the Pragmatic Optimal Platelet and Plasma Ratio (PROPPR) trial [65]. The PROPPR was designed as a randomized trial to be conducted in subjects with the highest level of trauma activation and predicted to have a massive transfusion. Twelve North American level 1 trauma centers were involved in the trial. The PROPPR aimed to look for a different outcome in patients randomized into one of two standard transfusion ratio interventions: 1:1:1 or 1:1:2 (FFP, PLT, and RBCs). Despite being able to randomize over 680 patients, the PROPPR trial was unable to reach definitive conclusions [66]. Patients treated with a 1:1:1 ratio, who therefore received PLT in a very early treatment stage, had a 5 % lower 24-h mortality and a 3.7 % lower hospital mortality if compared with those who initially received FFP (but no PLT) in a 1:2 ratio and were subsequently treated with a 1:1:2 PLT/FFP/RBCs ratio. However, these differences were not statistically significant. The early use of PLT was not associated with a higher rate of ARDS.

Transfusing patients based on an empirical ratio rather than guided solely by laboratory data (goal-directed) is considered controversial by some researchers [67]. Moreover there are still conflicting opinions among the experts on the choice of using FFP as the initial strategy for supporting coagulation. Severe tissue damage and hemorrhagic shock are frequently associated with a decreased fibrinogen. Administration of FFP to bleeding patients may stabilize fibrinogen levels, avoiding a further decrease, but FFP transfusions cannot result in a significant increase of fibrinogen levels unless very high volumes are infused [68]. The ACIT study [69] confirmed these findings showing that fibrinogen did not correct with standard damage control resuscitation.

There are indeed several limitations on the use of FFP to prevent and treat TIC. Both FFP and pathogen-inactivated plasma (industrial purified plasma) need to be group matched, thawed, and warmed before administration. Therefore, unless pre-thawed plasma is available, plasma transfusion cannot be started at the same time as RBCs. A delay of 93 min has been reported [61] possibly explaining why the targeted FFP/RBCs ratio is reached only a few hours after starting treatment. During this interval, fibrinogen level is likely to be lower than desired.

FFP transfusion has also been associated with an increased risk of post injury multiple organ dysfunction syndrome (MODS), ARDS, and infections. These complications increase with the volume of transfused FFP [70]. The risk of transfusion-related acute lung injury (TRALI) has been greatly reduced by avoiding the use of the FFP of women with pregnancy history [71]. In Italy the recent introduction of pathogen-inactivated plasma enabled to further minimize the risks of TRALI and virtually eliminate the risks of transmission of infective diseases. Although these measures are effective in reducing some of the adverse effects of FFP transfusions, there are data [72] showing that in patients who require less than 6 units of RBCs, the complications related to plasma transfusion may overcome the benefits.

Moreover the early and aggressive administration of plasma may result in diluting the blood cells with a decrease in hemoglobin level [73] and may further contribute to reduce platelet marginalization with a potentially negative impact on platelet activation. Therefore, dilutional anemia might bring to transfusing a higher amount of RBCs in order to adhere to the transfusion trigger recommended by the European Guidelines (7–9 g/dL) [17].

The balance between a rapid intervention to treat or prevent TIC and the risk related to unnecessary transfusion of plasma is difficult to achieve. Therefore, several authors prefer to start treatment with coagulation factors and in particular with fibrinogen.

The use of coagulation factor concentrates has been proposed as the strategy to reduce and even avoid plasma transfusion in patients with significant bleeding. In the Austrian guidelines [74], fibrinogen concentrate is the first-line treatment. Two retrospective studies comparing data from Austrian Trauma Centers with the German Trauma (TR-DGU) registry reported a significant reduction in platelet transfusion and a limited decrease in blood transfusion for bleeding patients treated with fibrinogen concentrate and PCC who did not receive FFP during initial resuscitation [75, 76]. However, these results have not been confirmed by prospective controlled studies.

Although very appealing, the "plasma-free" strategy proposed by Schöchl [75] may not be easily adopted by many trauma centers as it requires thromboelastometry monitoring to be started straight on patient's admission and not all the hospitals can adhere to this requirement at the moment. Moreover it may imply the use of a rather high amount of fibrinogen with considerable related costs.

7.2.4 Goal-Directed Correction of Specific Coagulation Abnormalities

The utility of the standard coagulation tests (PT, INR, activated partial thromboplastin time [aPTT], platelet count, and fibrinogen levels [Clauss method]) to guide the acute hemostatic treatment in trauma patients with significant bleeding is limited. First, their results are inevitably delayed. In addition, because they are not performed on whole blood but on plasma, they cannot analyze the entire process of coagulation as it occurs in vivo. Moreover, hyperfibrinolysis cannot be detected [77]. Although these conventional coagulation assays do not predict the future need for massive transfusion and have limited utility to direct ongoing blood component therapy in real time because of slow turnaround times, nevertheless all the guidelines still suggest they should be ordered to provide information that might be helpful in correcting abnormalities occurring during resuscitation. Recently, it has been suggested that point-of-care hemostasis assays, such as thromboelastography (TEG) and rotational thromboelastometry (ROTEM), might be better at assessing coagulopathy in patients with critical bleeding and TIC [78, 79]. These assays offer to clinicians a graphic representation of the coagulation process. In addition, the parameters obtained from TEG/ROTEM could provide a quantitative measure of individual components of the hemostatic process. Hence, the use of TEG/ROTEM can provide better information to guide blood component therapies in a more timely manner. There are several advantages of using TEG/ROTEM: first of all, the turnaround time for these assays is shorter compared with conventional assays; thus, they can be used in combination with clinical assessment for the decision-making process. Moreover the viscoelastic point-of-care

(POC) tests can detect severe hyperfibrinolysis that plays a major role in TIC. TEG/ROTEM can be performed at the patient's true temperature, which makes it more sensitive for detection of coagulopathy due to hypothermia. In a recent in vitro experimental study, Winsted et al. [80] observed that hypothermia affects coagulation more during hemodilution with starches than with crystalloids. Fibrinogen concentrate is effective in correcting dilutional coagulopathy induced by crystalloids irrespective of temperature. However, it is much less effective in case of hypothermia-induced coagulopathy associated with colloid-induced hemodilution. TEG/ROTEM has been shown to reduce the transfusion requirement and need for MT in patients undergoing cardiovascular surgery [81]. The early use of thromboelastometry to guide treatment is recommended by the Austrian Guidelines [19]. However, notwithstanding all these potential advantages, a Cochrane review suggested that there is no evidence that TEG/ROTEM reduced the morbidity and mortality in the massively transfused patients [82].

7.3 The Early Coagulation Support Protocol (ECS)

The updated European Guidelines [17] for management of bleeding and coagulopathy recommend that every trauma center implement an evidence-based treatment algorithm for the bleeding trauma patient and promote the use of treatment algorithms to guide clinical management. To adhere to these recommendations, the Italian Trauma Centers Network (TUN) has developed a treatment algorithm (early coagulation support or ECS) [83] aiming to improve and homogenize the early treatment of trauma patients with significant bleeding and at high risk of massive transfusion. The ECS has been formally adopted by several Italian Trauma Centers; to our knowledge, this is the first example in Europe of the adoption of the same step-by-step algorithm for the management of trauma-induced coagulopathy by a large number of trauma centers. The ECS protocol is summarized in Fig. 7.4. The ECS protocol is an integrated part of a comprehensive damage resuscitation strategy. It is also based on fluid restriction and the prohibition of colloids. As well as having the objective of ensuring an earlier coagulation support, the protocol also aims to limit the use of plasma in patients who are not likely to need it, in order to reduce plasma-related adverse effects.

- According to the ECS protocol, TA must be initiated on patient's admission immediately after the collection of a blood sample for laboratory tests, crossmatching, and basal clotting profile. TA must be initiated within the first 3 h after trauma. If for any reason, a patient has not received TA within this deadline, TA administration is not recommended. Recommendations for a quick reverse of drug-induced anticoagulation and/or antiplatelet treatment are summarized in Fig. 7.4.
- The ECS protocol suggests platelet transfusion for patients on antiplatelet drugs with critical bleeding and/or intracranial hemorrhage and/or undergoing emergency surgery. In patients with TICH on aspirin therapy, the protocol suggests the administration of 1 apheresis platelet concentrate (single donor) or 1 pool platelet concentrate (from pooling of 4–6 buffy coats). In patients with TICH or significant extracranial bleeding who are under the effects of P2Y12 inhibitors (ticlopidin, clopidogrel, prasugrel, ticagrelor), the administration of 2 apheresis platelet concentrates or 2 pool platelet concentrates is recommended [84–86].
- According to the ECS, coagulation support is started in patients presenting with signs of severe hypoperfusion even before the results of the first ROTEM test. Therefore, patients who met one or more of the following criteria ("clinical" criteria), SBP <100 mmHg, lactate ≥5 mmol/L, BE ≤6, or hemoglobin ≤9 g/dL, are expected to receive a standard dose of fibrinogen concentrates (2 g) together with the first units of RBCs. As soon as these patients start transfusion with universal RBCs, they should receive an initial dose of 2 g of fibrinogen concentrate. In the Brohi's study patients who did not receive any source

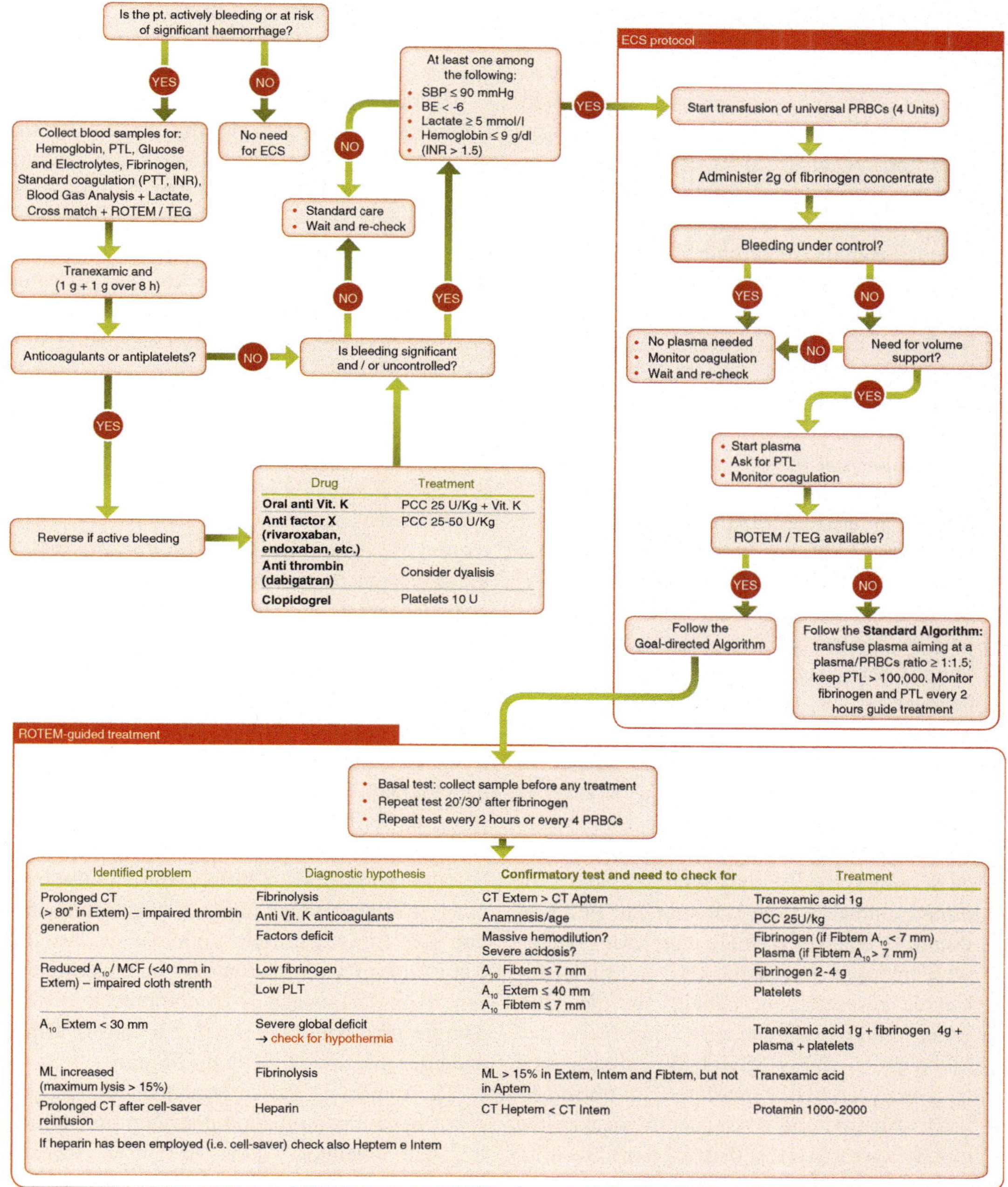

Drug	Treatment
Oral anti Vit. K	PCC 25 U/Kg + Vit. K
Anti factor X (rivaroxaban, endoxaban, etc.)	PCC 25-50 U/Kg
Anti thrombin (dabigatran)	Consider dyalisis
Clopidogrel	Platelets 10 U

Identified problem	Diagnostic hypothesis	Confirmatory test and need to check for	Treatment
Prolonged CT (> 80" in Extem) – impaired thrombin generation	Fibrinolysis	CT Extem > CT Aptem	Tranexamic acid 1g
	Anti Vit. K anticoagulants	Anamnesis/age	PCC 25U/kg
	Factors deficit	Massive hemodilution? Severe acidosis?	Fibrinogen (if Fibtem A_{10} < 7 mm) Plasma (if Fibtem A_{10} > 7 mm)
Reduced A_{10} / MCF (<40 mm in Extem) – impaired cloth strenth	Low fibrinogen	A_{10} Fibtem ≤ 7 mm	Fibrinogen 2-4 g
	Low PLT	A_{10} Extem ≤ 40 mm A_{10} Fibtem ≤ 7 mm	Platelets
A_{10} Extem < 30 mm	Severe global deficit → check for hypothermia		Tranexamic acid 1g + fibrinogen 4g + plasma + platelets
ML increased (maximum lysis > 15%)	Fibrinolysis	ML > 15% in Extem, Intem and Fibtem, but not in Aptem	Tranexamic acid
Prolonged CT after cell-saver reinfusion	Heparin	CT Heptem < CT Intem	Protamin 1000-2000
If heparin has been employed (i.e. cell-saver) check also Heptem e Intem			

Fig. 7.4 The Early Coagulation Support (ECS) Algorithm

of fibrinogen had a reduction in fibrinogen level to 1.2 g/L (1.0–1.8) as an average after the first 4 units of RBCs. The standard dose of 2 g of fibrinogen concentrate therefore aims to immediately provide the needed amount of fibrinogen to prevent its expected decrease following the first 4 units of RBCs. Four units of universal RBCs is the standard package for emergency transfusion immediately available in the trauma bay of the TUN trauma centers. Therefore, patients with ongoing critical bleeding and signs of hypoperfusion are expected to receive 4 units of RBCs and 2 g of fibrinogen as the first treatment step. POC tests (TEG/ROTEM) should subsequently guide the treatment algorithm (Fig. 7.4).

- FFP is not part of the early treatment stage. Permissive hypotension and moderate fluid restriction are recommended until surgical bleeding control is achieved. However in case of prolonged bleeding, if an increasing number of RBCs is required and high volume support is needed, FFP is indicated both for volume and coagulation support. Fibrinogen concentrate does not provide volume expansion; hence, higher amounts of crystalloids and/or colloids need to be infused to replace volume if a "plasma-free" strategy is adopted. Crystalloids and more importantly colloids significantly impair the clotting process, either by diluting clotting factors or directly impairing the clot strength. In a randomized controlled study comparing saline with hydroxyethyl starch (HES) 130/0.4 for trauma resuscitation, patients in the HES group required significantly more blood and blood products [87]. Synthetic colloids such as gelatins and HES interfere with fibrin network structure and consequently weaken the clot by a greater extent than explained by dilution of plasma proteins alone. If concentrates are employed instead of plasma, the higher amount of crystalloids and colloids needed to support volume might hamper the efficacy of this treatment strategy. This may explain the reason why, even in Schöchl series, a percentage of the bleeding patients still received plasma. As no proper study has compared yet the "factor-based" strategy with the "plasma-based" approach, this issue has not been settled.

The rationale of the ECS strategy is to provide a rapid support to the clotting process by the early administration of fibrinogen concentrate, with the aim to reduce plasma transfusion at least in patients who eventually will not need massive transfusion. These patients are the ones expected to get more harm than benefits from plasma. Patients who continue to present significant a bleeding notwithstanding early coagulation support and damage control surgery will usually require more than 10 units of RBCs and meet the definition of MT. The TUN expert committee that developed the protocol agreed there is still not enough evidence in the literature to adopt a "plasma-free" strategy for the patients who require MT. Moreover, it has been shown that in the severe uncontrolled bleeding, beside fibrinogen other coagulation factors as factor V and factor XIII may decrease. Some concern has therefore been raised about the potential risk of a "plasma-free" strategy, as administration of plasma might play a role in restoring factor XIII levels and factor V activity in the coagulopathic patients with severe hypoperfusion. It should be stressed that the choice of the ECS protocol to start coagulation support with 2 g of fibrinogen before plasma infusion differs substantially from other strategies which also consider administration of fibrinogen-rich components. In the Activation of Coagulation and Inflammation in Trauma (ACIT) study [69], cryoprecipitate was administered only after the first 6 units of RBCs and after infusion of the first FFP units.

The impact of the early coagulation support protocol on blood products consumption, mortality, and treatment costs has been recently addressed through a pre/post-cohort multicenter study [88]. Data from all severely injured patients (ISS >15) admitted to two Italian Trauma Centers during a 12-month period in 2013 were collected and compared with the same time period in 2011. In both periods, only patients transfused with at least three units of RBCs within 24 h of an accident were included in the study. The two groups were well matched (Table 7.2). In 2011 patients with significant hemorrhage were treated with "early" administration of plasma aiming at a high (≥1:2) FFP/RBCs ratio. In 2013 the ECS protocol was the treatment strategy. The adoption of the ECS protocol was associated with a 40 % overall reduction in RBCs transfusion, together with a statistically significant reduction in the use of FFP (−65 %) and platelet concentrates (−52 %) (Fig. 7.5). Hospital mortality for patients treated following the ECS protocol was 13.4 %, with a nonsignificant reduction if compared with the standard treatment group (20 %). Although these are only preliminary data, the observed mortality compares favorably with the recent data from the PROPPR study [66] where plasma at different ratio was used to support the failing hemostasis (22.4 % in the 1:1:1 group and 26.1 % in the 1:2 group).

Table 7.2 Matching of the two groups in the Italian multicenter study [88]

	Standard 1:1	ECS	
ISS >15	435	431	
ISS >15 e ≥3 PRBCs	130	96	
Age	48.8	51.1	Ns
Gender (f/m)	27 %	32 %	Ns
GCS	10.8	10.8	Ns
SBP	108.4	104.8	Ns
ISS	*32.92*	*33.58*	*Ns*
AIS head	2.19	2.49	Ns
AIS face	0.52	0.48	Ns
AIS chest	2.56	2.53	Ns
AIS abdomen	1.83	1.36	ns
AIS pelvis and limbs	2.15	2.51	Ns
AIS ext	0.36	0.20	Ns
PH	7.32	7.30	Ns
Lactate mmol/L	*3.15*	*3.2*	*Ns*
BE	−4.5	−4.8	Ns
Hb	10.8	11.3	Ns
PTL	196	205	Ns
INR	1.41	1.39	Ns
FIB (Clauss method)	184.6	196	Ns

One of the main concerns related to the use of concentrates in the treatment of trauma patients with critical bleeding is the economic impact of such a strategy. Data from the surgical and trauma intensive care units of the Innsbruck University show that a goal-directed coagulation management based on POC tests monitoring and the use of factors brought to a sharp reduction in FFP transfusions (−88 %) and RBCs requirement over a 5-year period [81]. The overall cost of blood products decreased by 200,000 Euro per year in spite of a significant increase in the cost of fibrinogen. However, these results are referred to the general population of patients requiring transfusions, including patients undergoing elective cardiac surgery; therefore, they might not be

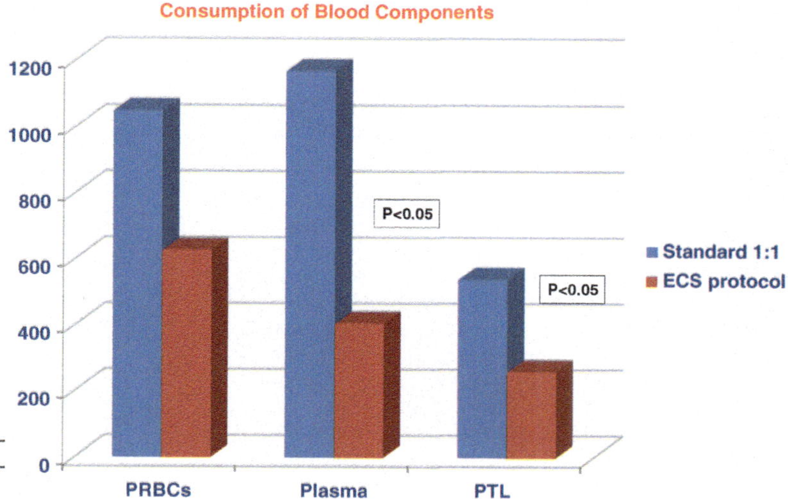

Fig. 7.5 Transfusion requirements reduction with the adoption ECS protocol

applicable to major bleeding in trauma victims. The impact of the ECS protocol on the global treatment cost in patients with clinical bleeding was also addressed by the Italian multicenter study: when costs for blood components, factors, and point-of-care tests were compared, a €76,340 saving in the ECS group (−23 %) was recorded.

Conclusions

Although our understanding of the pathophysiology of TIC is much improved in recent years, data in the literature are not sound enough to determine which is the best treatment. In the past 30 years, trauma hemorrhage has been evaluated through a limited number of trials. Many of these trials were poorly designed or numerically underpowered and did not produce reliable results. Recruitment to trauma RCTs can be difficult, not least because of the challenges of enrolling incapacitated patients, where informed consent is impossible to obtain. Low patient numbers affect study power and increase the risk of bias. Large, well-conducted studies with pragmatic endpoints are required to improve our understanding of the complex interplay between bleeding and coagulopathy, transfusion requirements, and mortality. However, these studies have extremely high costs, and this hinders their feasibility. For this reason, even the most recent recommendations for prevention and treatment of trauma coagulopathy could be only based on the results of observational studies.

References

1. Cohen MJ, Kutche MK, Redick B et al (2013) Clinical and mechanistic drivers of acute traumatic coagulopathy. J Trauma Acute Care Surg 75:S40–S47
2. Brohi K, Singh J, Heron M, Coats T (2003) Acute traumatic coagulopathy. J Trauma 54:1127–1130
3. Brohi K, Cohen MJ, Ganter MT et al (2008) Acute coagulopathy of trauma: hypoperfusion induces systemic anticoagulation and hyperfibrinolysis. J Trauma 64:1211–1217
4. Cohen MJ, Call M, Nelson M et al (2012) Critical role of activated Protein C in early coagulopathy and later organ failure, infection and death in trauma. Ann Surg 255:379–385
5. Bolliger D, Gorlinger K, Tanaka KA (2010) Pathophysiology and treatment of coagulopathy in massive hemorrhage and hemodilution. Anesthesiology 113:1205–1219
6. Theusinger OM, Madjdpour C, Spahn D (2012) Resuscitation and transfusion management in trauma patients: emerging concepts. Curr Opin Crit Care 18:661–670
7. Jansen JO, Scarpelini S, Pinto R, Tien HC, Callum J, Rizoli SB (2011) Hypoperfusion in severely injured trauma patients is associated with reduced coagulation factor activity. J Trauma 71:S435–S440
8. Duchesne JC, McSwain NE Jr, Cotton BA et al (2010) Damage control resuscitation: the new face of damage control. J Trauma 69:976–990
9. Dirkmann D, Gorlinger K, Gisbertz C et al (2012) Factor XIII and tranexamic acid but not recombinant factor VIIa attenuate plasminogen activator-induced hyperfibrinolysis in human whole blood. Anesth Analg 114:1182–1188
10. Pham HP, Shaz BH (2013) Update on massive transfusion. Br J Anaesth 111:i71–i82
11. Maegele M, Lefering R, Paffrath T et al Working Group on Polytrauma of the German Society of Trauma Surgery (DGU) (2008) Red blood cell to plasma ratios transfused during massive transfusion are associated with mortality in severe multiply injury: a retrospective analysis from the Trauma Registry of the Deutsche Gesellschaft für Unfallschirurie. Vox Sang 95:112–119
12. Johansson PI, Stensballe J (2010) Hemostatic resuscitation for massive bleeding: the paradigm of plasma and platelets — a review of the current literature. Transfusion 50:701–710
13. Cotton BA, Gunter OL, Isbell J et al (2008) Damage control hematology: the impact of a trauma exsanguination protocol on survival and blood product utilization. J Trauma 64:1177–1182
14. Gunter OL Jr, Au BK, Isbell JM, Mowery NT, Young PP, Cotton BA (2008) Optimizing outcomes in damage control resuscitation: identifying blood product ratios associated with improved survival. J Trauma 65:527–534
15. Magnotti LJ, Zarzaur BL, Fischer PE et al (2011) Improved survival after hemostatic resuscitation: does the emperor have no clothes? J Trauma 70:97–102
16. Patel SV, Kidane B, Klingel M, Parry N (2014) Risks associated with red blood cell transfusion in the trauma population, a meta-analysis. Injury 45:1522–1533
17. Spahn DR, Bouillon B, Cerny V et al (2013) Management of bleeding and coagulopathy following major trauma: an Updated European Guideline. Crit Care 17:R76
18. Kozek-Langenecker S, Afshari A, Albaladejo P et al (2013) Management of severe perioperative bleeding. Guidelines from the European Society of Anaesthesiology. Eur J Anaesthesiol 30:270–382
19. Recommendations of the working group on Perioperative Coagulation of the ÖGARI: coagulation

management in trauma-related massive bleeding. www.oegari.at
20. Yucel N, Lefering R, Maegele M (2006) Trauma associated severe hemorrhage (TASH)-Score: probability of mass transfusion as surrogate for life threatening hemorrhage after multiple trauma. J Trauma 60:1228–1236
21. Borgman MA, Spinella PC, Holcomb JB et al (2011) The effect of FFP: RBC ratio on morbidity and mortality in trauma patients based on transfusion prediction score. Vox Sang 101:44–54
22. Maegele M, Brockamp T, Nienaber U et al (2012) Predictive models and algorithms fort the need of transfusion including massive transfusion in severely injured patients. Transfus Med Hemother 39:85–97
23. Brockamp T, Nienaber U, Mutschler M et al (2012) Predicting on-going hemorrhage and transfusion requirement after severe trauma: a validation of six scoring systems and algorithms on the Trauma Register DGU(R). Crit Care 16:R129
24. Vandromme MJ, Griffin RL, McGwin G et al (2011) Prospective identification of patients at risk for massive transfusion: an imprecise endeavour. Am Surg 77:155–161
25. Ives C, Inaba K, Branco BC et al (2012) Hyperfibrinolysis elicited via thromboelastography predicts mortality in trauma. J Am Coll Surg 215:496–502
26. Schochl H, Frietsch T, Pavelka M, Jambor C (2009) Hyperfibrinolysis after major trauma: differential diagnosis of lysis patterns and prognostic value of thrombelastometry. J Trauma 67:125–131
27. Shakur H, Roberts I, Bautista R et al (2010) Effects of tranexamic acid on death, vascular occlusive events and blood transfusion in trauma patients with significant haemorrhage (CRASH-2): a randomized, placebo – controlled trial. Lancet 376:23–32
28. Raza I, Davenport R, Rourke C et al (2013) The incidence and magnitude of fibrinolytic activation in trauma patients. Thromb Haemost 11:307–314
29. The CRASH-2 Collaborators (2011) The importance of early treatment with tranexamic acid in bleeding trauma patients: an exploratory analysis of the CRASH-2 randomised controlled trial. Lancet 377:1096–1101
30. Moore H, Moore E, Gonzalez E et al (2014) Hyperfibrinolysis, physiologic fibrinolysis, and fibrinolysis shutdown: The spectrum of postinjury fibrinolysis and relevance to antifibrinolytic therapy. J Trauma Acute Care Surg 77:811–817
31. Dossett LA, Riesel JN, Griffin MR, Cotton BA (2011) Prevalence and implications of preinjury warfarin use. An analysis of the National Trauma Databank. Arch Surg 146:565–570
32. Guyatt GH, Akl EA, Crowther M et al (2012) American College of Chest Physicians Antithrombotic Therapy and Prevention of Thrombosis Panel Executive Summary. ACCP Evidence Based Clinical Practice Guidelines (9th Edition). Chest 141:7S–47S
33. Holbrook A, Schulman S, Witt DM et al (2012) American College of Chest Physicians. Evidence-based management of anticoagulant therapy: antithrombotic therapy and prevention of thrombosis (9th Edition). Chest 141:e152S–e184S
34. Keeling D, Baglin T, Tait C et al (2011) British Committee for Standards in Hematology. Guidelines on oral anticoagulation with warfarin – fourth edition. Br J Haematol 154:311–324
35. Appelboam R, Thomas EO (2009) Warfarin and intracranial haemorrhage. Blood Rev 23:1–9
36. McMillian WD, Rogers FB (2009) Management of prehospital antiplatelet and anticoagulant therapy in traumatic head injury: a review. J Trauma 66:942–950
37. Chapmann SA, Irwin ED, Beal AL, Kulinski NM, Hutson KE, Thorson MA (2011) Prothrombin complex concentrate versus standard therapies for INR reversal in trauma patients receiving warfarin. Ann Pharmacother 45:869–875
38. Imberti G, Barillari C, Biasioli M et al (2008) Prothrombin complex concentrate for urgent anticoagulation reversal in patients with intracranial haemorrhage. Pathophysiol Haemost Thromb 36:259–265
39. Pernod G, Godiér A, Gozalo C, Tremey B, Sié P, French National Authority for Health (2010) French clinical practice guidelines on the management of patients on vitamin K antagonists in at-risk situations (overdose, risk of bleeding, and active bleeding). Thrombosis Research 126:e167–e174
40. Prisco D (2005) Terapia anticoagulante orale, chirurgia e manovre invasive. Raccomandazioni della Federazione Centri per la Diagnosi della Trombosi e Sorveglianza della Terapie Antitrombotiche. Raccomandazioni FCSA. www.fcsa.it
41. Weitz JI (2012) New oral anticoagulants: a review from the laboratory. Am J Hematol 87:S133–S136
42. Schulman S, Crowther MA (2012) How I treat with anticoagulants in 2012: new and old anticoagulants, and when and how to switch. Blood 119:3016–3023
43. Dzik WS (2012) Reversal of drug-induced anticoagulation: old solutions and new problems. Transfusion 52:45S–55S
44. Kaatz S, Kouides PA, Garcia DA et al (2012) Guidance on the emergent reversal of oral thrombin and factor Xa inhibitors. Am J Hematol 87:S141–S145
45. Pengo V, Crippa L, Falanga A et al (2011) Questions and answers on the use of dabigatran and perspectives on the use of other new oral anticoagulants in patients with atrial fibrillation. A consensus document of the Italian Federation of Thrombosis Centers (FCSA). Thromb Haemost 106:868–876
46. Batchelor JS, Grayson A (2012) A meta-analysis to determine the effect on survival of platelet transfusion in patients with either spontaneous or traumatic antiplatelet medication-associated haemorrhage. BMJ 2:e000588
47. Washington CW, Schuerer DJ, Grubb R (2011) Platelet transfusion: an unnecessary risk for mild traumatic

brain injury patients on antiplatelet therapy. J Trauma 71:358–363
48. Downey DM, Monson B, Butler KL et al (2009) Does platelet administration affect mortality in elderly head-injured patients taking antiplatelet medication? Am Surg 75:1100–1103
49. Ivascu FA, Howells GA, Junn FS, Bair HA, Bendick PJ, Janczyk RJ (2008) Predictors of mortality in trauma patients with intracranial haemorrhage on pre-injury aspirin or clopidogrel. J Trauma 65:785–788
50. Fortuna GR, Mueller EW, James LE et al (2008) The impact of pre-injury antiplatelet and anticoagulant pharmacotherapy on outcomes in elderly patients with haemorrhagic brain injury. Surgery 144:598–603
51. Naidech AM, Liebling SM, Rosenberg NF et al (2012) Early platelet transfusion improves platelet activity and may improve outcomes for intracerebral haemorrhage. Neurocrit Care 16:82–87
52. Campbell PG, Sen A, Yadla S, Jabbour P, Jallo J (2010) Emergency reversal of antiplatelet agents in patients presenting with an intracranial haemorrhage: a clinical review. World Neurosurg 74:279–285
53. BCSH Guidelines for the use of platelet transfusions (2003) Br J Haematol 122:10–23. www.bcshguidelines.com
54. Schlimp CJ, Voelckel W, Inaba K, Maegele M, Ponschab M, Schochl H (2013) Estimation of plasma fibrinogen levels based on hemoglobin, base excess and ISS upon emergency room admission. Crit Care 17:R137
55. Rourke C, Curry N, Khan S et al (2012) Fibrinogen levels during trauma hemorrhage, response to replacement therapy and association with patient outcomes. J Thromb Haemost 10:1342–1351
56. Stinger HK, Spinella PC, Perkins JG et al (2008) The ratio of fibrinogen to red cells transfused affects survival in casualties receiving massive transfusions at an army combat support hospital. J Trauma 64:S79–S85
57. Spahn DR, Cerny V, Coats TJ et al (2007) Task Force for Advanced Bleeding Care in Trauma. Management of bleeding following major trauma: a European guideline. Crit Care 11:R17
58. Borgman MA, Spinella PC, Perkins JG et al (2007) The ratio of blood products transfused affects mortality in patients receiving massive transfusions at a combat support hospital. J Trauma 63:805–813
59. Duchesne JC, Hunt JP, Wahl G et al (2008) Review of current blood transfusions strategies in a mature level I trauma center: were we wrong for the last 60 years? J Trauma 65:272–276
60. Savage SA, Zarzaur BL, Croce MA, Fabian TC (2014) Time matters in 1:1 resuscitations: concurrent administration of blood: plasma and risk of death. J Trauma Acute Care Surg 77:833–838
61. Snyder CW, Weinberg JA, McGwin G Jr et al (2009) The relationship of blood product ratio to mortality: survival benefit or survival bias? J Trauma 66:358–362
62. Ho AM, Dion PW, Yeung JH et al (2012) Prevalence of survivors bias in observational studies on fresh frozen plasma: erythrocyte ratios in trauma requiring massive transfusion. Anesthesiology 116:716–728
63. Brown JB, Cohen MJ, Minei JP et al (2012) Debunking the survival bias myth: characterization of mortality during the initial 24 hours for patients requiring massive transfusion. J Trauma Acute Care Surg 73:358–364
64. Khan S, Davemport R, Raza I et al (2015) Damage control resuscitation using blood component therapy in standard doses has a limited effect on coagulopathy during trauma hemorrhage. Int Care Med 41:239–247
65. Baraniuk S, Tilley BC, del Junco DJ et al (2014) Pragmatic Randomized Optimal Platelet and Plasma Ratios (PROPPR) Trial: design, rationale and implementation. Injury 45:1287–1295
66. Holcomb JB, Tilley BC, Baraniuk S et al (2015) Transfusion of plasma, platelets, and red blood cells in a 1:1:1 vs a 1:1:2 ratio and mortality in patients with severe trauma: the PROPPR randomized clinical trial. JAMA 313:471–482
67. Kelly JM, Callum JL, Rizoli SB (2013) 1:1:1-warranted or wasteful? Even where appropriate, high ratio transfusion protocols are costly: early transition to individualized care benefits patients and transfusion services. Expert Rev Hematol 6:631–633
68. Chowdury P, Saayman AG, Paulus U, Findlay GP, Collins PW (2004) Efficacy of standard dose and 30 ml/kg fresh frozen plasma in correcting laboratory parameters of haemostasis in critically ill patients. Br J Haematol 125:69–73
69. Khan S, Brohi K, Chana M et al (2013) Hemostatic resuscitation is neither hemostatic nor resuscitative in trauma hemorrhage. J Trauma Acute Care Surg 76:561–568
70. Inaba K, Branco BC, Rhee P et al (2010) Impact of plasma transfusion in trauma patients who do not require massive transfusion. J Am Coll Surg 210:957–965
71. Pandey S, Vyas GN (2012) Adverse affects of plasma transfusion. Transfusion 52:65S–79S
72. Johnson JL, Moore EE, Kashuk JL et al (2010) Effect of blood products transfusion on the development of postinjury multiple organ failure. Arch Surg 145:973–977
73. Hess RJ (2013) Resuscitation of trauma induced coagulopathy. In: American Society of Hemathology, p 664–667
74. Fries D, Innerhofer P, Perger P et al (2010) Coagulation management in trauma-related massive bleeding. Recommendations of the Task Force for Coagulation (AGPG) of the Austrian Society of Anesthesiology, Resuscitation and Intensive Care Medicine (OGARI). Anasthesiol Intensivmed Notfallmed Schmerzther 45:552–561
75. Schöchl H, Nienaber U, Hofer G et al (2010) Goal-directed coagulation management of major trauma patients using thromboelastometry (ROTEM)-guided

administration of fibrinogen concentrate and prothrombin complex concentrate. Crit Care 14:R55
76. Nienaber U, Innerhofer P, Westermann I et al (2011) The impact of fresh frozen plasma vs coagulation factors concentrates on morbidity and mortality in trauma-associated haemorrhage and massive transfusion. Injury 42:697–701
77. Theusinger OM, Wanner GA, Emmert MY et al (2011) Hyperfibrinolisis diagnosed by rotational thromboelastometry (ROTEM) is associated with higher mortality in patients with severe trauma. Anesth Analg 113:1003–1012
78. Haas T, Görlinger K, Grassetto A (2014) Thomboelastometry for guiding bleeding management of the critically ill patient: a systematic review of the literature. Minerva Anestesiol 80:1–16
79. Da Luz LT, Nascimento B, Shankarakutty AK, Rizoli S, Adhikar NKJ (2014) Effect of thromboelastography (TEG®) and rotational thromboelastometry (ROTEM®) on diagnosis of coagulopathy, transfusion guidance and mortality in trauma: descriptive systematic review. Crit Care 18:R518
80. Winsted D, Thomas OD, Nisson F, Olanders K, Schött U (2014) Correction of hypothermic and dilutional coagulopathy with concentrates of fibrinogen and factor XIII: an in vitro study with ROTEM. Scand J Trauma Resusc Emerg Med 22:73
81. Görlinger K, Fries D, Dikmann D, Weber C, Hanke AA, Schöchl H (2012) Reduction of fresh frozen plasma requirements by perioperative point-of care coagulation management with early calculated goal-directed therapy. Transfus Med Hemother 39:104–113
82. Wikkelsø A, Lunde J, Johansen M (2013) Fibrinogen concentrate in bleeding patients (Review). Cochrane Database of Syst Rev 8:CD008864
83. Nardi G, Agostini V, Rondinelli MB et al (2013) Prevention and treatment of Trauma Induced Coagulopathy (TIC). An intended protocol from the Italian Trauma Update Research Group. J Anesthesiol Clin Sci www.hoajonline.com/jacs/2049-9752/2/22 (http://dx.doi.org/10.7243/2049-9752-2-22)
84. Sarode R (2012) How do I transfuse platelets (PLTS) to reverse anti-PLT drug effect. Transfusion 52:695–701
85. Vilahur G, Choi BG, Zafar MU et al (2007) Normalization of platelet reactivity in clopidogrel-treated subjects. J Thromb Haemost 5:82–90
86. Tosetto A, Balduini CL, Cattaneo M (2009) Management of bleeding and for invasive procedures in patients with platelet disorders and/or thrombocytopenia: Guidelines of the Italian Society for haemostasis and Throbosis (SISET). Thromb Res 124:e13–e18
87. James MF, Michell WL, Joubert IA et al (2011) Resuscitation with hydroxyethil starch improves renal function and lactate clearance in penetrating trauma in a randomized controlled study: the FIRST trial (Fluids Resuscitation of Severe Trauma). Br J Anaesth 107:693–702
88. Nardi G, Agostini V, Rondinelli MB et al (2015) Trauma induced coagulopathy: impact of the early coagulation support protocol on blood product consumption, mortality and costs. Crit Care 19:83

8 Management of Severe Bleeding in Cardiovascular Patients

Marco Ranucci, Blanca Martinez, Dionisio Colella, and Dorela Haxhiademi

8.1 Specific Aspects of Coagulopathy in Cardiac Surgery

Cardiac operations represent a clinical environment where a specific pattern of coagulopathy takes place in the majority of the cases. As a result, cardiac surgery is responsible for the majority of blood transfusions in many countries [1].

During cardiac operations, with or without cardiopulmonary bypass (CPB), an extensive amount of thrombin is generated [2]. Contrary to what generally thought in the first years of cardiac surgery, thrombin generated due to the contact of blood with foreign surfaces is a minor component, and the largest amounts of thrombin are generated due to tissue factor (TF) release [3]. TF is extensively formed from the surgical damages to tissues and accumulates in the pleuro-pericardial space, and, when shed blood is re-infused (especially during CPB), this activates the coagulation system and produces large amounts of thrombin [4, 5].

Separation of shed blood reduces thrombin generation: this may be achieved using closed circuits and shed-blood processing with a cell-saver before reinfusion [6]. Minimal invasive CPB circuits are associated with a decreased thrombin generation [7].

The nature of cardiac surgery-induced coagulopathy is complex and multifactorial. Cardiac surgery patients (especially coronary patients) are usually pretreated with anticoagulants and/or anti-platelet agents which may determine a pro-hemorrhagic status. Additionally, due to the extensive thrombin generation, unfractionated heparin is extensively used to guarantee anticoagulation during CPB. Heparin is then antagonized by protamine, but an incomplete antagonization may lead to bleeding, whereas protamine in excess is a bleeding factor as well [8].

The continuous activation of the coagulation system during surgery leads to consumption of coagulation factors and fibrinogen [9], and hemodilution further decreases coagulation factors and fibrinogen levels after surgery. These effects are even more pronounced in neonates and infants, where the role of hemodilution is more pronounced.

M. Ranucci, MD, FESC (✉)
Department of Cardiothoracic-Vascular Anesthesia and ICU, IRCCS Policlinico San Donato, San Donato Milanese, MI, Italy
e-mail: cardioanestesia@virgilio.it

B. Martinez, MD
Department of Anesthesia and Intensive Care Medicine, University Hospital of Udine, Udine, Italy

D. Colella, MD, PhD
Department of Cardiac Anesthesia, Policlinico Tor Vergata, University of Rome Tor Vergata, Rome, Italy

D. Haxhiademi, MD
Anesthesia and Intensive Care, G. Pasquinucci Hospital, G. Monasterio Foundation, Massa, Italy

M. Ranucci, P. Simioni (eds.), *Point-of-Care Tests for Severe Hemorrhage: A Manual for Diagnosis and Treatment*, DOI 10.1007/978-3-319-24795-3_8

Thrombocytopenia and platelet dysfunction are common findings in the context of postsurgical coagulopathy. Platelets are consumed due to adhesion/aggregation on the foreign surfaces of CPB; thrombin is a major source of platelet activation, leading to degranulation and loss of function. Additionally, platelets are often poorly working due to residual effects of antiplatelet agents.

Finally, hyperfibrinolysis is invariably found in cardiac surgery patients, due to the thrombin-mediated activation of the fibrinolytic system [10].

On top of all these mechanisms, post-cardiac surgery coagulopathy is associated with an endothelium disturbance that may lead even to a pro-coagulant condition. Due to the extensive thrombin generation, the endothelium reacts with a release of natural anticoagulants (protein C-S; tissue factor pathway inhibitor, antithrombin) [11], and circulating antithrombin is extensively consumed [12]. As a result, the endothelium loses its natural anticoagulant properties.

Overall, at the end of cardiac surgery, there is a sort of "downregulation" of the hemostatic system, with a reduced thrombin generation, platelet function, and fibrin(ogen)-derived clot firmness as pro-hemorrhagic mechanisms and loss of natural anticoagulants as pro-coagulant mechanism. This balance guarantees a mild-to-moderate bleeding, without the need for specific treatment in the majority of the cases. When the pro-hemorrhagic effects prevail, severe bleeding may occur, requiring a specific, targeted, and nonempirical treatment. A sound diagnostic of the bleeding state is mandatory, and point-of-care (POC) coagulation tests play an important role in this setting.

Nowadays, clinicians have a number of weapons to fight against major bleeding in cardiac surgery. Most of them are powerful and associated with potentially severe adverse events: in particular, excessive or inappropriate use of drugs increasing thrombin generation may determine thromboembolic complications.

The following sections will address the different mechanisms leading to bleeding in cardiac surgery patients, their diagnosis using POC coagulation tests, and their possible treatments.

8.2 The Bleeding Mechanisms in Cardiac Surgery

8.2.1 Residual Heparin Effect

Residual heparin and either poor or excessive reversal with protamine have been recognized as causes of microvascular bleeding after cardiopulmonary bypass.

Heparin is a glycosaminoglycan that exerts its coagulant effect by binding to antithrombin. Heparin presents a sophisticated anticoagulant effect. The heparin-AT complex inactivates thrombin factor (IIa) and factors Xa, IXa, XIa, and XIIa. By inhibiting thrombin, heparin also inhibits thrombin-induced activation of factor V and factor VIII. Furthermore, heparin presents other anticoagulant effects as it induces secretion of tissue factor pathway inhibitor (TFPI) by vascular endothelial cells that reduces the pro-coagulant activity of TF-FVIIa complex and releases t-PA from endothelial cells, triggering hyperfibrinolysis [13].

Incomplete heparin neutralization could obviously cause bleeding after cardiopulmonary bypass [14]. On the other hand, also an excessive dose of protamine could lead to bleeding, whereas protamine sulfate alters the interaction between the platelet receptor glycoprotein Ib and the von Willebrand factor interfering with platelet adhesion as assessed by ristocetin-induced platelet agglutination test [15–17].

Several methods have been proposed in order to assess the residual effect of heparin after cardiopulmonary bypass. The main are the activated clotting time (ACT), the measurement of plasma heparin concentration, and the heparinase-modified viscoelastic tests such as the heparinase-modified thromboelastography and thromboelastometry.

The ACT presents several limits after CPB weaning. The ACT depends on temperature and hemodilution, so a prolonged level of ACT may not exactly reflect the extent of anticoagulation by heparin leading to inappropriate further administration of protamine that can paradoxically exacerbate the anticoagulant state [18].

The heparin concentration-based anticoagulation system (Hepcon HMS; Medtronic,

Minneapolis, MN) titrates the presence of heparin using different concentrations of protamine, so this method confirms the complete in vitro reversal of heparin after CPB weaning [19, 20].

The viscoelastic tests TEG (Haemoscope Corporation, Niles, IL, USA) and ROTEM (Tem International, Munich, Germany) evaluate the presence of heparin in the sample comparing the reaction time (R) or clotting time (CT) of a test that analyzes the intrinsic pathway (kaolin-TEG and INTEM, respectively), with and without adding heparinase to the cuvette. Heparinase is derived from the *Flavobacterium heparinum* and neutralizes heparin by enzymatic cleavage of alpha-glycosidic linkages at the antithrombin III binding site [21–25].

Another potential cause of bleeding related to heparin is the heparin rebound [26] or recurrence of heparin anticoagulant effect. It has been observed up to 6 h after adequate protamine administration following cardiopulmonary bypass and, according to some authors, could lead to postoperative bleeding [27]. The mechanism of heparin rebound is still discussed and not well understood. The main hypothesis includes a release of heparin from fat cells several hours after surgery, a rapid protamine elimination from plasma, and the presence of plasma proteins that bind heparin subsequently released at a later time [28]. The clinical importance of heparin-rebound phenomena remains unclear [29].

8.2.2 Decreased Thrombin Generation

Dilution and consumption are mechanisms leading to decreased activity of coagulation factors after cardiac surgery. The great majority of coagulation factors (with the exception of factors I and XIII) concur in the mechanism of thrombin generation.

There are different views with respect to reduced thrombin generation as a mechanism leading to postoperative bleeding. The activity of coagulation factors may decrease down to 30 % without giving course to a significant bleeding tendency, and the decrease of any coagulation factor involved in thrombin generation was not associated with increased bleeding in a prospective study [9]. Conversely, other authors [30] could find that direct thrombin generation measurement during CPB provides clinically relevant data and that there is an inverse relationship between thrombin generation and postoperative bleeding. In general terms, it is unlikely that a reduced thrombin generation may lead to clinically relevant bleeding in the setting of routine cardiac surgery; however, there are conditions that are associated to a greater consumption/dilution of coagulation factors, and in this setting, a reduced thrombin generation may be considered within the possible mechanisms leading to bleeding. These conditions include prolonged (>2 h) CPB, preoperatively reduced levels of coagulation factors activity, preoperative consumption due to thrombi formation (aortic dissection), and extensive use of cell-saver. Additionally, preoperative use of drugs inhibiting vitamin K-dependent factors (warfarin) or direct factor Xa (rivaroxaban and apixaban) or thrombin inhibitors (dabigatran) creates an environment of poor thrombin generation.

8.2.2.1 Thrombin Generation Tests

Thrombin generation may be measured in plasma samples by calibrated automated thrombography (CAT, Fig. 8.1). After activation with TF, thrombin generation is defined by a peak level, a time to peak, and the endogenous thrombin potential. At present, CAT cannot be considered as a POC test, even if new devices (based on whole blood thrombin generation assessment) are entering the market.

Conventional tests offer a limited information on thrombin generation, even if prothrombin time and international normalized ratio are related to extrinsic pathway-dependent thrombin generation and activated partial thromboplastin time to intrinsic pathway-dependent thrombin generation.

Viscoelastic tests (thromboelastography, TEG®, and rotational thromboelastometry ROTEM®) may offer a contribution to indirect assessment of thrombin generation. In TEG and ROTEM, whole blood may be activated by kaolin

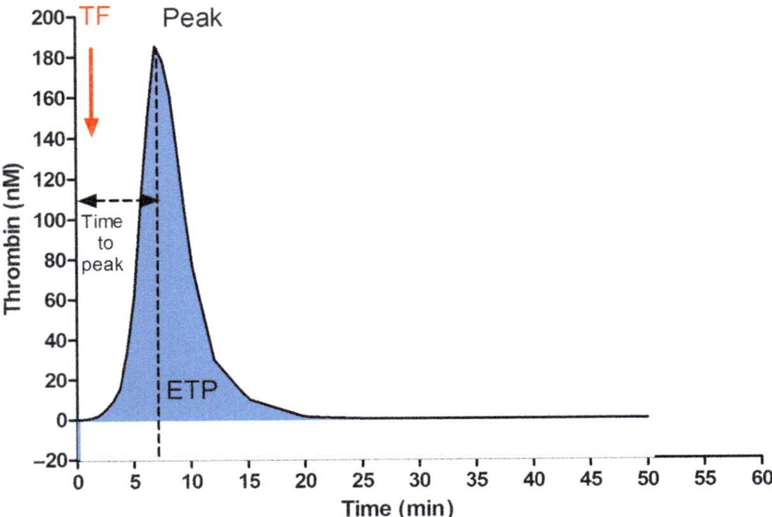

Fig. 8.1 Calibrated automated thrombography. *ETP* endogenous thrombin potential; *TF* tissue factor

(classical TEG) and ellagic acid (INTEM) or by TF (rapid TEG and EXTEM). The time required to change the physical properties of blood from the liquid phase to the gel phase (time to gel point [31]) is expressed as reaction time (R-time, TEG) or clotting time (CT, ROTEM) and may be considered as a surrogate for thrombin generation through the intrinsic or extrinsic pathway. However, it should be considered that the main determinant of a poor thrombin generation after cardiac surgery is a residual heparin activity [32]. Whereas some tests are insensitive to heparin (EXTEM), other tests like classical TEG should be run with and without heparinase to rule out the heparin role and address heparin-independent thrombin generation.

The main problem of viscoelastic tests in the setting of cardiac surgery is their very low positive predictive power for severe postoperative bleeding. In particular, there is a poor or even null relationship between R-time or CT and postoperative bleeding (Fig. 8.2). However, once there is the evidence for microvascular bleeding, viscoelastic tests may provide some information suggestive for poor thrombin generation. After cardiac surgery, a certain degree of reduced thrombin generation is usual and acceptable. Empirically, an R-time or CT time up to 20 % longer than the upper normal range may be considered a routine value. At present, we are lacking clear cutoff values suggestive for a bleeding mechanism related to poor thrombin generation. In the setting of pediatric cardiac surgery, a CT value >111 s was suggested [33], whereas other algorithms in adult cardiac surgery empirically suggest shorter values, around 80–90 s [34–36]. Given the low positive predictive power of these tests, and the multifactorial nature of postoperative bleeding in cardiac surgery, these cutoff values make sense only in the bleeding patient and once heparin effects or other reasons for bleeding are ruled out.

8.2.2.2 Therapeutic Interventions

Bleeding related to a poor thrombin generation may be corrected using fresh frozen plasma (FFP), 3–4 factors prothrombin complex concentrates (PCCs), activated factors like factor eight inhibitors bypassing activity (FEIBA), or recombinant activated factor VII (rFVIIa).

FFP is the most "natural" source of coagulation factors; however, large doses are required to restore thrombin generation. The dose ranges from 10 to 15 mL/kg in mild patterns of decreased thrombin generation to larger doses (30 mL/kg) in the most severe cases [37]. FFP is still largely used in the setting of cardiac surgery, basically due to its low cost and to its nature of "balanced" solution, containing both pro-coagulant and anti-

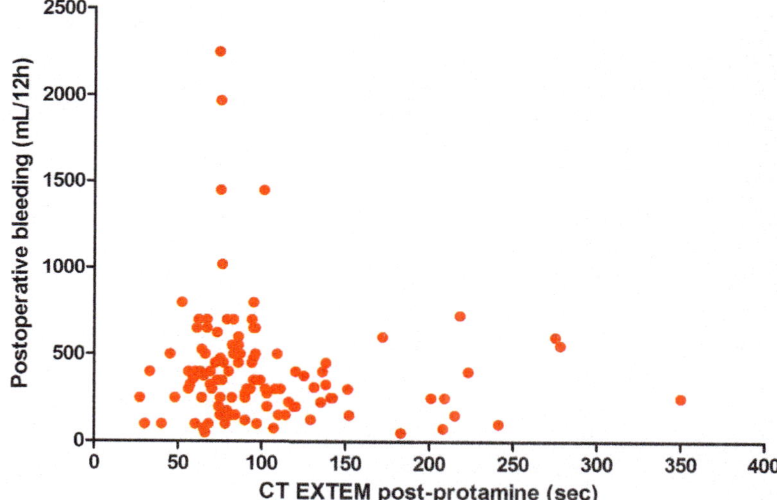

Fig. 8.2 Relationship between clotting time at ROTEM (after protamine administration) and postoperative bleeding. No significant association was found (personal data). *CT* clotting time

coagulant factors. However, FFP is associated with a number of possible adverse reactions (see Chap. 6) and to fluid overload.

PCCs are certainly more effective in terms of thrombin generation recovery. Their use for the treatment of dilution/consumption coagulopathy has been successfully tested in cardiac surgery patients [38, 39]. However, there are reports of increased thromboembolic complications linked to the use of PCCs [40].

Due to its ability to bypass the other coagulation factors, rFVIIa is able to induce a thrombin burst. The suggested dose ranges from 60 to 90 μg/kg i.v. rFVIIa is certainly effective in reducing bleeding in cardiac surgery as well as in other scenarios [41, 42]. However, there is a well-established risk of thromboembolic complications [41].

As a general rule, every correction leading to increased thrombin generation (with the exception of FFP) has been linked to an increased risk of thromboembolic events. Additionally, it should be considered that thrombin alone is unable to induce the formation of a stable clot unless adequate amounts of fibrinogen and well-working platelets (together with FXIII) are available. Therefore, a prerequisite for interventions aimed to increase thrombin generation is the presence of adequate levels of the abovementioned hemostatic factors.

8.2.3 Low Fibrinogen Levels

Fibrinogen is converted into fibrin by thrombin and binds platelets through the platelet receptor GPIIbIIIa, leading to a stable clot after the intervention of factor XIII.

After cardiac surgery, low levels of fibrinogen are a common finding [9]. Low levels of fibrinogen after surgery have been associated with postoperative bleeding in a number of studies [9, 43–45]. Additionally, other studies have found an association between preoperative fibrinogen levels and postoperative bleeding [46–49].

The clinical conditions leading to low fibrinogen levels after cardiac surgery are similar to those leading to a consumption of coagulation factors.

8.2.3.1 Functional Fibrinogen Tests

Low fibrin(ogen) levels lead to a poor clot firmness. In general, there is presently a general opinion that clot firmness may be most relevant than thrombin generation in the pathophysiology of severe postoperative bleeding in cardiac surgery.

Viscoelastic tests provide a measure of clot firmness based on the viscoelastic properties of the clot, namely, expressed in terms of "amplitude" (mm) of the formed clot. For TEG, this is represented by the maximum amplitude (MA) and for ROTEM as maximum clot firmness (MCF). However, these measures provide a combined assessment of the interaction between fibrin(ogen) and platelets and are therefore not specific for fibrin(ogen) contribution to clot firmness. To achieve this specific measure, the platelet contribution must be eliminated, and modified TEG/ROTEM assays are available. Basically, platelet contribution is blunted by a GPIIbIIIa inhibitor in functional fibrinogen (FF) TEG and by cytochalasin D in FIBTEM (ROTEM).

The resulting values of MA and MCF at FF-TEG or FIBTEM are representative of fibrin(ogen) alone contribution to clot firmness.

There is an acceptable correlation between viscoelastic tests measure of fibrin(ogen) contribution to clot firmness and fibrinogen levels as measured with the conventional Clauss method [50] (Fig. 8.3). However, the two measures are not interchangeable, since one represents fibrinogen concentration, the other a functional fibrinogen activity.

At present, it is still unclear which levels of postoperative fibrinogen should lead to fibrinogen supplementation. Some authors suggest trigger values of 1.0–2.0 g/L [51–53], while others suggest higher values in the setting of cardiac surgery [54].

A specific issue is represented by the possibility of prophylactic correction of low preoperative fibrinogen levels. The recently released guidelines for the management of severe perioperative bleeding (European Society of Anaesthesiology) [54] consider the possibility of correcting values <3.8 g/L, based on a single, small randomized controlled trial [47]. However, an analysis of the existing literature [55] has demonstrated that preoperative fibrinogen levels have a very poor (about 10 %) positive predictive power for prediction of severe postoperative bleeding. A trigger value of 3.8 g/L would lead to an unacceptable 90 % rate of superfluous treatments. Trigger values settled around 2.0 g/L seems more adequate, but however a strategy based on postoperative values is certainly more reasonable.

8.2.3.2 Therapeutic Interventions

Fibrinogen can be supplemented using three different strategies. FFP contains fibrinogen but actually at a very variable concentration. A reasonable value can be settled at about 2 g/L [56], and therefore, the amount of FFP to increase fibrinogen levels by 1 g/L is about 30 mL/kg. Therefore, the same considerations applied to FFP as a source of factors increasing thrombin generation may be applied to FFP as a source of fibrinogen, the main problem remaining the large dose required to achieve a clinically relevant benefit.

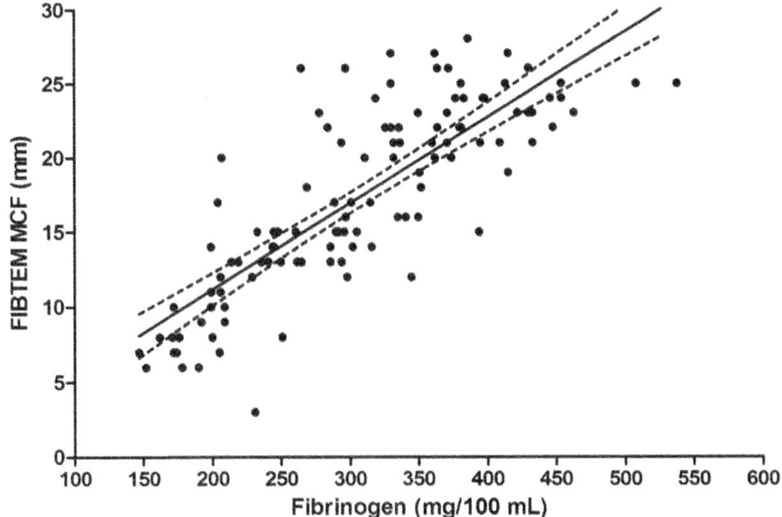

Fig. 8.3 Linear regression relationship between fibrinogen concentration (Clauss method) and maximum clot firmness at the FIBTEM ROTEM test (personal data). Dashed lines are 95 % confidence interval. *MCF* maximum clot firmness

A second source of fibrinogen is represented by cryoprecipitates. The fibrinogen content in cryoprecipitates is variable, but a value of 12 g/L seems reasonable [57]. In some countries, cryoprecipitates are the standard of care for fibrinogen supplementation in case of acquired bleeding; however, they are not available in many European countries [58].

Fibrinogen concentrate is probably the most effective treatment for fibrinogen deficiency. The high concentration (20 g/L) allows treatment without volume overload, and its purified nature limits the risks associated with FFP and cryoprecipitates. The suggested dose is 25–50 mg/kg [54]. Fibrinogen concentrate is not licensed for acquired bleeding in the UK and USA [58].

Many studies suggest to settle the fibrinogen dose on the value of MCF at FIBTEM [17–19]. A target value of 22 mm at FIBTEM is suggested, and an equation to achieve the target has been proposed [59, 60]:

$$\text{Fibrinogen concentrate dose}(\text{g}) = \left(\begin{array}{l}\text{target FIBTEM MCF}[22\ \text{mm}]\\ -\text{actual FIBTEM MCF}[\text{mm}]\end{array}\right) \times (\text{bodyweight}[\text{kg}]/140).$$

However, following this equation leads to administration of large doses of fibrinogen concentrate. At present, we are lacking an evidence-based information with respect to the exact fibrinogen trigger values, targets, and dosage.

A recent RCT on postoperative fibrinogen concentrate administration demonstrated the efficacy of this strategy in reducing postoperative bleeding and transfusions [61]. This study suggested that a target MCF at FIBTEM in the range of 15–17 mm is enough to avoid severe bleeding.

Finally, FXIII has been proposed to increase clot firmness in the setting of the bleeding patient. However, a recent randomized controlled trial of FXIII supplementation in cardiac surgery failed to demonstrate any effect on bleeding and transfusions [62].

8.2.4 Thrombocytopenia

After cardiac surgery with CPB, a certain degree of thrombocytopenia is inevitable. Different factors concur in its determinism: platelet activation and adhesion to the CPB circuit, hemodilution, extensive use of cell-saver, platelet activation due to the elevated shear stress in critical parts of the CPB circuit, and thrombin-induced platelet activation.

Platelet counts about 30–40 % lower than the preoperative value are common findings and are not necessarily associated with bleeding. In adults, platelet count rarely reaches critical levels unless in case of preoperative thrombocytopenia. This last condition can be found in patients operated under septic conditions or in patients with congenital cyanotic heart disease.

8.2.4.1 POC Tests and Platelet Count

The diagnosis of thrombocytopenia is based on conventional cell count. However, thrombocytopenia may be suspected in case of low values of clot firmness (MA-MCF) with normal values of functional fibrinogen. When applying this concept, however, it should be considered that the values of MA/MCF are not linearly correlated with the real viscoelastic properties of the clot.

8.2.4.2 Therapeutic Options

The only therapeutic option is transfusion of platelet concentrates. Compensating a low platelet count with large doses of fibrinogen is a theoretical option which has never been confirmed in large studies.

8.2.5 Platelet Dysfunction

There are basically two mechanisms leading to acquired platelet dysfunction in cardiac surgery patients. The first is related to the preoperative use of antiplatelet agents (aspirin and P2Y12 receptor inhibitors); the second depends on the effects of surgery and CPB (platelet activation by the extensive thrombin generation and adhesion to foreign surfaces). As a result of these combined effects, after cardiac surgery, platelet dysfunction is an invariable finding. Both adhesion and aggregation are blunted, in a time-dependent fashion, by CPB [63].

Platelet function tests (PFTs) in this setting have an important role. However, they are still poorly diffused in the clinical practice, and their role in preventing and treating postoperative bleeding is still a matter of debate.

8.2.5.1 Platelet Function Tests before Surgery

Before surgery, coronary patients are usually treated with aspirin and/or P2Y12-inhibitors (ticlopidine, clopidogrel, prasugrel, and ticagrelor). Aspirin determines a mild increase in postoperative bleeding [64]; conversely, P2Y12-inhibitors are associated with patterns of severe bleeding and risk of reoperation [65, 66].

The existing guidelines suggest 5 days of drug discontinuation before surgery [67, 68], but it is admitted that even three days may be enough [67]. Platelet recovery after antiplatelet drug discontinuation is highly individual and somehow unpredictable [69]; for this reason, the use of PFTs to assess the correct timing of surgery after P2Y12-inhibitors discontinuation is considered a reasonable option [54, 70]. Conventional tests confirm that preoperative assessment of platelet function may predict postoperative bleeding: a value <40 % of ADP-dependent platelet activation at light transmission aggregometry was found predictive of severe bleeding in clopidogrel-treated patients [71].

Multiple-electrode aggregometry (MEA) has been proposed to assess ADP-dependent platelet reactivity in P2Y12-inhibitors treated patients. A study based on the Multiplate technology (Roche Diagnostics GmbH, Mannheim, Germany) proposed a minimal value of 31 [U] at the ADP test as a suitable cutoff level for admitting patients to surgery, with a negative predictive power of 92 % [72]. Subsequently, a combination of ADP test and TRAP test was found to offer better accuracy: a minimal value of TRAP test of 75 [U] in patients with an ADP test <22 [U] was associated with a 100 % negative predictive power for severe bleeding [73] MEA was found useful even to detect patients that may be operated after a time from drug discontinuation shorter than five days [74].

Other POC-PFTs have shown an association between ADP-dependent preoperative platelet function and postoperative bleeding. Modified TEG (TEG platelet mapping) may predict postoperative bleeding in clopidogrel pretreated patients [75]. A preoperative value of MAadp <42.5 mm had a 78 % sensitivity and 84 % specificity for predicting excessive bleeding [75].

The VerifyNow (Accumetrics Inc, San Diego, CA, USA) is another POC-PFT which can aid in determining the timing of cardiac surgery: preoperative values of ADP-dependent platelet inhibition >21 % in clopidogrel-treated patients have been found associated with a higher surgical revision rate and blood use in off-pump coronary surgery [76]. A previous study demonstrated an association between preoperative VerifyNow P2Y12 platelet inhibition and blood loss and blood use in coronary patients under double antiplatelet therapy until three days before surgery [77].

Recently, ROTEM has provided a ROTEM platelet device based on multielectrode aggregometry, but no data are available at present.

8.2.5.2 Platelet Function Tests after Surgery

After surgery, PFTs show different degrees of platelet dysfunction, depending on the preoperative use of antiplatelet agents, the type of surgery, and the duration of CPB. Low levels of platelet function after surgery have been associated with postoperative bleeding [78, 79]. Algorithms including PFTs for the diagnosis of postoperative bleeding exist, including trigger values for desmopressin infusion or platelet concentrate transfusions. A recent study proposed MEA test values for triggering interventions aimed to increase platelet function: a TRAP test <50 [U] and/or an ASPI test <30 [U] and/or an ADP test <30 [U] [34]. Previously, another study suggested the following values: TRAP test <50 [U] and/or an ASPI test <20 [U] and/or an ADP test <30 [U] to trigger platelet concentrates transfusions in actively bleeding patients after cardiac surgery

[36]. These values, however, are empirical and not yet validated; they have been proposed within algorithms including other POC tests to rule out other possible causes of bleeding. The combination of drug-related factors with operation-related factors makes difficult a clear determination of a specific value of postoperative platelet activity responsible for severe bleeding.

8.2.5.3 Therapeutic Interventions

The most reasonable approach to the treatment of drug-related platelet dysfunction bleeding is the transfusion of platelet concentrates. In patients treated with ticagrelor, the transfused platelets may be attacked by the still active forms of the drug, given the pharmacokinetic of ticagrelor.

Desmopressin (0.3 μg/kg) may be used to treat surgical bleeding due to acquired platelet dysfunction, especially in the setting of acquired von Willebrand disease (aortic stenosis patients) [80] and after CPB. Despite a low level of evidence, this approach is included in the European Guidelines [54].

8.2.6 Hyperfibrinolysis

Hyperfibrinolysis has been identified as a cofactor of hemostatic impairment during cardiac surgery contributing to cardiopulmonary bypass coagulopathy and microvascular bleeding [81].

Fibrinolysis is responsible for fibrin degradation and consequently for clot breakdown. Fibrinolysis starts when plasmin cleaves fibrin and fibrinogen. The process is triggered by the plasminogen activators as tissue plasminogen activator (t-PA) released by the Weibel-Palade bodies of endothelial cells and urokinase plasminogen activator synthesis by monocytes, macrophages, and fibroblasts. The process is regulated by the plasminogen activator inhibitors (PAI) type 1 and 2, the thrombin activatable fibrinolytic inhibitor (TAFI), and the α-2-antiplasmin. The most important systemic plasminogen inhibitor PAI 1 is mainly released by platelets at the site of a forming thrombus. Hyperfibrinolysis occurs when the balance between fibrinolysis activators and inhibitors is altered [82, 83].

Activation of fibrinolysis depends on several simultaneous mechanisms [84], and both intrinsic and extrinsic coagulation pathways can initiate fibrinolysis [14].

Cardiac surgery using CPB is associated with increased fibrinolytic activity compared to off-pump cardiac surgery. During cardiopulmonary bypass, excessive fibrinolysis can due to either primary or secondary fibrinolysis (i.e., as related to reduced fibrinolysis inhibitors such as PAI-1, alpha 2-antiplasmin) [83]. Before weaning from CPB, a discrepancy between plasma levels of plasmin and alpha 2-antiplasmin is observed due to alpha 2-antiplasmin absorption to extracorporeal surfaces [85]. The high thrombin generation throughout CPB associated with the contributions of high levels of epinephrine, bradykinin and vasopressin trigger a high fibrinolytic activity [2]. Almost immediately after CPB initiation, t-PA levels rise 6-fold and plasmin generation suffers a 100-fold increase [86]. Besides, alternative pathways of fibrinolysis as neutrophil elastase-mediated fibrin digestion may also contribute to hyperfibrinolysis during CPB demonstrating that the systemic inflammatory response syndrome induced by CPB is closely related to hemostatic phenomena [87]. Plasmin interacts also with the inflammatory system triggering the complement cascade and kallikrein [14].

The fibrinolytic response to CPB is heterogeneous, and large interindividual variations in fibrinolytic response have been observed during CPB. The most frequent (40 %) pattern or typical response consists in a rapid rise in active and total t-PA during CPB followed postoperatively by elevated PAI-1 and reduced t-PA. Approximately one-third of patients show no change in fibrinolytic parameters. When present, the t-PA response is rapid, occurring within the first 30 min of CPB and is more common in patients undergoing valve surgery than in coronary artery bypass grafting [88, 89]. Some studies have described the influence of genetic factors as 675 (4G75G) polymorphism, on the plasma levels of PAI 1, t-PA, and t-PA/PAI-1 complex [90]. The main factors contributing to fibrinolysis are the t-PA released from CPB-mediated contact activation of factor XII, thrombin, or hypothermia or released from the traumatized shocked endothelial cells or returned from the blood suctioned from the pericardial cavity [91–93].

Moreover, hyperfibrinolysis could affect other aspects of hemostasis. For instance, plasmin may reduce platelet adhesion and aggregation by degradation of von Willebrand receptor glycoprotein Ib and platelet fibrinogen receptor glycoprotein IIb/IIIa, respectively [94].

Hyperfibrinolysis can be classified as primary and secondary hyperfibrinolysis. Primary is independent to high amounts of thrombin generation, whereas secondary hyperfibrinolysis is the consequence of activation of coagulation and thrombin formation. Secondary hyperfibrinolysis is not always harmful as it prevents end organ damage caused by microvascular fibrin deposition during disseminated intravascular coagulation [81].

8.2.6.1 Therapeutic Interventions

When bleeding is associated to primary hyperfibrinolysis, the use of an antifibrinolytic agent is appropriate. Several studies and meta-analyses have shown the synthetic lysine analogues and aprotinin to be effective in reducing bleeding and the need for blood transfusion during high-risk cardiac surgery, as compared with placebo [95–99]. However, the blood conservation using antifibrinolytics in a randomized trial (BART) demonstrated a strong and consistent negative mortality trend associated with aprotinin compared to lysine analogues, leading to aprotinin withdrawal worldwide by manufacturer in 2007 [100]. The synthetic lysine analogues tranexamic acid (TXA) and epsilon-aminocaproid acid (EACA) inhibit in a reversible way the fibrinolytic enzyme plasmin. Both are indicated to reduce the number of patients who require blood transfusion and to reduce total blood loss after cardiac operations. However, these agents are slightly less potent drugs, and the safety profile of these drugs is less well studied compared with aprotinin [66].

A wide range of dosages of antifibrinolytic drugs has been proposed [101]. Suggested TXA doses during cardiac surgery varies from a loading dose of 12.5 mg/kg followed by an infusion of 6.5 mg/kg/h [102] up to higher doses such as 20 g administered during a period of 12 h [103]. Often, the chosen regime is not denoted by pharmacokinetic studies. It has been observed that plasma levels are maintained over the therapeutic level for most of the duration of cardiopulmonary bypass with a regime of 10 mg/kg loading dose followed by an infusion of 1 mg/kg/h for up to 2 h after arrival in intensive care unit. The dosing of TXA is important because its side effects are dose related [104]. The administration of high doses of TXA has been associated to a higher rate of seizures in the postoperative period [104, 105]. The safer scheme and optimal dosing regimen for lysine analogues in cardiovascular surgery has still to be established [101]. Currently, a new antifibrinolytic drug CU-2010 is in clinical development [106].

Monitoring the fibrinolytic activity can be made by the determination of D-dimers, FDP, and XDP plasma levels or using viscoelastic tests. The D-dimer, FDP, an XDP levels are not quickly and immediately available. Besides, D-dimers are not useful to determine the etiology of coagulopathy in situations of perioperative bleeding, as its concentration is usually increased postoperatively in all patients [81]. Viscoelastic hemostatic assays such as TEG and ROTEM are the current most useful clinical hemostatic test used in perioperative setting to determine hyperfibrinolytic status in bleeding patients. However, it has been argued that the viscoelastic tests only detect the most severe forms of systemic hyperfibrinolysis, but lower degrees of fibrinolysis may critically influence the outcome too [107].

The TEG parameters of lysis are the Ly30 and Ly60 (percentage of lysis 30 and 60 min after maximum amplitude respectively) and the EPL (estimated percent lysis parameter). Both parameters measure the decrease in amplitude of the trace as a function of time and reflect the loss of clot integrity due to clot lysis [108]. ROTEM parameters of lysis are maximum lysis (ML) [%] and clot lysis index 30 or 60 min after maximum clot firmness (CLI30; CLI60) [%]. Monitoring can be performed in EXTEM or HEPTEM tests that allow for timely detection of hyperfibrinolysis even under the conditions of anticoagulation with heparin during cardiopulmonary bypass. In addition, the APTEM test consists in a specific ROTEM assays that test the in vitro effect of antifibrinolytics (i.e., aprotinin) in a whole blood sample of a bleeding patient [109]. According to some published protocols in cardiac surgery, hyperfibrinolytic state needing antithrombotic therapy is diagnosed in the presence of EPL >7.5 % in TEG analysis [110] or CLI60 <85 % according to ROTEM analysis during or after CPB [36].

8.2.7 Surgical Sources

The nature itself of cardiac surgery involves the risk of surgical sources of bleeding (suture lines, small arteries, collateral vessels, and others). In this setting, the value of POC tests relies on their high negative predictive value. In the setting of the bleeding patient, each test should be applied to rule out residual heparin effects, poor thrombin generation, poor clot firmness, and hyperfibrinolysis. Once none of these factors appear to be involved, surgical revision of the patient is warranted.

8.3 Bleeding in Pediatric Cardiac Surgery

Children that undergo cardiac surgery are particularly prone to surgical and CPB effects on the coagulation system. Early postoperative hemorrhage is independently associated with increased mortality in infants after cardiac surgery [111]. Besides the alterations of coagulation due to exposure to CPB, the risk for postoperative coagulation disorders in this population is increased by small age and body weight, as well as preexisting congenital and acquired coagulation disorders, specific for cardiac congenital heart disease.

8.3.1 Preoperative Conditions

8.3.1.1 Developmental Hemostasis

The concept of developmental hemostasis, introduced by Andrew and colleagues [112–115], states that the hemostatic system of newborns and infants is effective and they do not suffer from spontaneous hemorrhagic complications, but their concentration of the majority of coagulation proteins, as measured by functional assays, varies significantly with age. At birth. plasma concentrations of the vitamin K-dependent and contact factors are decreased, whereas fibrinogen, FV, FVIII, and FXIII are similar or increased compared with adults. Plasma concentrations of plasminogen are decreased, whereas tissue plasminogen activator and plasminogen activator inhibitor are increased. The hemostatic system of the young is a dynamic process. Within the first 6 months of life, at times even later, the concentration of the coagulation factors reaches the adult levels. Reference ranges for ROTEM and TEG are determined for all pediatric age groups [116–118].

8.3.1.2 Congenital Heart Disease (CHD) and Coagulation

In patients with CHD, the heart defect itself compromises coagulation. Neonates and infants with single-ventricle or two-ventricle physiology have lower levels of pro-coagulant and anticoagulant factors compared to healthy children of the same age group [119, 120]. POC-based studies (TEG and ROTEM) indicate that children of less than 1 year affected by congenital heart disease have a lesser balance between coagulation and fibrinolysis compared to healthy children of the same age [121, 122] and that cyanosis and/or polycythemia has the major negative impact on hemostasis [123].

The shear stress-induced degradation of VWF might be the cause of the high frequency of acquired von Willebrand disease in pediatric patients with a shunt defect or valve stenosis associated with increased shear [124, 125].

8.3.1.3 Special Considerations in Children with Cyanotic Heart Disease

Cyanotic heart disease is associated with a significant tendency to bleeding. Platelet count reduction in cyanotic children is an ongoing process. In 25 % of the patients of a study that included Eisenmenger syndrome patients, the authors found thrombocytopenia. They hypothesized that platelets are reduced due to right-to-left intracardiac shunts that bypass the lungs where megakaryocytes are fragmented into platelets [126]. Born aggregometry studies have shown a higher platelet reactivity compared to controls in children with cyanotic heart disease [127]. At hematocrit levels over 60 %, due to blood hyperviscosity, there is an overproduction of platelet microparticles and suppression of platelet aggregation [128]. Recently, some authors reported impaired fibrinogen functionality (detected by TEG and TEG FF) in patients with cyanotic heart disease [129, 130].

8.3.2 Intraoperative Bleeding Mechanisms in Pediatric Cardiac Surgery

Exposure to CPB puts in jeopardy the fragile hemostatic balance of the young. The mechanisms of intraoperative coagulation alterations are the same as for adult patients, but the impact they have on the children hemostasis is more pronounced. On CPB levels of coagulation, factors and platelet counts are lower than the adult ones because the preoperative coagulation alterations sum up with coagulation factors consumption and massive dilution by CPB priming. In an average adult, the CPB priming volume is 1/3–1/4 of total blood volume (i.e., 1000–1500 mL of priming to 4200–4500 mL of total blood volume). For a newborn, it can be 1–1.5 times the total blood volume (i.e., 250–300 mL of priming volume to 200–250 mL of total blood volume). In a study in neonates, at the initiation of CPB, the authors found 50 % decrease in circulating coagulation factors and antithrombin levels, as well as 70 % of platelet count reduction [131].

8.3.2.1 Low Thrombin Generation

In pediatric cardiac surgery, thrombin generation has been studied with the markers of thrombin generation such as TAT and F 1.2 and recently with calibrated automated thrombography [132]. Preoperative thrombin generation is a predictive risk factor for postoperative bleeding [133], but intraoperative data is lacking. The information that viscoelastic tests give on thrombin generation is used in the perioperative settings for its evaluation. To date, there are no cutoff values that can guide therapy. In a recent algorithm, CT $\geq$111 s was suggested to trigger hemostatic therapy [33].

FFP and cryoprecipitates are the sources of coagulation factors more used in pediatric patients. Where available, especially in small patients, cryoprecipitate (0.5–1 Unit/kg) is a much more efficient source of coagulation factors than FFP.

PCCs have been successfully used in pediatric cardiac surgery, but concern still remains about thromboembolic events reported in adult patients. In a recent study, infusion of a PCC (0.1 mg/kg of 4-factor PCC) in infants younger than 1 year reduced postoperative bleeding and red blood cell transfusion [134].

There is little evidence to guide clinicians on the most effective or safe dose of rFVIIa for off-label indications of rFVIIa. In the hemostasis registry of Australia and New Zealand, FVIIa was administered in 202 cardiac surgery patients, the first dose ranging from 90 to 193 mcg/kg, and 8 % of patients experienced a thromboembolic event [135, 136].

8.3.2.2 Low Fibrinogen Level

Hemodilution and consumption are the leading causes for low fibrinogen level after pediatric cardiac surgery. Recently, there is an increasing awareness on the role of fibrinogen and clot firmness in the postoperative hemostasis even in this group of patients. Fibrinogen concentrations of less than 1.5 g/L and a MCF less than 3 mm predict excessive blood loss in pediatric cardiac surgery [45]. Cutoff levels to trigger pharmacological intervention are not yet established. In a recent TEM-based algorithm, the authors propose A10 $\leq$3 mm on FIBTEM to be the guiding level for hemostatic therapy [33]. Fibrinogen supplements can be provided by FFP, cryoprecipitate, and fibrinogen concentrations. FFP is traditionally used in pediatric cardiac surgery, especially in newborns, for CPB priming, and in the post-CPB period, to avoid and treat hypofibrinogenemia. Fibrinogen concentrates (60 mg/kg) were as effective as cryoprecipitate in the treatment of postoperative bleeding in a study in pediatric cardiac surgery [137]. Although low levels of fibrinogen are found to correlate with postoperative blood loss, prophylactic use of FFP in the priming solution does not provide the presumed clinical benefits [138, 139].

8.3.2.3 Decreased Platelet Count and Function

Both platelet count and platelet aggregation are markedly reduced during surgery with the greatest reduction on CPB. The duration of CPB and hypothermia are associated with significant changes in platelet function [140, 141].

Due to the complexity of platelet function and heterogeneity of platelet testing assays, data on intraoperative platelet testing should be interpreted carefully. Platelet function tested with MEA TRAP test and cone and platelet analyzer have shown no correlation with postoperative blood loss [142, 143]. Other authors find correlation between platelet function tested with MEA and platelet function analyzer and transfusion requirements [140, 144, 145].

Platelet transfusions of 0.5–1.0 unit/kg is the first-line therapy for the low platelet count and platelet dysfunction.

8.3.2.4 Hyperfibrinolysis

Besides the demonstrated importance of fibrinolysis in adult patients, a few studies have investigated fibrinolysis during CPB surgery in children. Hyperfibrinolysis accompanying CPB in children can cause significant bleeding in this population after CPB [146].

Fibrinolysis defined at TEG as A30/MA less than 0.85 was found in 16 % of children during CPB. It occurred in young children undergoing complex surgery with prolonged CPB and deep hypothermia [147].

Prevention of hyperfibrinolysis with lysine analogues, especially with tranexamic acid, is given routinely in pediatric cardiac surgery. Different infusion protocols and dosages are in use nowadays. In a dose-ranging study of TXA, the authors found the most effective dosing scheme, a 10 mg/kg load, 10 mg/kg in the pump prime, and 10 mg/kg after protamine [148].

In conclusion, POCs can be used in pediatric cardiac surgery to detect coagulation abnormalities in the preoperative period [124–130], to predict postoperative bleeding and to guide its treatment [149–152].

References

1. Wells AW, Llewelyn CA, Casbard A et al (2009) The EASTR Study: indications for transfusion and estimates of transfusion recipient numbers in hospitals supplied by the National Blood Service. Transfus Med 19:315–328
2. Edmunds LH, Colman RW (2006) Thrombin during cardiopulmonary bypass. Ann Thorac Surg 82:2315–2322
3. Boisclair SJ, Lane DA, Philippou H (1993) Mechanisms of thrombin generation during surgery and cardiopulmonary bypass. Blood 82:3350–3357
4. Chung JH, Gikakis N, Rao AK et al (1996) Pericardial blood activates the extrinsic coagulation pathway during clinical cardiopulmonary bypass. Circulation 93:2014–2018
5. De Somer F, Van Belleghem Y, Caes F et al (2002) Tissue factor as the main activator of the coagulation system during cardiopulmonary bypass. J Thorac Cardiovasc Surg 123:951–958
6. Albes JM, Stohr IM, Kaluza M et al (2003) Physiological coagulation can be maintained in extracorporeal circulation by means of shed blood separation and coating. J Thorac Cardiovasc Surg 126:1504–1512
7. Wippermann J, Albes JM, Hartrumpf M et al (2005) Comparison of minimally invasive closed circuit extracorporeal circulation with conventional cardiopulmonary bypass and with off-pump technique in CABG patients: selected parameters of coagulation and inflammatory system. Eur J Cardiothorac Surg 28:127–132
8. Khan NU, Wayne CK, Barker J, Strang T (2010) The effects of protamine overdose on coagulation parameters as measured by the thrombelastograph. Eur J Anaesthesiol 27:624–627
9. Ternström L, Radulovic V, Karlsson M et al (2010) Plasma activity of individual coagulation factors, hemodilution and blood loss after cardiac surgery: a prospective observational study. Thromb Res 126:e128–e133
10. Teufelsbauer H, Proidl S, Havel M, Vukovich T (1992) Early activation of hemostasis during cardiopulmonary bypass: evidence for thrombin mediated hyperfibrinolysis. Thromb Haemost 68:250–252
11. Boyle EM Jr, Verrier ED, Spiess BD (1996) Endothelial cell injury in cardiovascular surgery: the

procoagulant response. Ann Thorac Surg 62:1549–1557
12. Ranucci M, Frigiola A, Menicanti L, Ditta A, Boncilli A, Brozzi S (2005) Postoperative antithrombin levels and outcome in cardiac operations. Crit Care Med 33:355–360
13. Hirsch J, Warkentin TE, Shaughnessy SG et al (2001) Heparin and Low-molecular-weight heparin. Mechanisms of action, pharmacokinetics, dosing, monitoring, efficacy and safety. Chest 119:64S–94S
14. Paparella D, Brister SJ, Buchanan MR (2004) Coagulation disorders of cardiopulmonary bypass: a review. Intensive Care Med 30:1873–1881
15. AmmaT FCF (1997) The effects of heparinase I and protamine on platelet reactivity. Anesthesiology 86:1382–1386
16. Lindblad B, Wakefield TW, Whitehouse WM Jr, Stanley JC (1998) The effects of protamine sulfate on platelet function. Scand J Thorac Cardiovasc Surg 22:55–59
17. Barstad RM, Stephens RW, Hamers MJ, Sakariassen KS (2000) Protamine sulphate inhibits platelet membrane glycoprotein Ib-von Willebrand factor activity. Thromb Haemost 83:334–337
18. Despotis GJ, Joist JH (1991) Anticoagulation and anticoagulation reversal with cardiac surgery involving cardiopulmonary bypass: an update. J Cardiothorac Vasc Anesth 13(suppl 1):18–29
19. Koster A, Fischer T, Praus M et al (2002) Hemostatic activation and inflammatory response during cardiopulmonary bypass: impact of heparin management. Anesthesiology 97:837–841
20. Despotis GJ, Joist JH, Hogue CW Jr et al (1996) More effective suppression of hemostatic system activation in patients undergoing cardiac surgery by heparin dosing based on heparin blood concentrations rather than ACT. Thromb Haemost 76:902–908
21. Tuman KJ, McCarthy RJ, Djuric M, Rizzo V, Ivankovich AD (1994) Evaluation of coagulation during cardiopulmonary bypass with a heparinase-modified thromboelastographic assay. J Cardiothorac Vasc Anesth 8:144–149
22. Gertler R, Wiesner G, Tassani-Prell P, Braun SL, Martin K (2011) Are the point-of-care diagnostics MULTIPLATE and ROTEM valid in the setting of high concentrations of heparin and its reversal with protamine? J Cardiothorac Vasc Anesth 25: 981–986
23. Mittermayr M, Velik-Salchner C, Stalzer B et al (2009) Detection of protamine and heparin after termination of cardiopulmonary bypass by thrombelastometry (ROTEM): results of a pilot study. Anesth Analg 108:743–750
24. Mittermayr M, Margreiter J, Velik-Salchner C et al (2005) Effects of protamine and heparin can be detected and easily differentiated by modified thrombelastography (Rotem): an in vitro study. Br J Anaesth 95:310–316
25. Gronchi F, Perret A, Ferrari E et al (2014) Validation of rotational thromboelastometry during cardiopulmonary bypass: a prospective, observational in-vivo study. Eur J Anaesthesiol 31:68–75
26. Hyun BH, Pence RE, Davila JC, Butcher J, Custer RP (1962) Heparin rebound phenomenon in extracorporeal circulation. Surg Gynecol Obstet 124:191–198
27. Purandare SV, Parulkar GB, Panday SR, Bhattacharya S, Bhatt MM (1979) J Postgrad Med 25:70–74
28. Teoh KHT, Young E, Bradley CA, Hirsh J (1993) Heparin binding proteins. Contribution to heparin rebound after cardiopulmonary bypass. Circulation 88(suppl II):420–425
29. Martin P, Horkay F, Gupta NK et al (1992) Heparin rebound phenomenon-much ado about nothing? Blood Coagul Fibrinolysis 3:187–191
30. Bosch YP, Al Dieri R, ten Cate H et al (2014) Measurement of thrombin generation intra-operatively and its association with bleeding tendency after cardiac surgery. Thromb Res 133:488–494
31. Ranucci M, Laddomada T, Ranucci M, Baryshnikova E (2014) Blood viscosity during coagulation at different shear rates. Physiol Rep 2: pii: e12065. doi:10.14814/phy2.12065
32. Radulovic V, Hyllner M, Ternström L et al (2012) Sustained heparin effect contributes to reduced plasma thrombin generation capacity early after cardiac surgery. Thromb Res 130:679–687
33. Faraoni D, Willems A, Romlin BS, Belisle S, Van der Linden P (2015) Development of a specific algorithm to guide haemostatic therapy in children undergoing cardiac surgery: a single-centre retrospective study. Eur J Anaesthesiol 32:320–329
34. Weber CF, Görlinger K, Meininger D et al (2012) Point-of-care testing: a prospective, randomized clinical trial of efficacy in coagulopathic cardiac surgery patients. Anesthesiology 117:531–547
35. Görlinger K, Dirkmann D, Weber CF, Rahe-Meyer N, Hanke AA (2011) Algorithms for transfusion and coagulation management in massive haemorrhage. Anästh Intensivmed 52:145–159
36. Görlinger K, Dirkmann D, Hanke AA et al (2011) First-line therapy with coagulation factor concentrates combined with point-of-care coagulation testing is associated with decreased allogeneic blood transfusion in cardiovascular surgery. A retrospective, single-center cohort study. Anesthesiology 115:1179–1191
37. Puetz J (2013) Fresh frozen plasma: the most commonly prescribed hemostatic agent. J Thromb Haemost 11:1794–1799
38. Tanaka KA, Mazzeffi MA, Grube M, Ogawa S, Chen EP (2013) Three-factor prothrombin complex concentrate and hemostasis after high-risk cardiovascular surgery. Transfusion 53:920–921
39. Arnékiana V, Camousa J, Fattalb S, Rézaiguia-Delclauxa S, Nottinc R, Stéphana F (2012) Use of prothrombin complex concentrate for excessive bleeding after cardiac surgery. Interact Cardiovasc Thorac Surg 15:382–389
40. White R, Rushbrook J, McGoldrick J (2008) The dangers of prothrombin complex concentrate administra-

tion after heart surgery. Blood Coagul Fibrinolysis 19:609–610
41. Gill R, Herbertson M, Vuylsteke A et al (2009) Safety and efficacy of recombinant activated factor VII: a randomized placebo-controlled trial in the setting of bleeding after cardiac surgery. Circulation 120:21–27
42. Levi M, Peters M, Buller HR (2005) Efficacy and safety of recombinant factor VIIa for treatment of severe bleeding: a systematic review. Crit Care Med 33:883–890
43. Kindo M, Hoang Minh T, Gerelli S et al (2014) Plasma fibrinogen level on admission to the intensive care unit is a powerful predictor of postoperative bleeding after cardiac surgery with cardiopulmonary bypass. Thromb Res 134:360–368
44. Pillai RC, Fraser JF, Ziegenfuss M, Bhaskar B (2014) The influence of circulating levels of fibrinogen and perioperative coagulation parameters on predicting postoperative blood loss in cardiac surgery: a prospective observational study. J Card Surg 29: 189–195
45. Faraoni D, Willems A, Savan V, Demanet H, De Ville A, Van der Linden P (2014) Plasma fibrinogen concentration is correlated with postoperative blood loss in children undergoing cardiac surgery. A retrospective review. Eur J Anaesthesiol 31:317–326
46. Waldén K, Jeppsson A, Nasic S, Backlund E, Karlsson M (2014) Low preoperative fibrinogen plasma concentration is associated with excessive bleeding after cardiac operations. Ann Thorac Surg 97:1199–1206
47. Karlsson M, Ternström L, Hyllner M et al (2009) Prophylactic fibrinogen infusion reduces bleeding after coronary artery bypass surgery. A prospective randomised pilot study. Thromb Haemost 102:137–144
48. Karlsson M, Ternstrom L, Hyllner M, Baghaei F, Nilsson S, Jeppsson A (2008) Plasma fibrinogen level, bleeding, and transfusion after on-pump coronary artery bypass grafting surgery: a prospective observational study. Transfusion 48:2152–2158
49. Aljassim O, Karlsson M, Wiklund L, Jeppsson A, Olsson P, Berglin E (2006) Inflammatory response and platelet activation after off-pump coronary artery bypass surgery. Scand Cardiovasc J 40:43–48
50. Kalina U, Stohr HA, Bickhard H et al (2008) Rotational thromboelastography for monitoring of fibrinogen concentrate therapy in fibrinogen deficiency. Blood Coagul Fibrinolysis 19:777–783
51. O'Shaughnessy DF, Atterbury C, Bolton Maggs P et al (2004) Guidelines for the use of fresh-frozen plasma, cryoprecipitate and cryosupernatant. Br J Haematol 126:11–28
52. Rossaint R, Bouillon B, Cerny V et al (2010) Management of bleeding following major trauma: an updated European guideline. Crit Care 14:R52
53. Rahe-Meyer N (2011) Fibrinogen concentrate in the treatment of severe bleeding after aortic aneurysm graft surgery. Thromb Res 128(Suppl 1):S17–S19
54. Kozek-Langenecker SA, Afshari A, Albaladejo P et al (2013) Management of severe perioperative bleeding: guidelines from the European Society of Anaesthesiology. Eur J Anaesthesiol 20:270–382
55. Ranucci M, Jeppsson A, Bayshnikova E (2015) Preoperative fibrinogen supplementation in cardiac surgery patients: an evaluation of different trigger values. Acta Anaesthesiol Scand 59:427–433
56. Theusinger OM, Baulig W, Seifert B, Emmert MY, Spahn DR, Asmis LM (2011) Relative concentrations of haemostatic factors and cytokines in solvent/detergent-treated and fresh-frozen plasma. Br J Anaesth 106:505–511
57. Pantanowitz L, Kruskall MS, Uhl L (2003) Cryoprecipitate. Patterns of use. Am J Clin Pathol 119:874–881
58. Ranucci M, Solomon C (2012) Supplementation of fibrinogen in acquired bleeding disorders: experience, evidence, guidelines, and licences. Br J Anaesth 109:135–137
59. Rahe-Meyer N, Pichlmaier M, Haverich A et al (2009) Bleeding management with fibrinogen concentrate targeting a high-normal plasma fibrinogen level: a pilot study. Br J Anaesth 102:785–792
60. Rahe-Meyer N, Solomon C, Winterhalter M et al (2009) Thromboelastometry-guided administration of fibrinogen concentrate for the treatment of excessive intraoperative bleeding in thoracoabdominal aortic aneurysm surgery. J Thorac Cardiovasc Surg 138:694–702
61. Ranucci M, Baryshnikova E, Crapelli GB et al (2015) Randomized, double-blinded, placebo-controlled trial of fibrinogen concentrate supplementation after complex cardiac surgery. J Am Heart Assoc 4(6). pii: e002066. doi:10.1161/JAHA.115.002066
62. Karkouti K, von Heymann C, Jespersen CM et al (2013) Efficacy and safety of recombinant factor XIII on reducing blood transfusions in cardiac surgery: a randomized, placebo-controlled, multicenter clinical trial. J Thorac Cardiovasc Surg 146:927–939
63. Greilich PE, Brouse CF, Beckham J, Jessen ME, Martin EJ, Carr ME (2002) Reductions in platelet contractile force correlate with duration of cardiopulmonary bypass and blood loss in patients undergoing cardiac surgery. Thromb Res 105:523–529
64. Ferraris VA, Brown JR, Despotis GJ et al (2011) 2011 update to the society of thoracic surgeons and the society of cardiovascular anesthesiologists blood conservation clinical practice guidelines. Ann Thorac Surg 91:944–982
65. Pickard AS, Becker RC, Schumock GT, Frye CB (2008) Clopidogrel-associated bleeding and related complications in patients undergoing coronary artery bypass grafting. Pharmacotherapy 28:376–392
66. Berger JS, Frye CB, Harshaw Q, Edwards FH, Steinhubl SR, Becker RC (2008) Impact of clopidogrel in patients with acute coronary syndromes requiring coronary artery bypass surgery: a multicenter analysis. J Am Coll Cardiol 52:1693–1701
67. Ferraris VA, Ferraris SP, Saha SP et al (2007) Perioperative blood transfusion and blood conservation in cardiac surgery: the society of thoracic sur-

geons and the society of cardiovascular anesthesiologists clinical practice guideline. Ann Thorac Surg 83(5 Suppl):S27–S86
68. Fitchett D, Eikelboom J, Fremes S et al (2009) Dual antiplatelet therapy in patients requiring urgent coronary artery bypass grafting surgery: a position statement of the Canadian Cardiovascular Society. Can J Cardiol 25:683–689
69. Di Dedda U, Ranucci M, Baryshnikova E, Castelvecchio S; Surgical and Clinical Outcome Research (SCORE) Group (2014) Thienopyridines resistance and recovery of platelet function after discontinuation of thienopyridines in cardiac surgery patients. Eur J Cardiothorac Surg 45:165–170
70. Ferraris VA, Saha SP, Oestreich JH et al (2012) 2012 update to the Society of Thoracic Surgeons guideline on use of antiplatelet drugs in patients having cardiac and noncardiac operations. Ann Thorac Surg 94:1761–1781
71. Chen L, Bracey AW, Radovancevic R et al (2004) Clopidogrel and bleeding in patients undergoing elective coronary artery bypass grafting. J Thorac Cardiovasc Surg 128:425–431
72. Ranucci M, Baryshnikova E, Soro G, Ballotta A, De Benedetti D, Conti D; Surgical and Clinical Outcome Research (SCORE) Group (2011) Multiple electrode whole-blood aggregometry and bleeding in cardiac surgery patients receiving thienopyridines. Ann Thorac Surg 91:123–129
73. Ranucci M, Colella D, Baryshnikova E, Di DeddaU; Surgical and Clinical Outcome Research (SCORE) Group (2014) Assessment of preoperative P2Y12 and thrombin platelet receptor inhibition and their relationships with post-cardiac surgical bleeding. Br J Anaesth 113:970–976
74. Mahla E, Suarez TA, Bliden KP et al (2012) Platelet function measurement-based strategy to reduce bleeding and waiting time in clopidogrel-treated patients undergoing coronary artery bypass graft surgery: the timing based on platelet function strategy to reduce clopidogrel-associated bleeding related to CABG (TARGETCABG) study. Circ Cardiovasc Interv 5:261–269
75. Preisman S, Kogan A, Itzkovsky K, Leikin G, Raanani E (2010) Modified thromboelastography evaluation of platelet dysfunction in patients undergoing coronary artery surgery. Eur J Cardiothorac Surg 37:1367–1374
76. Brizzio ME, Shaw RE, Bosticco B et al (2012) Use of an objective tool to assess platelet inhibition prior to off-pump coronary surgery to reduce blood usage. J Invasive Cardiol 24:49–52
77. Alström U, Granath F, Oldgren J, Ståhle E, Tydén H, Siegbahn A (2009) Platelet inhibition assessed with VerifyNow, flow cytometry and PlateletMapping in patients undergoing heart surgery. Thromb Res 124:572–577
78. Schimmer C, Hamouda K, Sommer SP, Özkur M, Hain J, Leyh R (2013) The predictive value of multiple electrode platelet aggregometry (multiplate) in adult cardiac surgery. Thorac Cardiovasc Surg 61:733–743
79. Orlov D, McCluskey SA, Selby R et al (2014) Platelet dysfunction as measured by a point-of-care monitor is an independent predictor of high blood loss in cardiac surgery. Anesth Analg 118:257–263
80. Steinlechner B, Zeidler P, Base E et al (2011) Patients with severe aortic valve stenosis and impaired platelet function benefit from preoperative desmopressin infusion. Ann Thorac Surg 91:1420–1426
81. Teuselsbauer H, Proidi S, Havel M, Vukovich T (1992) Early activation of hemostasis during cardiopulmonary bypass: evidence for thrombin mediated hyperfibrinolysis. Thromb Haemost 68:250–252
82. Hunt BJ, Segal H (1996) Hyperfibrinolysis. J Clin Pathol 49:958
83. Despotis G, Eby C, Lublin DM (2008) A review of transfusion risks and optimal management of perioperative bleeding with cardiac surgery. Transfusion 48(1 Suppl):2S–30S
84. Despotis GJ, Hogue CW (1999) Pathophysiology, prevention, and cardiac surgery: a primer for cardiologists and an update for the cardiothoracic team. Am J Cardiol 83:15B–30B
85. Edmunds LH (1993) Blood surface interactions during cardiopulmonary bypass. J Card Surg 8:404–410
86. Chandler WL, Velan T (2003) Secretion of tissue plasminogen activator and plasminogen activator inhibitor 1 during cardiopulmonary bypass. Thromb Res 112:185–192
87. Gando S, Kameue T, Sawamura A, Hayakawa M, Hoshino H, Kubota N (2007) An alternative pathway for fibrinolysis is activated in patients who have undergone cardiopulmonary bypass surgery and major abdominal surgery. Thromb Res 120:87–93
88. Chandler WL, Fitch JC, Wall MH, Verrier ED, Cochran RP, Sollow LO, Spiess BD (1995) Individual variations in the fibrinolytic response during and after cardiopulmonary bypass. Thromb Haemost 74:1293–1297
89. Ozolina A, Strike E, Jaunalksne I, Krumina A et al (2012) PAI-1 and t-PA/PAI-1 complex potential markers of fibrinolytic bleeding after cardiac surgery employing cardiopulmonary bypass. BMC Anesthesiol 12:27
90. Iribarren JL, Jimenez JJ, Hernandez D, Brouard M, Riverol D, Lorente L et al (2008) Postoperative bleeding in cardiac surgery: the role of tranexamic acid in patients homozygous for the 5G polymorphism of the plasminogen activator inhibitor-1 gene. Anesthesiology 108:596–602
91. de Haan J, Boonstra PW, Monnik SH, Ebels T, van Oeveren W (1995) Retransfusion of suctioned blood during cardiopulmonary bypass impairs hemostasis. Ann Thorac Surg 59:901–907
92. Stibbe J, Kluft C, Brommer EJ, Gomes M, de Jong DS, Nauta J (1984) Enhanced fibrinolytic activity during cardiopulmonary bypass in open heart surgery in main caused by extrinsic (tissue-type) plasminogen activator. Eur J Clin Invest 14:375–382

93. Tabuchi N, de Haan J, Boonstra PW, van Oeveren W (1993) Activation of fibrinolysis in the pericardial cavity during cardiopulmonary bypass. J Thorac Cardiovasc Surg 106:828–833
94. Adelman B, Michelson AD, Loscalzo J, Greenberg J, Handin RI (1985) Plasmin effect on platelet glycoprotein Ib-von Willebrand factor interactions. Blood 65:32–40
95. Laupacis A, Fergusson D (1997) Drugs to minimize perioperative blood loss in cardiac surgery: meta-analyses using perioperative blood loss transfusion as the outcome. Anesth Analg 85:1258–1267
96. Fremes SE, Bi W, Lee E et al (1994) Meta-analysis of prophylactic drug treatment in the prevention of postoperative bleeding. Ann Thorac Surg 58:1580–1588
97. Fergusson D, Glass KC, Hutton B, Shapiro S (2005) Randomized controlled trials of aprotinin in cardiac surgery: could clinical equipoise have stopped the bleeding? Clin Trials 2:218–229
98. Henry DA, Carless PA, Moxey AJ et al (2007) Antifibrinolytic use for minimizing perioperative allogenic blood transfusion. Cochrane Database Syst Rev 4:CD001886
99. Ngaage DL, Bland JM (2010) Lessons from aprotinin: is the routine use and inconsistent dosing of tranexamic acid prudent? Meta-analysis of randomized and large matched observational studies. Eur J Cardiothorac Surg 37:1375–1383
100. Fergusson DA, Hebert PC, Mazer CD et al (2008) A comparison of aprotinin and lysine analogues in high-risk cardiac surgery. N Engl J Med 358(22):2319–2331
101. Koster A, Schimer U (2011) Re-evaluation of the role of antifibrinolytic therapy with lysine analogs during cardiac surgery in the post aprotinin era. Curr Opin Anaesthesiol 24:92–97
102. Dowd NP, Karski JM, Cheng DC et al (2002) Pharmacokinetics of tranexamic acid during cardiopulmonary bypass. Anesthesiology 97:390–399
103. Fiechtner BK, Nuttal GA, Johnson ME et al (2001) Plasma Tranexamic acid concentrations during cardiopulmonary bypass. Anesth Analg 92:1131–1136
104. Ender J, Brüning J, Mukherjee C et al (2010) Tranexamic acid increases the risk of postoperative seizures in adults undergoing on-pump cardiac surgery. J Cardiothorac Vasc Anesth 24(Suppl):P-78
105. Sander M, Spies C, Martiny V et al (2010) Mortality associated with administration of high-dose tranexamic acid and aprotinin in primary open-heart procedures: a retrospective analysis. Crit Care 14:R148
106. Dietrich W, Nicklisch S, Koster A, Spannagl M, Giersiefen H, van de Locht A (2009) CU-2010--a novel small molecule protease inhibitor with antifibrinolytic and anticoagulant properties. Anesthesiology 110:123–130
107. Stensballe J, Ostrowski RS, Johansson PI (2014) Viscoelastic guidance of resuscitation. Curr Opin Anaesthesiol 27:212–218
108. O'Shaughnessy D, Gill R (2009) Cardiothoracic surgery. In: Key N, Markis M, O'Shaughnessy D et al (eds) Practical hemostasis and thrombosis. Wiley-Blackwell, Chichester, pp 194–208
109. Luddington RJ (2005) Thrombelastography/thromboelastometry. Clin Lab Haematol 27:81–90
110. Diprose P, Herbertson MJ, O'Shaughnessy D, Deakin CD, Gill RS (2005) A randomized double-blind placebo-controlled trial of antifibrinolytic therapies used in addition to intraoperative cell savage. Br J Anaesth 94:271–278
111. Wolf M, Maher K, Kanter K, Kogon B, Guzzetta N, Mahle W (2014) Early postoperative bleeding is independently associated with increased surgical mortality in infants after cardiopulmonary bypass. J Thorac Cardiovasc Surg 148:631–636
112. Andrew M, Paes B, Milner R et al (1998) Development of the human coagulation system in the healthy premature infant. Blood 72:1651–1657
113. Monagle P, Massicotte P (2011) Developmental haemostasis: secondary haemostasis. Semin Fetal Neonatal Med 16:294–300
114. Monagle P, Ignjatovic V, Savoia H (2010) Hemostasis in neonates and children: pitfalls and dilemmas. Blood Rev 24:63–68
115. Guzzetta NA, Miller BE (2010) Principles of hemostasis in children: models and maturation. Paediatr Anaesth 21:3–9
116. Oswald E, Stalzer B, Heitz E et al (2010) Thromboelastometry (ROTEM) in children: age-related reference ranges and correlations with standard coagulation tests. Br J Anaesth 105: 827–835
117. Chan KL, Summerhayes RG, Ignjatovic V, Horton SB, Monagle PT (2007) Reference values for kaolin-activated thromboelastography in healthy children. Anesth Analg 105:1610–1613
118. Miller BE, Bailey JM, Mancuso TJ et al (1997) Functional maturity of the coagulation system in children: an evaluation using thrombelastography. Anesth Analg 84:745–748
119. Odegard KC, Zurakowski D, DiNardo JA et al (2009) Prospective longitudinal study of coagulation profiles in children with hypoplastic left heart syndrome from stage I through Fontan completion. J Thorac Cardiovasc Surg 137:934–941
120. Odegard KC, Zurakowski D, Hornykewycz S et al (2007) Evaluation of the coagulation system in children with two-ventricle congenital heart disease. Ann Thorac Surg 83:1797–1804
121. Haizinger B, Gombotz H, Rehak P, Geiselseder G, Mair R (2006) Activated thrombelastogram in neonates and infants with complex congenital heart disease in comparison with healthy children. Br J Anaesth 97:545–552
122. Osthaus WA, Boethig D, Johanning K et al (2008) Whole blood coagulation measured by modified thrombelastography (ROTEM) is impaired in infants with congenital heart diseases. Blood Coagul Fibrinolysis 19:220–225

123. Faraoni D, Van der Linden P (2014) Factors affecting postoperative blood loss in children undergoing cardiac surgery. J Cardiothorac Surg 9:32
124. Arslan MT, Ozyurek R, Kavakli K et al (2007) Frequency of acquired von Willebrand's disease in children with congenital heart disease. Acta Cardiol 62:403–408
125. Wiegand G, Hofbeck M, Zenker M, Budde U, Rauch R (2012) Bleeding diathesis in Noonan syndrome: Is acquired von Willebrand syndrome the clue? Thromb Res 130:e251–e254
126. Lill MC, Perloff JK, Child JS (2006) Pathogenesis of thrombocytopenia in cyanotic congenital heart disease. Am J Cardiol 98:254–258
127. Kierzkowska B, Stanczyk J, Wiectawska B et al (2001) Activation of circulating platelets and platelet response to activating agents in children with cyanotic congenital heart disease: their relevance to palliative systemic-pulmonary shunt International. Int J Cardiol 79:49–59
128. Horigome H, Hiramatsu Y, Shigeta O, Nagasawa T, Matsui A (2002) Overproduction of platelet microparticles in cyanotic congenital heart disease with polycythemia. J Am Coll Cardiol 39:1072–1077
129. Jensen AS, Johansson PI, Bochsen J (2013) Fibrinogen function is impaired in whole blood from patients with cyanotic congenital heart disease. Int J Cardiol 167:2210–2214
130. Jensen AS, Johansson PI, Idorn L (2013) The haematocrit - an important factor causing impaired haemostasis in patients with cyanotic congenital heart disease. Int J Cardio 167:1317–1321
131. Kern FH, Morana NJ, Sears JJ, Hickey PR (1992) Coagulation defects in neonates during cardiopulmonary bypass. Ann Thorac Surg 54:541–546
132. Koestenberger M, Cvirn G, Nagel B et al (2008) Thrombin generation determined by calibrated automated thrombography (CAT) in pediatric patients with congenital heart disease. Thromb Res 122:13–19
133. Bosch Y, Al Dieri R, ten Cate H et al (2013) Preoperative thrombin generation is predictive for the risk of blood loss after cardiac surgery: a research article. J Cardiothorac Surg 8:154
134. Giorni C, Ricci Z, Iodice F et al (2014) Use of Confidex to control perioperative bleeding in pediatric heart surgery: prospective cohort study. Pediatr Cardiol 35:208–214
135. McQuilten ZK, Barnes C, Zatta A, Phillips LE (2012) Off-Label use of recombinant Factor VIIa in pediatric patients. Pediatrics 129:e1533–e1540
136. Warren OJ, Rogers PL, Watret al et al (2009) Defining the role of recombinant activated factor VII in pediatric cardiac surgery: where should we go from here? Pediatr Crit Care Med 10:572–582
137. Galas FR, de Almeida JP, Fukushima JT et al (2014) Hemostatic effects of fibrinogen concentrate compared with cryoprecipitate in children after cardiac surgery: a randomized pilot trial. J Thorac Cardiovasc Surg 148:1647–1655
138. Miao X, Liu J, Zhao M et al (2015) Evidence-based use of FFP: the influence of a priming strategy without FFP during CPB on postoperative coagulation and recovery in pediatric patients. Perfusion 30:140–147
139. Faraoni D, Sanchez Torres C (2014) No evidence to support a priming strategy with FFP in infants. Eur J Pediatr 173:1445–1446
140. Romlin BS, Soderlund F, Wahlander H, Nilsson B, Baghaei F, Jeppsson A (2014) Platelet count and function in paediatric cardiac surgery: a prospective observational study. Br J Anaesth 113:847–854
141. Andreasen B, Hvas AM, Ravn HB (2014) Marked changes in platelet count and function following pediatric congenital heart surgery. Paediatr Anaesth 24:386–392
142. Ranucci M, Carlucci C, Isgrò G, Baryshnikova E (2012) A prospective pilot study of platelet function and its relationship with postoperative bleeding in pediatric cardiac surgery. Minerva Anestesiol 78:556–563
143. Tirosh-Wagner T, Strauss T, Rubinshtein M et al (2011) Point of care testing in children undergoing cardiopulmonary bypass. Pediatr Blood Cancer 56:794–798
144. Hofer A, Kozek-Langenecker S, Schaden E, Panholzer M, Gombotz H (2011) Point-of-care assessment of platelet aggregation in paediatric open heart surgery. Br J Anaesth 107:587–592
145. Mujeeb Zubair M, Bailly DK, Lantz G (2015) Preoperative platelet dysfunction predicts blood product transfusion in children undergoing cardiac surgery. Interact Cardiovasc Thorac Surg 20:24–30
146. Ignjatovic V, Chandramouli A, Than J et al (2012) Plasmin generation and fibrinolysis in pediatric patients undergoing cardiopulmonary bypass surgery. Pediatr Cardiol 33:280–285
147. Williams GD, Bratton SL, Nielsen NJ, Ramamoorthy C (1988) Fibrinolysis in pediatric patients undergoing cardiopulmonary bypass. J Cardiothorac Vasc Anesth 12:633–638
148. Eaton MP (2008) Antifibrinolytic therapy in surgery for congenital heart disease. Anesth Analg 106:1087–1100
149. Niebler R, Gill JC, Brabant CP (2012) Thromboelastography in the assessment of bleeding following surgery for congenital heart disease. World J Pediatr Congenit Heart Surg 3:433–438
150. Faraoni D, Fenger-Eriksen C, Gillard S et al (2015) Evaluation of dynamic parameters of thrombus formation measured on whole blood using rotational thromboelastometry in children undergoing cardiac surgery: a descriptive study. Paediatr Anaesth 25:573–579
151. Romlin B, Wåhlander H, Synnergren M, Baghaei F, Jeppsson A (2013) Earlier detection of coagulopathy with thromboelastometry during pediatric cardiac surgery: a prospective observational study. Paediatr Anaesth 23:222–227
152. Romlin B, Wåhlander H, Berggren H et al (2011) Intraoperative thromboelastometry is associated with reduced transfusion prevalence in pediatric cardiac surgery. Anesth Analg 112:30–36

9 Clinical Management of Postpartum Hemorrhage

Vanessa Agostini, Maria Pia Rainaldi, Maria Grazia Frigo, Massimo Micaglio, and Agostino Brizzi

Postpartum hemorrhage (PPH) is the leading cause of severe maternal morbidity and mortality worldwide.

Its management is complex and requires timely interventions, skilled personnel, human, technological and financial resources, and well-organized maternity services. A treatment failure or near misses could be the results of misdiagnosis or a delay in diagnosis of the underestimation of the bleeding rate and of a lack of adequate education and training together with a deficiency in the organization.

This chapter focuses the attention on the hemostatic management of severe obstetric hemorrhage.

9.1 Definitions and Epidemiology

A satisfactory definition of PPH does not exist, but traditionally, primary PPH is defined as a blood loss of 500 mL or more from the genital tract within 24 h from the birth of a baby, and it can be minor (500–1000 mL), moderate (1000–2000 mL), or severe (more than 2000 mL). Massive PPH has been defined as a bleeding >2500 mL and is associated with significant morbidity such as hysterectomy and need for intensive care admission (http://www.healthcareimprovementscotland.org). The amount of blood loss is very difficult to clinically assess and is usually underestimated [1]. Other definitions of PPH are the following: a decline in hemoglobin of 4 g/dL or more, transfusion of at least 4 units of red blood cells, or the need for embolization or operative intervention.

A recent systematic review [2] has estimated a global prevalence of PPH to be 10.8 % and severe PPH to be 2.8 %.

It is well known that there is a regional variation of postpartum hemorrhage (≥500 mL) ranging from 7.2 % in Oceania to 25.1 % in Africa, while the prevalence of a blood loss equal or above 1000 mL is higher in Africa (5.1 %) and lower in Asia (1.9 %).

V. Agostini, MD (✉)
Transfusion Medicine Cesena/Forlì and Blood Establishment, Clinical Pathology Department-Cesena Azienda U.S.L Romagna, Romagna, Italy
e-mail: vani.agostini@gmail.com

M.P. Rainaldi, MD
Department of Obstetrics and Gynecology, Sant'Orsola Malpighi University Hospital, University of Bologna, Bologna, Italy

M.G. Frigo, MD
Obstetric Anesthesia, Fatebenefratelli Hospital Isola Tiberina Rome, Rome, Italy

M. Micaglio, MD
Department of Anesthesia and Intensive Care, Careggi University Hospital, Florence, Italy

A. Brizzi, MD
Department of Anesthesia and Intensive Care, Santa Maria Hospital, Bari, Italy

M. Ranucci, P. Simioni (eds.), *Point-of-Care Tests for Severe Hemorrhage: A Manual for Diagnosis and Treatment*, DOI 10.1007/978-3-319-24795-3_9

In developed countries such as Europe and North America, the prevalence is around 13 %, being higher for multiple pregnancies (32.4 % compared with 10.6 % for singletons) and for first-time mothers (12.9 % compared with 10.0 % for women in subsequent pregnancies). Furthermore there are some evidences of an increased incidence in PPH in Canada, the UK, Australia, and the USA between 2001 and 2006 related to a rise in obesity.

On the contrary it is possible that the lower prevalence of PPH in Asian women is related to regional differences in genetics or underlying risk factors such as a lower incidence of obesity in Asia.

9.2 The Pathogenesis of PHH

There are several causes of PPH, classified according to their underlying pathophysiology: tone (uterine atony), tissue (placenta accreta, percreta, increta, previa), trauma (laceration of cervix, vagina), and thrombin (congenital coagulation disorders). Uterine atony is the leading cause of massive obstetric hemorrhage, difficult to be predicted.

9.2.1 Pregnancy-Induced Coagulation Changes

It is important to highlight that at term the hemostatic system is unbalanced toward a prothrombotic state, due to an increase of procoagulant factors VII, VIII, IX, X, XII, von Willebrand, and fibrinogen. In particular the fibrinogen level is markedly increased, reaching 4–6 g/L compared with the nonpregnant normal range of 2–4 g/L. Prothrombin (FII) and factor V remain unchanged, while factor XI is somewhat reduced [3, 4]. On the other hand, there is a decrease of the natural anticoagulant protein S level. These changes are responsible for the shorter prothrombin time (PT) and activated partial thromboplastin time (aPTT) and for the increase of thromboelastometric parameters such as maximum amplitude (MA) and maximum clot firmness (MCF) [5].

Plasma fibrinolytic activity is reduced during pregnancy, remains low during labor, and increases at the time of delivery due to the reduction of the fibrinolytic inhibitors (PAI-1 and 2) and to the high levels of plasminogen tissue factor (t-PA).

Five different studies with different entry criteria demonstrated that low fibrinogen levels in the early stages of PPH have similar predictive values. In particular, a fibrinogen level <2 g/L is associated with progression to severe PPH.

Charbit and associates [6] showed that in women at the time of a second-line uterotonic for atony, a fibrinogen level <2 g/L had a positive predictive value (PPV) of 100 % for progression to severe PPH, while a level >4 g/L had a negative predictive value of 79 %.

Collins and associates [7] recently investigated the utility of FIBTEM A5 and Clauss fibrinogen as predictors of progression of PPH in a consecutive cohort of 356 women in a 1-year period (2012–2013), all experiencing a bleeding >1000 mL. Entry criteria were a bleeding of 1000–1499 plus cesarean section or uterine atony or placental abruption or placenta previa or microvascular bleeding or cardiovascular instability or any bleeding >1500 mL. Blood samples were collected before any administration of prohemostatic drugs or blood component therapy.

The primary outcome was to evaluate the utility of FIBTEM A5 and/or Clauss fibrinogen as predictors of progression to massive hemorrhage (>2500 mL). Other outcomes were transfusion of <4 or ≥ 4 units of red blood cells, transfusion <8 or ≥ 8 of any blood product (red blood cells, fresh frozen plasma, or platelets), need for an invasive procedure, bleeding duration, and length of stay in the high-dependency unit.

The positive predictive value for progression to any transfusion of a fibrinogen <2 g/L or FIBTEM A5 <10 mm was 75 and 71 %, respectively; these values reached 100 % in women with ongoing bleeding at study entry. For progression to massive PPH (>2500 mL) in the final multivariate analysis, only FIBTEM A5 was an independent predictor.

The median fibrinogen level of women transfused with ≥ 4 units RBCs was 2.6 g/L compared with 3.9 g/L for those not transfused.

During PPH, coagulopathies may develop secondary to the dilution related to volume replacement and to the loss and consumption of coagulation factors. All these factors lead to a fall in fibrinogen levels and platelet count and affect thrombin generation.

9.3 Coagulation Monitoring

To date there are mainly two different strategies to monitor coagulation changes during PPH: the first is based on standard laboratory tests (PT/aPTT and Clauss fibrinogen) and the second on point-of-care coagulation testing devices such as thromboelastometry/thromboelastography.

Despite the hemostatic derangement, standard coagulation tests (PT/aPTT) remain normal until the blood loss reaches 4000–5000 mL, while the fibrinogen levels fall earlier than the other coagulation factors [8]. Recent data show that a low Clauss fibrinogen (<2 g/L) and a reduced maximum amplitude at the ROTEM device are accurate biomarkers for the progression to severe PPH, and the recent ESA guidelines [9] recommend thromboelastometric measurements in order to identify the contribution of fibrinogen to clot strength.

Conventional coagulation tests typically require 45–60 min to be available; they are not adequate to diagnose hyperfibrinolysis, and their results may not influence the initial resuscitation although they are a useful baseline for later management of blood component therapy.

Viscoelastic tests such as rotational thromboelastometry or thromboelastography are dynamic tests which give information on the whole coagulation process from the initiation of clot formation through fibrinolysis. The major advantages of point-of-care testing are that the clinicians can rapidly identify if the bleeding has a coagulopathic or a surgical origin. Furthermore there is good evidence that the ROTEM FIBTEM A5 assay can be used as a surrogate for Clauss fibrinogen during PPH [7, 10, 11].

In a prospective observational study, Houissoud and associates [11] compared 51 women with PPH to a control group and demonstrated that in ROTEM, FIBTEM clotting amplitudes were lower in the PPH group in comparison with the control group. Furthermore a strong correlation between fibrinogen levels and the FIBTEM parameters was present in both groups. The Clauss fibrinogen threshold of 2 g/L corresponded to a FIBTEM A5 of 6 mm and to a FIBTEM A15 of 8 mm with a sensitivity of 100 % both and a specificity of 87 and 84 %, respectively. It is important to consider that thromboelastometry normal ranges at the time of delivery differ from the nonpregnant normal range. Armstrong and associates [12] studied ROTEM parameters from 60 healthy pregnant women presenting for elective cesarean section and 60 matched nonpregnant female controls presenting for elective surgery and demonstrated that pregnant women had significant lower INTEM CT, CFT, and EXTEM CFT ($p<0.001$) and higher MCF in INTEM, EXTEM, and FIBTEM ($p<0.001$) in comparison to the control nonpregnant group.

De Lange et al. [5] in a Dutch multicenter study reported ROTEM reference values after having collected blood samples from 161 women at two different times: time 1 during labor between 6 and 10 cm cervical dilatation or before elective cesarean section and time 2 within 1 h of delivery of the placenta. They found a shorter CT and CFT in EXTEM and INTEM and larger A10, A20, and MCF in INTEM and FIBTEM in pregnant women in comparison with reference values in nonpregnant adults. Parameters before and after labor were not different, and there was a strong correlation between ROTEM FIBTEM and fibrinogen concentration.

All these data are extremely important because of the increasing use of viscoelastic tests in postpartum hemorrhage management and in order to define specific triggers for hemostatic therapy in this setting.

9.4 The Hemostatic Management of PPH

Rapid diagnosis and early treatment of PPH are critical for a favorable patient outcome. It is well known that the underestimation of the speed and extent of hemorrhage, delay in blood transfusion, lack of treatment algorithm, lack of adequate education and training, poor communication, and deficiencies in organization [13] are responsible for failures in treatment.

The hemostatic management of PPH is challenging, and current guidelines rely on experience from the nonpregnant population and expert opinion.

Three different approaches are used to date for the management of PPH: a laboratory-driven approach, a formula-driven one, and, more recently, a goal-directed strategy based on viscoelastic coagulation monitoring.

9.4.1 Laboratory-Driven Strategy

This approach derived from the past guidelines [14–16] recommends to start red blood cell (RBC) transfusion as soon as possible together with warm crystalloid and colloid solutions for the volume replacement.

Fresh frozen plasma (FFP) should be used when the results of PT/aPTT are available and >1.5 × normal at the standard dose of 12–15 mL/kg or a total of 1 l every 6 units of RBC. Platelet concentrates (PLT) should be transfused if platelet count $<50\times10^9$/L and cryoprecipitated (2 pools) if fibrinogen level <1 g/L with the goal to keep:

- Hemoglobin >8 g/dl
- Platelet count $>75\times10^9$/L
- PT/aPTT <1.5 × normal control
- Fibrinogen >1 g/L

This kind of approach is now considered unsatisfactory especially in case of severe/massive PPH and in case of hemodynamically unstable patients, when there is no time to wait for the result of standard laboratory test.

9.4.2 The Formula-Driven Approach

In order to save time, most centers have recently adopted the strategy used for the management of trauma-induced coagulopathy based on the delivery of predefined "shock packs" (the so-called formula-driven approach).

This strategy, derived from trauma experiences, consists in the adoption of formulaic protocols based on the release of blood component therapy in fix ratio 1:1 RBC/FFP or 1:1:1 RBC/FFP/PLT, adding cryoprecipitate later on during resuscitation. A number of retrospective studies, in the last decade, have reported a correlation between earlier and higher FFP to RBC transfusion ratios and improved survival and outcomes. In comparison to traumatology data, fewer studies have been conducted in obstetric setting.

In 2007 Burtelow and associates [17] described the implementation of a massive transfusion protocol for life-threatening primary postpartum hemorrhage consisting in the release of 6 units of group 0 D-negative RBC, 4 units of FFP, and 1 apheresis unit of platelets (fixed ratio 6:4:1). This fixed pack allowed the blood bank to quickly release blood component therapy during the acute phase of resuscitation and the clinicians to anticipate and probably prevent dilutional coagulopathy. After the first pack (6:4:1), the protocol consisted in the release of other FFP, platelets, and cryoprecipitate units on the basis of the standard coagulation laboratory results. The same group in 2011 [18] analyzed the impact of their massive transfusion protocol (fix pack 6:4:1) on blood inventory and the wastage rates of blood components.

The rationale for a fixed ratio approach is to recapitulate whole blood and to maintain thrombin generation and fibrinogen concentration by the replacement of coagulation factors as soon as possible.

However recent data from trauma research demonstrated the inability of this strategy to maintain good levels of fibrinogen.

Moreover the major disadvantage of a formulaic unmonitored approach is the risk of an overtreatment of women with a normal coagulation profile at admission and a dilution effect on fibrinogen level, if it is considered that plasma derived from donors contains approximately 2 g/L of fibrinogen.

Early empirical transfusion of FFP might be justified in cases:

- Of consumption (e.g., amniotic fluid embolism)
- Of expected very large volumes of blood loss (placenta abnormalities, e.g., placenta accreta)
- Of hemodynamically instability

9.4.3 The Goal-Directed Approach

This strategy was started in German-speaking countries since 20 years ago, and it can be considered a tactical approach to the problem. It is based on the rapid differential diagnosis of coagulopathies through the use of viscoelastic coagulation monitoring devices (ROTEM, TEG) with the possibility to step by step treat the coagulation abnormality without using an empirical or formulaic approach, avoiding unnecessary blood component transfusions and using prohemostatic drugs such as antifibrinolytic agents, fibrinogen concentrate, and prothrombin complex concentrates.

Different algorithms were recently published from different groups.

Girard and associates in 2014 [19] proposed an algorithm from a German-speaking countries' (Austria, Germany, and Switzerland) working group of obstetricians, anesthesiologists, and hemostasis specialists.

The algorithm is based on four steps:

- Step 1 (no more than 30 min): recognize PPH, establish monitoring measures, identify the source of bleeding, and try to increase the uterine tone.
- Step 2 (no more than 30 min): is focused on the interdisciplinary management of obstetricians, anesthesiologists, and hemostasis specialists. During this step every effort should be done to anticipate the development of coagulopathy. Point-of-care coagulation monitoring (ROTEM or TEG) should be scheduled, and tranexamic acid (2g IV) and fibrinogen concentrate (2–4 g) should be administered; RBC, FFP, and platelet concentrates are requested.
- Step 3: the goal is to maintain hemodynamic stability and to stop bleeding.
- Step 4: if the bleeding persists, invasive measures are necessary such as interventional radiology procedures or surgery.

At any time it is mandatory to avoid acidosis, hypothermia, and hypocalcemia.

In 2014 Mallaiah and associates [20] published the results of a prospective study at the Liverpool Women's Hospital comparing the transfusion requirements and patient outcomes using the traditional "shock pack" containing 4 RBC units, 4 FFP units, and 1 adult dose of platelets versus a pack containing fibrinogen (fibrinogen phase) in place of FFP and platelets. The fibrinogen phase consisted in the administration of 3 g of fibrinogen concentrate if fibrinogen <1.5 g/L or as guided by ROTEM. The authors chose a conservative trigger for the administration of fibrinogen concentrate: FIBTEM A5 <7 mm indicative of a fibrinogen level of 1.5–2 g/L. The algorithm suggests to quickly reassess the response to treatment in order to administer more fibrinogen in case of persistence of FIBTEM abnormalities and patient still bleeding.

The results showed a reduction in transfused RBC, FFP, platelets, and cryoprecipitate and transfusion-associated cardiac overload. There was also a nonsignificant reduction in hysterectomy.

Carvalho and associates [21] for the Share Network Group, a multidisciplinary Portuguese group, published their algorithm for the management of coagulopathy during postpartum hemorrhage based on ROTEM monitoring. It is a vertical algorithm considering five steps: hyperfibrinolysis, fibrinogen deficiency, thrombocytopenia, deficiency in other coagulation factors, and lastly factor XIII deficiency.

In the Share Network Group algorithm, a trigger of fibrinogen <3–4 g/L or FIBTEM MCF <18 mm was chosen for fibrinogen concentrate supplementation.

Collis and associates [22] have recently published their pragmatic protocol for the management of postpartum hemorrhage in Cardiff using

ROTEM. The protocol is activated in case of bleeding of 1000 mL or more by the delivery suite staff. On activation, blood samples are taken together with a sample for a FIBTEM assay, and fibrinogen concentrate is infused if FIBTEM <7 mm.

9.5 Pharmacologic Treatment of PPH

All the above algorithms for the management of postpartum hemorrhage include the utilization of a pharmacological approach.

In fact in recent years there has been an increasing and renewed interest in antifibrinolytic therapy (tranexamic acid, TA) and fibrinogen supplementation, mainly after trauma studies.

9.5.1 Tranexamic Acid

The new interest in fibrinolysis during bleeding and in antifibrinolytic therapy in reducing bleeding derives from the large randomized control trial CRASH-2, published in 2010 [23]. This study included more than 20,000 adult trauma patients received empirically TA and demonstrated a reduction in all-cause mortality (14.5 % vs 16 %, relative risk: 0.91, 95 % CI:0.85–0.97, $p=0.0035$) as well as mortality due to hemorrhage (4.9 % vs 5.7 %) in the TA group, without a significant increase in thromboembolic complications.

The role of TA in postpartum hemorrhage is not well established although a Cochrane systematic review [24] established that TA reduces postpartum blood loss after vaginal delivery and cesarean section.

Current guidelines on postpartum hemorrhage recognize a role of tranexamic acid in control of bleeding.

The Royal College of Obstetricians and Gynecologists guidelines [14] confirm that "there is a consensus that fibrinolytic inhibitors (such as tranexamic acid) seldom, if ever, have a place in the management of obstetric hemorrhage."

The ESA guidelines "recommend the administration of tranexamic acid in obstetric bleeding to reduce the blood loss, bleeding duration and the number of units transfused" (level 1B) [9]. The World Health Organization (WHO) guidelines [25] recognize a role of tranexamic acid in uterine atony in case of failure to control bleeding of uterotonics, and NICE guidelines (2007) [26] consider tranexamic acid an additional option.

There are several prospective randomized trials demonstrating a small and not clinically significant reduction in estimated blood loss obtained by prophylactic administration of TA before elective cesarean section or routine vaginal delivery [27–31].

A controlled, multicentered, open-label trial, published in 2011 [32], randomized women experiencing a blood loss >800 mL following vaginal delivery to receive TA loading dose 4 g over 1 h and a maintenance dose of 1 g/h over 6 h (TA group) versus no antifibrinolytic treatment (control group). The primary end point was to verify the efficacy of TA in the reduction of blood loss, while secondary end points were to assess the efficacy of TA on duration of bleeding, anemia, need for invasive procedures (surgery and interventional radiology), and need for transfusions.

The high dose of TA was mutated from studies in high-risk cardiac surgery [33, 34].

A total of 144 women completed the study protocol.

The evaluation of blood loss was scheduled at four time points: at inclusion (T1), after 30 mins (T2), after 2 h from T2 (T3), and after 6 h from inclusion (T4).

The blood loss between T1 and T4 was lower in the TA group (median 170 mL, interquartile range 58 mL to 323 mL) compared to the control group (median 221 mL, interquartile range 110–543 mL) ($p=0.041$). The duration of bleeding was also lower in the TA group ($p=0.004$), and bleeding was stopped in 63 % of patients in TA group by T2 in comparison to 46 % in the control group.

Furthermore there was a reduction in severe PPH progression, hemoglobin drop >4 g/dL, and number of RBC units transfused throughout day 42.

The study has some limitations: firstly it is unblinded, secondly it was not designed to evaluate the reduction in maternal death, and lastly it was not powered to evaluate thromboembolic complications although an increase in thrombosis in the treatment group was not observed.

The pragmatic, randomized, double-blinded placebo-controlled WOMAN trial [35] is ongoing with the aim to evaluate the role of TA in early PPH in reducing death, hysterectomy, and other morbidities (surgical intervention, blood transfusion, and risk of nonfatal vascular event) (www.thewomantrial.lshtm.ac.uk accessed 05/01/2015).

Finally, a systematic review and meta-analysis on prophylactic tranexamic acid in women at low risk for postpartum hemorrhage have been recently published [36]. It included seven studies [29–31, 37–40] on 1760 patients at low risk for PPH (excluded women with multiple gestations or preterm deliveries), of which six reported on cesarean sections under spinal anesthesia and one on vaginal delivery.

The dosages of TA used were different in the studies analyzed, ranging from 1 g to 15 mg/kg. The analysis found that TA reduced blood loss (weighted mean difference: −140 mL, 95 % CI −189 to −91 mL; $p<0.00001$) and the risk for blood transfusion (RR 0.34, 95 % CI 0.20–0.60). However data on the incidence of blood transfusion must be confirmed in further studies because the transfusion policy was described only in one study; additionally, there were wide differences in the transfusion rate in the placebo group (between 1.4 and 33 %). The study also demonstrated that TA did not increase the rate of thrombosis.

9.5.2 Fibrinogen Supplementation

Recent studies demonstrated a correlation between severe PPH and hypofibrinogenemia [6, 8, 41–43] and the role of fibrinogen level as good biomarker of PPH progression. These evidences opened the possibility for a potential therapeutic role of fibrinogen administration to correct the acquired hypofibrinogenemia.

Three main sources are available for fibrinogen supplementation: FFP, cryoprecipitate, and fibrinogen concentrates, with FFP containing lesser amount of fibrinogen in comparison with the other two products.

With respect to cryoprecipitate, fibrinogen concentrate has the advantage of being pathogen reduced, of containing a more standardized dose of fibrinogen, and of being used as an infusion over 10–15 min without thawing.

To date there are no randomized control trials comparing the efficacy of cryoprecipitate and fibrinogen concentrates for the management of hypofibrinogenemia during PPH.

Ahmed and associates (2012) [44] reported a prospective audit on 21,614 women during a 2.5-year period, identifying 77 cases of major obstetric hemorrhage, of which 34 developed hypofibrinogenemia (<2 g/L) and required treatment with cryoprecipitate ($n=14$) and fibrinogen concentrate ($n=20$).

Cryoprecipitate had been produced by the Irish Blood Transfusion Service and supplied in pools of five donor units. The minimum fibrinogen content was >700 mg/pool, and the mean fibrinogen content was 1470 mg/pool.

The mean dose of cryoprecipitate was 2.21 ± 0.35 pools, and the mean dose of fibrinogen concentrate was 4 ± 0.8 g.

Hypofibrinogenemia was corrected by both products; the fibrinogen level achieved with the two treatments was the same although the correlation between the level of increase and the dose administered was stronger for fibrinogen concentrate than for cryoprecipitate.

The study demonstrated the non-inferiority of fibrinogen concentrate compared to cryoprecipitate in correcting hypofibrinogenemia leading to the decision of the Irish Blood Transfusion Service to replace cryoprecipitate with fibrinogen concentrate.

A Japanese single-center study [45] reported the efficacy of fibrinogen concentrate in the management of 18 cases of massive postpartum hemorrhage, defined as bleeding >1000 mL, with hypofibrinogenemia (fibrinogen level <150 mg/

dL) due to consumption (placental abruption and amniotic fluid embolism) and dilution (uterine atony, uterine inversion, placenta previa, and vaginal trauma). The fibrinogen level increased approximately by 40 mg/dL, and the response rate was considered good (bleeding <1000 mL after drug administration and no interventional procedures required) or moderate (bleeding >1000 mL after drug infusion and no interventional procedures performed) in 88 % of dilution coagulopathy and 89 % in case of consumptive coagulopathy. The authors did not report serious adverse events related to fibrinogen concentrate infusion.

The FIB-PPH trial [46] is ongoing in Denmark with the aim to investigate if early fibrinogen concentrate supplementation reduces transfusions in PPH. The study is randomized, placebo controlled, and double blinded including patients experiencing blood loss after vaginal delivery. The patients are randomly assigned to receive 2 g of fibrinogen concentrate or placebo, and the primary end point is the reduction of allogeneic blood transfusion.

9.5.3 Recombinant Factor VIIa

Recombinant activated factor VII (rFVIIa, NovoSeven, Novo Nordisk A/S, Bagsvaerd, Denmark) is licensed for the treatment of hemorrhage in patients with congenital hemophilia A and B and who have developed inhibitors to factor VIII and IX, in patients with FVII deficiency, and in patients suffering Glanzmann's thrombasthenia with anti-GpIIb/IIIa.

Data on its use in the management of PPH are anecdotal or derived from national and international registries or from systematic review [47–50]. There are no dose-finding studies in obstetric hemorrhage, but there is a general agreement on a standard dose of 90 μg/kg.

To date rFVIIa is considered a rescue therapy in case of refractory PPH when all the other measures have failed and hemoglobin level is >8 g/dL, platelet count is $>70 \times 10^9$/L, fibrinogen level is >2 g/L, and the patient is not acidotic and hypothermic.

Conclusions

An optimal management of postpartum hemorrhage requires:

- A team-working approach
- The existence of transfusion protocols based on local organization in order to ensure the availability of blood products
- Point-of-care technologies, such as rotational thromboelastometry or thromboelastography, to obtain timely information on clot formation and lysis and to guide an early coagulation support

References

1. Stafford I, Dildy GA, Clark SL et al (2008) Visually estimated and calculated blood loss in vaginal and cesarean delivery. Am J Obstet Gynecol 199:519.e1–519.e7
2. Calvert C, Thomas SL, Ronsmans C et al (2012) Identifying regional variation in the prevalence of postpartum haemorrhage: a systematic review and meta-analysis. PLoS One 7:e 41114
3. Hellgren M (2003) Hemostasis during normal pregnancy and puerperium. Semin Thromb Hemost 29:125–130
4. O'Riordan MN, Higgins JR (2003) Haemostasis in normal and abnormal pregnancy. Best Pract Res Clin Obstet Gynaecol 17:385–396
5. De Lange NM, van Rheenen-Flach LE, Lancè MD et al (2014) Peri-partum reference ranges for ROTEM thromboelastometry. Br J Anaesth 112:852–859
6. Charbit B, Mandelbrot L, Samain E et al (2007) The decrease of fibrinogen is an early predictor of the severity of postpartum haemorrhage. J Thromb Haemost 5:266–273
7. Collins PW, Lilley G, Bruynseels D et al (2014) Fibrin-based clot formation an early and rapidly biomarker for progression of postpartum hemorrhage: a prospective study. Blood 124:1727–1736
8. de Lloyd L, Bovington R, Kaye A et al (2011) Standard haemostatic tests following major obstetric hemorrhage. Int J Obstet Anesth 20:135–141
9. Kozeck-Langenecker SA, Afshari A, Albalajedo P et al (2013) Management of perioperative bleeding. Guidelines from the European Society of Anesthesiology. Eur J Anaesthesiol 30:270–382
10. Solomon C, Collis RE, Collins PW (2012) Haemostatic monitoring during postpartum haemorrhage and implications for management. Br J Anaesth 109:851–853

11. Houissoud C, Carabin N, Audibert F et al (2009) Bedside assessment of fibrinogen level in postpartum haemorrhage by thromboelastometry. BJOG 116:1097–1102
12. Armstrong S, Fernando R, Ashpole K et al (2011) Assessment of coagulation in the obstetric population using ROTEM thromboelastometry. Int J Obstet Anesth 20:293–298
13. Upadhyay K, Scholefiel H (2008) Risk management and medico-legal issues related to postpartum hemorrhage. Best Pract Res Clin Obstet Gynaecol 75:875–882
14. Royal College of Obstetricians and Gynaecologists (2009) Prevention and management of postpartum hemorrhage. Green-top guideline No. 52. http://www.rcog.org.uk/files/rcog-corp/GT52postpartumHaemorrhage0411.pdf. Accessed 01 Jan 2015
15. Association of Anesthetist of Great Britain and Ireland (2010) Blood transfusion and the anesthetist: management of massive haemorrhage. Anaesthesia 65:1153–1161
16. British Committee for Standards in Haematology (2006) Guidelines on the management of massive blood loss. Br J Haematol 135:634–641
17. Burtelow M, Riley E, Druzin M et al (2007) How we treat: management of life-threatening primary postpartum hemorrhage with a standardized massive transfusion protocol. Transfusion 47:1564–1572
18. Goodnough LT, Daniels K, Wong AE et al (2011) How we treat: transfusion medicine support of obstetric services. Transfusion 51:2540–2548
19. Girard T, Morti M, Schlembach D (2014) New approaches to obstetric hemorrhage: the postpartum hemorrhage consensus algorithm. Curr Opin Anaesthesiol 27:267–274
20. Mallaiah S, Barclay P, Harrod I et al (2014) Introduction of an algorithm for ROTEM-guided fibrinogen concentrate administration in major obstetric haemorrhage. Anaesthesia. doi:10.1111/anae.12859
21. Carvalho M, Rodrigues A, Gomes M, et al (2014) Interventional algorithms for the control of coagulopathic bleedin in surgical, trauma and postpartum setting: recommendations from the Share Network Group. Clin Appl Thromb Hemost. 1–17 DOI: 101177/1076029614559773
22. Collis RE, Collins PW (2015) Haemostatic management of obstetric haemorrhage. Anaesthesia 70(Suppl 1):78–86
23. Shakur H, Roberts I, Bautista R et al (2010) Effects of tranexamic acid on death, vascular occlusive vents, and blood transfusion in trauma patients with significant hemorrhage (CRASH-2): a randomized, placebo-controlled trial. Lancet 376:23–32
24. Novikova N, Hofmeyer GL et al (2010) Tranexamic acid for preventing postpartum haemorrhage. Cochrane Database Syst Rev 7:CD007872
25. World Health Organization. WHO guidelines for the management of postpartum hemorrhage and retained placenta. http://apps.who.int/iris/bitstream/10665/75411/1/9789241548502
26. Kenyon S (2007) Intrapartum Care: Care of healthy women and their babies during childbirth. National institute for health and care excellence FVII in postpartum hemorrhage. Clin Obstet Gynecol 53:219–227
27. Gay MY, Wu LF, Su QF et al (2004) Clinical observation of blood loss reduced by tranexamic acid during and after cesarean section: a multi-center, randomized trial. Eur J Obstet Gynecol Reprod Biol 112:154–157
28. Sekhavat L, Tabatabaii A, Dalili M et al (2009) Efficacy of tranexamic acid in reducing blood loss after cesarean section. J Matern Fetal Neonatal Med 22:72–75
29. Movafegh A, Esalmian L, Dorabadi A (2011) Effect of intravenous tranexamic acid administration on blood loss during and after cesarean delivery. Int J Gynaecol Obstet 115:224–226
30. Gungorduk K, Yildirm G, Asicioglu O et al (2011) Efficacy of intravenous tranexamic acid in reducing blood loss after elective cesarean section: a prospective, randomized double-blind, placebo-controlled study. Am J Perinatol 28:233–240
31. Gungorduk K, Asicioglu O, Yildirim G et al (2013) Can intravenous injection of tranexamic acid be used in routine practice with active management of the third stage of labor in vaginal delivery? A randomized controlled study. Am J Perinatol 30:407–413
32. Ducloy-Bouthors AS, Jude B, Duhamel A et al; for The Exadeli Study Group (2011) High-dose tranexamic acid reduces blood loss in postpartum hemorrhage. Crit Care 15:R117
33. Karski JM, Teasdale SJ, Norman PH et al (1993) Prevention of post bypass bleeding with tranexamic acid and e-aminocaproic acid. J Cardiothorac Vasc Anesth 7:431–435
34. Karski JM, Teasdale SJ, Norman PH et al (1995) Prevention of bleeding after cardiopulmonary bypass with high-dose tranexamic acid: double-blind, randomized clinical trial. J Cardiothorac Vasc Anesth 110:835–842
35. Shakur H, Elbourne D, Gulmezoglu M et al (2010) The WOMAN trial (World Maternal Antifibrinolytic Trial): tranexamic acid for the treatment of postpartum hemorrhage: an international randomized, double blind placebo controlled trial. Trials 11:40
36. Heesen M, Bohmer J, Klohr S et al (2014) Prophylactic tranexamic acid in parturients at low risk for postpartum hemorrhage: systematic review and meta-analysis. Acta Anaesthesiol Scand 58:1075–1085
37. Senturk MB, Cakmak Y, Yildiz G et al (2013) Tranexamic acid for cesarean section: a double-blind, placebo-controlled, randomized clinical trial. Arch Gynecol Obstet 287:641–645
38. Shahid A, Khan A (2013) Tranexamic acid in decreasing blood loss during and after cesarean section. J Coll Physicians Surg Pak 23:459–462
39. Xu J, Gao W, Ju Y (2013) Tranexamic acid for the prevention of postpartum hemorrhage after cesarean

section: a double-blind randomized trial. Arch Gynecol Obstet 287:463–468
40. Goswani U, Sarangi S, Gupta S et al (2013) Comparative evaluation of two doses of tranexamic acid used prophylactically in anemic parturients for lower segment cesarean section: a double-blind randomized control prospective trial. Saudi J Anaesth 7:427–431
41. Cortet M, Deneux-Tgaraux C, Dupont C et al (2012) Association between fibrinogen level and severity of postpartum hemorrhage: secondary analysis of a prospective trial. Br J Anaesth 108:984–989
42. Butwick AJ (2013) Postpartum hemorrhage and low fibrinogen levels: the past, present and future. Int J Obstet Anesth 22:87–91
43. Levy JH, Welsby I, Goodnough LT (2014) Fibrinogen as a therapeutic target for bleeding: a review of critical levels and replacement therapy. Transfusion 54:389–405
44. Ahmed S, Harrity C, Johnson S et al (2012) The efficacy of fibrinogen concentrate compared with cryoprecipitate in major obstetric haemorrhage-an observational study. Transfus Med 22:344–349
45. Kikuchi M, Itakura A, Miki A et al (2013) Fibrinogen concentrate therapy for obstetric hemorrhage complicated by coagulopathy. J Obstet Gynecol Res 39:770–776
46. Wikkelsoe AJ, Afshari A, Stensballe J et al (2012) The FIB-PPH trial: fibrinogen concentrate as initial treatment for postpartum haemorrhage: study protocol for a randomised controlled trial. Trials 13:110
47. Barillari G, Frigo MG, Casarotto M et al (2009) Use of recombinant activated factor VII in massive postpartum hemorrhage: data from the Italian registry. A multi centric observational study. Thromb Res 124:e41–e47
48. Phillips LE, McLintock C, Pollock W et al (2009) Recombinant activated factor VII in obstetric hemorrhage: experiences from the Australian and New Zealand hemostasis registry. Anesth Analg 109:1908–1915
49. Franchini M, Franchi M, Bergamini V et al (2008) A critical review of the use of recombinant factor VIIa in life-threatening obstetric postpartum hemorrhage. Semin Thromb Hemost 34:104–112
50. Franchini M, Franchi M, Bergamini V et al (2010) The use of recombinant activated FVII in postpartum haemorrhage. Clin Obstet Gynecol 53:219–227

Management of Severe Bleeding in Liver Disease and Transplantation

10

Lesley De Pietri, Andrea De Gasperi, Paolo Feltracco, Gianni Biancofiore, Marco Senzolo, and David Sacerdoti

10.1 Hemostasis in Chronic Liver Disease

The liver plays key roles in blood coagulation being involved in both primary and secondary hemostasis [1]. It is the site of synthesis of most coagulation factors and their inhibitors except for von Willebrand factor (vWf) [2]. Liver failure is accompanied by multiple changes in the hemostatic system, because of reduced plasma levels of procoagulative and anticoagulative clotting factors synthesized by the intact liver [3]. The hemostatic system is then in a delicate balance between prothrombotic and antithrombotic processes, the final aim being to prevent both excessive blood loss from injured vessels and spontaneous thrombosis. In case of liver failure, there is a reduced capacity to clear both activated hemostatic proteins and protein inhibitor complexes from the circulation. Since the global effect of liver disease on the hemostatic system is complex, patients with end-stage liver disease (ESLD) can experience severe bleeding or, at the opposite, thrombotic complications. Finally, together with marked portal hypertension with secondary splenomegaly, thrombocytopenia develops. Decreased platelet function could be counteracted by the concomitant increase level of vWf. This delicate hemostatic balance can be easily tip towards bleeding or thrombosis by superimposed conditions such as infections.

While in classical coagulation disorders such as hemophilia A or B, or von Willebrand disease, a specific coagulation factor (namely, factor VIII, factor IX, or von Willebrand factor, respectively) is missing or defective, making bleeding predictable based on the absent factor; cirrhosis represents a far more complex scenario, where multiple aspects of hemostasis are deeply altered, making the prediction of bleeding much more challenging.

L. De Pietri, MD (✉)
Division of Anaesthesiology and Intensive Care Unit, Azienda Ospedaliero-Universitaria di Modena-Policlinico, Modena, Italy
e-mail: lesley.depietri@yahoo.it

A. De Gasperi, MD
2nd Service Anesthesia Critical Care Medicine, Ospedale Niguarda Ca' Granda, Milan, Italy

P. Feltracco, MD
Department of Medicine, Anesthesia and Intensive Care Unit, Padova University Hospital, Padova, Italy

G. Biancofiore, MD
Liver Transplant Anaesthesia and Critical Care, Azienda Ospedaliera Universitaria Pisana, Pisa, Italy

M. Senzolo, MD
Multivisceral Transplant Unit, Gastroenterology, Department of Surgery, Oncology and Gastroenterology, Padua University Hospital, Padua, Italy

D. Sacerdoti, MD, PhD
Department of Medicine, 5th Chair of Internal Medicine, University of Padua Medical School, Padua, Italy

M. Ranucci, P. Simioni (eds.), *Point-of-Care Tests for Severe Hemorrhage: A Manual for Diagnosis and Treatment*, DOI 10.1007/978-3-319-24795-3_10

Progressive worsening of the ESLD is characterized by varying degrees of alterations of the different hemostatic components, but in general, cirrhosis entails modifications both in the pro-thrombotic and the pro-hemorrhagic components.

Although it is becoming clear that standard hemostatic tests (SHT) are inadequate to evaluate the so-called rebalanced hemostatic profile of the cirrhotic patient and are poor predictors of bleeding, they are still widespread used and may provide misleading information regarding the risk of bleeding: in particular, clinicians have to be aware that unneeded, useless, or even dangerous pro-hemostatic factors might be administered with no demonstrated benefit.

Thrombocytopenia is very frequent (77 % in compensated cirrhosis, even higher in more advanced stages of cirrhosis) [4] ranking first among the altered hematological tests [5]. Thrombocytopenia is probably due to the combination of decreased hepatic thrombopoietin synthesis [6, 7], splenic pooling/sequestration and destruction due to hypersplenism [8]; relative bone marrow suppression [9, 10], according to the available literature, is a predictor of mortality in cirrhosis [11]. Moreover, platelet adherence to the subendothelium of an injured vessel is altered, sharing similarities with the uremic thrombocitopathy [12].

Von Willebrand factor is elevated and ADAMTS-13 (the protease that cleaves von Willebrand factor) instead decreased, counterbalancing/compensating in some way the thrombocytopenia [13, 14]. Bleeding time (much less used now) is regarded as the global test for primary hemostasis: it is prolonged in up to 40 % of cirrhotic patients; the longer the time, the greater the severity of liver disease. When tested in Child-Pugh C patients, it shows an inverse (significant) correlation both with platelet count and with fibrinogen levels [15].

Reflecting the impaired synthetic function of the liver, proteins involved in coagulation are diminished in plasma. Reduced levels of procoagulant factors like factors V, VII, IX, X, XI, and XIII, as well as fibrinogen and prothrombin, are offset by elevated levels of procoagulant factor VIII and reduced levels of the anticoagulants antithrombin, protein C, protein S, and tissue factor pathway inhibitor [16]. In vitro thrombin generation is maintained or even increased in patients with cirrhosis and platelet counts >75 × 10³/dL, because of the above-cited simultaneous decrease in coagulation inhibitors (protein C, protein S, and antithrombin) and increased procoagulant factor VIII.

Fibrinolysis is also altered two-sidedly: elevated levels of plasminogen activator (tPA), decreased levels of thrombin-activated fibrinolysis inhibitor (TAFI), and low levels of plasmin inhibitors are balanced by reduced levels of plasminogen and high levels of plasminogen activator inhibitor (PAI) [17, 18]. Aside from a delayed conversion of fibrinogen to the fibrin clot under the influence of thrombin, the occurrence of abnormal fibrin polymerization in ESLD, characterized by an acceleration of fibrinolysis and prolonged presence of cross-linked fibrin degradation products, is frequent [19–22]. However, whether fibrinolytic activation is primary or secondary in response to disseminated intravascular coagulation is still controversial [23]. The role that these abnormalities play in the clinical risk of bleeding is still unclear.

10.2 Bleeding during Invasive Procedures

Bleeding risk associated with invasive procedures in patients with cirrhosis, albeit small, is significant [24]. The most frequent procedures performed in patients with cirrhosis include paracentesis, liver biopsy, and dental extraction. Traditionally, platelet count and prothrombin time (PT) international normalized ratio (INR) have been used to evaluate the bleeding risk during invasive procedures and surgery. Although PT/INR correlates with severity of liver disease and is usually considered a prognostic indicator in this regard, the usefulness of INR in assessing the bleeding risk in patients with cirrhosis is limited [25–27]. Thrombocytopenia, present in nearly half of the advanced cirrhotic patients [2], seems to be the major determinant of procedural bleeding: a threshold between 50 and 75 × 10³/dL [28] is significantly associated with a negative outcome. Patients with platelet count above this limit are generally not at risk for bleeding during minor invasive procedures. Instead, platelet transfusion prior to more invasive procedures (liver biopsy) or in case of bleeding is frequent in patients with platelet counts below this threshold [29]. In vitro studies on platelet-rich plasma from patients with cirrhosis demonstrated that platelet count of 60×10^3/dL is sufficient to sustain normal thrombin generation [30].

Patients with severe thrombocytopenia ($<75 \times 10^3$/dL) who require invasive procedures are at higher risk of bleeding. In a series of 121 candidates to OLT undergoing nonsurgical invasive procedures (e.g., endoscopic variceal ligation, transcatheter arterial chemoembolization, transjugular intrahepatic portosystemic shunt, dental extraction, large volume paracentesis, endoscopic polypectomy radiofrequency thermal ablation (RFTA), thyroid biopsy, endoscopic gastric biopsies, and liver biopsies), procedure-related bleeding events occurred significantly more frequently in patients with platelet count $<75 \times 10^3$/dL [28]. Bleeding-related deaths or surgical interventions to correct bleeding were not reported. Notably, "significant coagulopathy" (defined as INR >1.5) was similar in patients who bled (30 %) and those who did not (35 %) [31]. In the same study, severe thrombocytopenia and MELD and Child-Pugh scores and other biochemical, hematological, or clinical variables were not predictive of bleeding. Even uremia, without abnormal creatinine, was not associated with bleeding risk.

Major bleeding episodes after paracentesis are reported in two landmark studies. Platelet count below 50×10^3/dL and a therapeutic (vs. diagnostic) procedure were the only two factors significantly associated at univariate analysis with major complications (bleeding, small bowel perforation, and secondary bacterial peritonitis) in the first study [32]. In the second [33] during a 10-year period, the occurrence of severe hemorrhage was recorded in 0.19 % of all procedures, with a death rate of 0.016 %. Interestingly, bleeding was unrelated to operator experience, elevated INR, or thrombocytopenia but rather occurred in patients with high Child-Pugh and MELD scores, underscoring the impact of multiple factors (including the disease severity) on bleeding. The lack of correlation between INR, platelet count, and bleeding complications in paracentesis performed in cirrhotic patients was also reported by other authors [34]. Data from an evidence-based review demonstrate that altered parameters (including prolonged PT/INR and platelet count $<50 \times 10^3$/dL) do not predict bleeding, particularly in case of central vein cannulation [35]. A prospective study analyzing complications following central venous cannulation in patients with acute or chronic liver disease (with an INR ranging from 2.4 to 2.7 and median platelet count of $81–83 \times 10^3$/dL) documented 1 major bleeding event (related to accidental subclavian arterial puncture) out of 638 procedures [36]. Superficial hematoma formation was significantly and independently associated with a high INR and low platelet count, while oozing from the puncture site was associated with low platelet count and local heparin therapy.

Liver biopsy is a common procedure in patients with cirrhosis: bleeding complications are reported in 0.35–0.5 %, with a mortality rate of 0.1 % [37]. Bleeding risk after laparoscopic liver biopsy is not correlated with standard coagulation factors but rather with local factors including elasticity of the hepatic tissue. Notwithstanding INR and platelet count are still considered key to assess the bleeding risk during percutaneous liver biopsy [38, 39]. Experts' opinion suggests keeping platelet count above 50×10^3/dL to safely perform a liver biopsy to avoid a major bleeding risk [38–40]. In spite of being considered useful in predicting bleeding risk before a planned liver biopsies, bleeding time in the actual clinical practice is not routinely performed, being cumbersome, partly reflecting platelet count, and of unclear value in predicting bleeding.

10.3 Bleeding Risk Associated with Surgery

In cirrhotic patients, outcomes of major surgery, which are largely dependent upon the severity of portal hypertension, are best predicted by the

Child-Pugh score [41–43]: postoperative complications are more frequent than in the general population and include renal failure, bleeding, postoperative ascites, and infection [44–46]. However, there are no large prospective studies able to predict the bleeding risk (mainly but not exclusively from the surgical site or the GE tract) which can seriously affect morbidity and mortality [47]. As a matter of fact, in cirrhotic patients undergoing surgery, increased morbidity and mortality [48, 49] are associated with increased bleeding in 60 % of cases [50, 51]. Another author states that prolonged PT (>1.5 s and >2.5 s) was associated with 47 and 87 % mortality, respectively [52], while platelet count below 50×10^3/dL correlated with an increased risk of bleeding during surgery. Severity of liver disease itself is another predictor of bleeding associated with surgery in cirrhosis patients: recently, the severity of liver disease has been shown to correlate with the risk of bleeding complications during brain surgery, mortality rate reaching 63 % in Child C patients [53].

In a study dealing with outcomes of open heart surgery (both emergency and elective surgery) in 24 cirrhotic patients, a large part of the postoperative complications were related to bleeding: mediastinal bleeding occurred in 25 % of patients, while cardiac tamponade occurred in 17 %. Moreover, the principal causes of death in Child B patients (4/6) were hemorrhage and infection, while the cause of death in Child A and C patients (1/17 and 1/17, respectively) was infection. In this study, platelet count was not different in survivors versus nonsurvivors, and other parameters related to coagulation and hemostasis were not explored in relation to survival or to frequency of complications [54]. In another study reporting on outcomes of 12 cirrhotic patients (6 Child A and 6 Child B) who underwent open heart surgery, major complications (including hemorrhage and hepatic decompensation) were associated with platelet count, and mortality (5/12) was associated with bleeding complications in three cases [55]. In another study, Hayashida and associates, reporting on open heart surgery in cirrhotic patients, found infection complications in 33 % and major bleeding in 17 % of patients [56]. INR does not predict catheterization-related bleeding complications, as was shown in one study in which, however, no patient had an INR greater than 2.35 [57].

Under physiological conditions, the hemostatic system in patients with cirrhosis reaches a new equilibrium, determined by a parallel decline of the pro- and anticoagulants factors, but this balance is not as stable as that present in healthy persons, who have an excess of both procoagulants and anticoagulants: the actual definition of this condition is "rebalanced hemostasis,"a new concept recently introduced by Tripodi, Mannucci, and Lisman [26, 58].

The fact that ESLD patients, in spite of the elevated INR and the sometimes very severe thrombocytopenia, rarely bleed outside of the consequences of portal hypertension should be attributed to the parallel reduction of procoagulant and anticoagulant factors realizing the abovementioned "rebalanced hemostasis."

The acquisition of this new concept has allowed therefore overcoming the assumption that patients with ESLD have a natural bleeding tendency ("naturally anticoagulated") and has introduced new knowledge with regard to the management of hemostasis. These new concepts discourage prophylactic transfusion of blood products prior to invasive procedures and underline the unreliability of laboratory routine tests in predicting the risk of bleeding. As very recently reported by van Veen and associates [59] and Weeder and associates [60], bleeding tendency is not predicted by the extent of the alterations of both PT and INR neither in medical nor in surgical setting. On the contrary, global coagulation assays, such as thrombin generation and more global techniques based on whole blood, such as thromboelastometry/graphy (ROTEM or TEG), may be used to assess and manage the hemostasis in cirrhotic patients [26, 60]. This new viscoelastic testing such as thromboelastometry/graphy seems to be the best method to reflect the interaction between plasmatic and cellular components of hemostasis [61]. Moreover, these methods can also be used for the reliable and fast detection of hyperfibrinolysis and hypofibrinogenemia [62–64]. Fibrinogen levels vary greatly among cirrhotic patients. The Clauss method is currently considered the gold standard for determination of fibrinogen, but it can be affected by multiple factors. The infusion of colloidal solutions (starch and gelatins) and the administration of direct thrombin inhibitors may alter the results of this test, making it less reliable [65, 66]. Since the early clinical experiences of human orthotopic liver transplantation (OLT), it was clear that an already impaired hemostatic system was further stressed by complex and multiple changes occurring during the various phases of the transplant procedure [67] and still now OLT can be accompanied by severe bleeding [68–70]. As the coagulation balance in the cirrhotic is unstable, the early recognition of the cause of the severe bleeding (technical, surgical, not surgical/medical) is important in order to start an appropriate and timely intervention.

10.4 Severe Bleeding in Liver Transplant (OLT): An Open Problem

Liver transplantation is actually the treatment of choice for patients with acute or ESLD not responding to medical treatment. Since the late 1963 when the first recipients of liver allografts transplanted by Thomas E. Starzl died mainly by uncontrolled bleeding, great progresses have been made in surgical and anesthesia techniques and in bleeding management: in spite of that, liver transplantation can be associated with catastrophic and life-threatening hemorrhagic complications as yet. Major blood losses are a consequence of pre-existing hemostatic abnormalities, previous abdominal surgery, portal hypertension with multiple collateral vessels, portal vein thrombosis, and poor functional recovery of the new liver. Even if important both for research purposes and to define strategies to manage bleeding and transfusion in clinical practice, an accepted common definition of perioperative massive bleeding/massive transfusion in this setting is still lacking.

In trauma setting, massive blood transfusion (MBT) is the transfusion of 10 or more red blood cell (RBC) units within a period of 24 h [71, 72] even if several other definitions are available, due to the arbitrary definition of the length of the period during which acute blood loss and resuscitation occur.

Other definitions of massive bleeding used in other settings are the following:

- Loss of 100 % of blood volume within 24 h [73, 74]
- Loss of 50 % of blood volume within 3 h [73, 74]
- A rate of blood loss of 150 mL/min [74]

Same concerns are present in the liver transplant setting. MBT is still defined as the transfusion of >6 units of packed RBC within the first 24 h of surgery [75] even if more practical could be to limit the definition to a period ranging from bleeding due to injury to control of hemorrhage [76]. The most recent and convincing definition of MBT in the perioperative period of OLT, defined as the first 48 h after the first cut, has been proposed by Reichert and associates [77] according to the clinical outcome (significantly worse patient survival and significantly worse dialysis-free survival). In this definition, the cutoff values for massive transfusion are packed red blood cells (PRCs) >17.5 units, fresh frozen plasma (FFP) >12.5 units, and platelets >1.5 unit (not specified if pooled or from apheresis). This definition includes both the timespan (48 h since the first cut) and the transfusion needs.

Beside MBT definition, in OLT, it is crucial to identify any perioperative condition that might facilitate a possible severe bleeding during the transplant. In general, the prediction of bleeding during OLT is based on the severity of liver disease, preoperative coagulation function (under discussion, see below), recipient's clinical status (mainly nutritional status, very recently assessed with the psoas diameter), quality of the donor liver, and experience of the transplantation team: contributing factors to blood loss during OLT can be categorized as *preoperative* and *intraoperative*.

10.4.1 Preoperative Factors Contributing to Bleeding [78]

There are several preoperative important variables affecting transfusion requirements during OLT:

1. Baseline platelet count [79], preoperative hematocrit value, baseline hemoglobin value [80].
2. Severity of disease (MELD, Child-Turcotte-Pugh score, United Network for Organ Sharing priority for transplantation) [81]. On the contrary, coagulation parameters at the time of surgery (preoperative prothrombin time, activated partial thromboplastin time) do not predict the risk of bleeding in OLT candidates [78, 82].
3. Hyperdynamic circulation and the portal hypertension [83].
4. The type of liver disease (primary biliary cirrhosis, primary sclerotizing cholangitis, and fatty liver disease, characterized by a procoagulant imbalance) [84, 85].
5. Quality of the donor liver (ischemia time, the use of a partial liver graft, the use of extended criteria donors).
6. Experience of the surgical and anesthetic transplantation team [86].
7. The length of cold ischemia time and poor graft preservation have also been associated with short-term graft dysfunction and negative effects on perioperative red blood cell (RBC) [75, 86].

10.4.2 Intraoperative Factors Contributing to Bleeding [78]

Complex coagulation disorders may occur during liver transplantation and can derive from:

1. Possible platelet and coagulation factors consumption. Platelets are implicated in reperfusion injury in the ischemic liver [87]. Adhesion to the sinusoidal endothelium with a concomitant increase of vWf expression in the reperfused liver is one of the main deleterious effects of cold preservation of liver allografts, amplifying the reperfusion injury independently of their procoagulant properties and contributing to their decrease in number [88].
2. Hemodilution and reduction of coagulation factor synthesis and clearance (anhepatic phase). Visceral congestion may play a relevant role in bleeding during the anhepatic phase.
3. Fibrinolysis: bleeding is greatly potentiated by the activation of the fibrinolytic system, which occurs both during the anhepatic and reperfusion phases. During the anhepatic and reperfusion phases, circulating levels of t-PA are increased respectively for PAI-1 level reduction and for tPA release from the reperfused graft [68]. The fibrinolytic process may fade spontaneously within hours of reperfusion in a well-functioning allograft or may have a more protracted course associated with marginal functional recovery [89, 90]. In the liver transplant settings, hyperfibrinolysis may occur in up to 60–70 % of the cases, a third of which are self-limiting without antifibrinolytic treatment [58, 91].
4. Surgical technical problems during hepatic dissection and vascular anastomoses.
5. The release of exogenous heparin from the harvested graft after donor heparinization or endogenous heparin-like substances from the damaged ischemic graft endothelium may also play a role in the coagulopathy at reperfusion [92]. Even if the heparin-like effect (HLE) is detected in many liver transplant patients both before and after reperfusion of the donor graft, it is still a matter of debate whether HLE contributes to bleeding during OLT and requires to be treated [84, 91, 93].
6. Acidosis, hypothermia, hypocalcemia, and citrate toxicity.

Transplantation of an optimal graft restores the patient's clotting function, while a dysfunctional graft leads to a prolonged coagulopathy usually associated with and increase transfusion requirement [82]. Given the poor predictive value of a single preoperative variable even in a homogeneous population, some authors recommend a center-oriented transfusion practice to identify the center-specific risk factors and patients at high risk for perioperative blood losses [94].

10.5 Transfusion Practice during OLT: Intraoperative Blood and Blood Component Management with Viscoelastic Tests (TEG/ROTEM)

SHT such as prothrombin time (PT/INR), activated partial thromboplastin time (aPTT), fibrinogen level, and D-dimer have long been the standard laboratory indicators of patients' coagulation status. According to the cell-based model of hemostasis, these tests do not take into account the important interactions between platelets, clotting factors, and other cellular components in the generation of thrombin nor the balance between coagulation and fibrinolysis. Because of the limits of conventional coagulation tests in recognizing significant coagulopathies or guiding transfusion, in recent years, the viscoelastic tests (VET) have gained increasing importance. A more dynamic and targeted approach to the overall hemostatic process is at the base of their success providing a visual information on fibrinolysis and tendency to hypercoagulability: these characteristics make these tests ideal for a rapid diagnosis of the type of coagulopathy and for an appropriate (and rationale) choice of the therapeutic option.

A recent review of Yeung and associates [95], including the original and major review articles related to the use of VET in different surgical settings including trauma, cardiac surgery, and liver transplantation, came to the conclusion that VET, as compared with conventional coagulation tests, are relevant for the detection of coagulopathy and are the only tests able to provide a rapid diagnosis of hyperfibrinolysis. Goal-directed administration of blood products based on the results of viscoelastic hemostatic assays was furthermore associated with reduction in allogeneic blood product transfusions in liver transplantation cases [95]. Similarly, Mallet and associates performed a systematic review of all relevant studies that used VET of coagulation in patients with liver disease: although many studies are observational and small sized, VET provide additional information compared to SHT in patients with liver disease and should be used to monitor coagulation changes and to guide hemostatic therapy during liver transplantation [96]. In another study analyzing 303 liver graft recipients, the use of operating room ROTEM resulted in better definition of coagulation changes and reliable indication of the need for FFP, prothrombin concentrate complex (PCC), and fibrinogen and platelet (PLT) requirements. Furthermore, the use of ROTEM during the OLT was able to reduce the postoperative mortality in polytransfused patients [97]. A Cochrane review which included all randomized clinical trials that were performed to compare various methods of decreasing blood loss and blood transfusion requirements during liver transplantation (1913 patients studied) concluded that VET may potentially reduce blood loss and transfusion requirements during liver transplantation [98].

These point-of-care devices, providing a rapid and reliable diagnostic test, are able to support the clinician in the differential diagnosis between surgical bleeding and coagulation alteration, to guide the therapeutic interventions in case of hyperfibrinolysis, thus contributing in the reduction of intraoperative blood loss and transfusion requirements [86, 99]. Since Kang's TEG-based algorithm, several other algorithms (TEG or ROTEM based) have been developed to guide intraoperative blood component transfusion during OLT [99–101]: recently, the European Society of Anesthesia (ESA) has recommended the use of perioperative coagulation monitoring using ROTEM/TEG for targeted management of coagulopathy. According to these guidelines, implementation of transfusion and coagulation management algorithms (based on ROTEM/TEG) can reduce transfusion-associated costs in trauma, cardiac surgery, and liver transplantation [102].

10.5.1 Red Blood Cell Transfusion

The decision to transfuse RBCs is still a matter of debate. General guidelines for patients with liver disease are not available so far, and several approaches have been proposed/reported by different centers. Erythrocytes contribute to hemostasis, influencing the biochemical and functional responsiveness of activated platelets, via the rheological effect on platelet margination and supporting thrombin generation [103]. RBCs release adenosine diphosphate, which promotes platelet aggregation and stimulates platelet synthesis of thromboxane-A2, a platelet activator, thus reducing platelet activation in anemia [104]. Theoretically, RBC transfusion is needed only when the hemoglobin concentration decreases to a level below which oxygen demand cannot be met. As a matter of fact in cirrhotic patients, RBC transfusion until the restitution of the whole blood volume may induce a rebound increase in portal pressure, able to precipitate portal hypertension-related bleeding. In this line, a restrictive strategy (transfusion only for Hb concentration below 7 g/dL) was safe in acute gastrointestinal bleeding [105]. In Jehovah's witnesses undergoing surgery, postoperative morbidity and mortality increased for each gram of Hb decrement only in cases where the hemoglobin concentration was less than 7 g/dL [106]. Massicotte and associates showed that phlebotomy prior to the anhepatic phase of OLT was effective in limiting blood losses, thus leading to a decreased transfusion rate [107].

In spite of multiple trials evaluating transfusion thresholds on patient outcome, the evidence in the literature is insufficient to define a transfusion trigger in surgical patients [108, 109].

In case of massive bleeding, ESA guidelines [102] recommend aggressive and timely stabilization of the cardiac preload throughout the surgery but insist against crystalloids or colloids overload. During active bleeding, the ESA guidelines suggest a hemoglobin concentration of 7–9 g/dL as a transfusion threshold, while in a recent prospective survey in the OLT setting, an extreme trigger for packed RBC transfusion was a hemoglobin level below 6 g/dL [110]. Probably, more than a fixed Hb threshold as a transfusion trigger, a combination of physiologic parameters able to describe the need for an increased oxygen-carrying capacity, is to be considered also in OLT. Repeated measurements of a combination of hematocrit/hemoglobin, serum lactate, and base deficit in order to monitor tissue perfusion, tissue oxygenation, and the dynamics of blood loss during acute bleeding are perhaps the parameters to be considered. In the liver transplant setting, serum lactate concentration and base deficit reflect not only global tissue perfusion and oxygenation during hemorrhagic shock but are also influenced by the ischemic injury to the graft during harvesting, the post-reperfusion acute acid load secondary to the visceral and pelvic congestion during the anhepatic phase, and the quality of functional recovery of the graft [111]. As stated by Niemann and Liu [68, 109], the peculiar context of OLT (possible acute blood loss and consequent hemodynamic instability) makes unlikely a strict standardization, as proposed for other clinical settings.

10.5.2 Fresh Frozen Plasma Transfusion

Along with RBCs, both PLT and FFP [112] transfusions have been associated with adverse outcomes.

Even if the standard indication for FFP administration is a clotting process improvement, every hemostatic intervention should be reserved for the bleeding patients and not just to correct laboratory results ("numbers") [113]. Many guidelines including the recent ESA ones recommend against pre-procedural correction with FFP in case of mild-to-moderate elevated INR [60, 96] and in not-bleeding patients when INR is ≤2. As conventional laboratory methods (PT/INR, aPTT) do not predict bleeding risk/complications in these patients [84, 114], the perioperative use of ROTEM/TEG (VET), as point-of-care coagulation monitors for a targeted and dynamic management of coagulopathies, is becoming a relevant alternative in patients with cirrhosis [102].

In the ESLD patients, FVIII and vWf blood levels are elevated (up to 200 % of the reference value) [13, 113]: aggressive efforts to normalize the coagulation profile with volumes of blood products as high as 30 mL/kg are probably not necessary due to a more than possible creation of a hypervolemic state, responsible for an increased portal pressure and bleeding risk. The use of VET-based algorithm has shown to reduce FFP use [115]: however, its administration remains the only valid option in all coagulopathies caused by factors V and XI and vWf deficiencies. Although an isolated decreased activity of coagulation factors V and XI down to 10–20 % does not compromise thrombin generation [116], these are the only factors replaced solely by FFP and not by coagulation factor concentrates [84]. During an ongoing massive bleeding, the activity of coagulation factors V, VIII, or XI may limit thrombin generation in patients treated exclusively with fibrinogen and PCC: these are the cases in which FFP should be administered at a dose of 15–30 mL/kg body weight [101, 117].

Currently, no consensus exists on the volume or rate of infusion of FFP required to prevent or treat intraoperative liver transplant persistent bleeding: in the common practice, volumes close to 10–15 mL/kg are usually administered. Because of the lack of universally shared guidelines, beside some center-specific indications, both the amount and timing of FFP administration during OLT are still guided by experienced clinical judgment or local practices: the assistance of VET is becoming the best alternative option to optimize and verify the efficacy of correction/supplementation.

10.6 TEG-/ROTEM-Guided Indication for FFP Transfusions and PCC Administration

The implementation of perioperative algorithms for coagulation management based on early goal-directed therapy with VET-guided supplementation of fibrinogen concentrate and PCC has been associated with a reduction in the transfusion requirements for FFP, RBC, and PLT as well as with a reduced incidence of massive transfusion [99, 115, 118, 119].

10.6.1 TEG-Based Indications

Recommendations for correction of TEG parameters are often not standardized across transplant centers and usually refer to kaolin-activated assay. Wang and associates suggest a FFP titration to provide an r-time of less than 10 min at kaolin-activated TEG assay [99]. The same authors in a more recent paper adopted a TEG-guided transfusion protocol using higher threshold values to start transfusions [120]:

2 units of FFP if the r-time was >15 min
1 unit of apheresis platelets if the MA was <40 mm
6 units of cryoprecipitate (6 pooled units) for an alpha angle <45°
Another transfusion algorithm (kaolin-activated TEG assay) proposed by Larsen [121] suggests to transfuse:
2 units of FFP or 10 mL/kg if $11 \geq R \leq 14$ min
4 units of FFP or 20 mL/kg if R >14 min

Although not standardized across transplant centers, recommendations to correct TEG parameters on native (without activators) TEG assays are often those suggested by Kang and associates. In the late 1980s, during OLT [100]:

2 units of plasma for an *r*-time >15 min.
10 units of platelets for a maximum amplitude <40 mm.
6 units of cryoprecipitate for an α-angle <40–45°.
Unfortunately, these indications refer to 1985. Compared to the abovementioned period, improvements in surgical techniques and anesthetic management led to a revision of the Kang's algorithm.

If TEG is performed on native blood, FFP is titrated to provide a reaction time of <40 min according to a single-center experience. The use of native blood allows to avoid the risk of alterations of the test results secondary to the addition of citrate and calcium, in particular of the *r*, *k*, and alpha angle parameters, as observed by Roche and Zambruni [122, 123]. Native blood avoids the possible alteration associated to kaolin as well. Kaolin, in fact, not only initiates the intrinsic coagulation pathway but has complex effects on platelets. It activates platelets by releasing platelet factor 3 [124] and can also affect the clot retraction mimicking the fibrinolysis pattern [125].

In case of long reaction time (r>40 min, native blood; r>15 min, kaolin), active bleeding, and circulatory overload, the administration of 25 IU/kg PCC is perhaps the best alternative to FFP.

10.6.2 ROTEM-Based Indications

An EXTEM clotting time of >80 s in a bleeding patient triggers PCC administration at a dose of 25 IU/kg. If patients continue to bleed after correction with factor concentrates and show signs of FV and/or FXI deficiency (indicated by prolonged INTEM clotting time, cutoff value of ≥240 s), FFP is administered at a dose of 15–20 mL/kg [101, 126].

All the ROTEM-based algorithms' apply a goal-directed strategy with a first-line administration of fibrinogen concentrate and prothrombin complex concentrate (PCC) instead of the use of FFP and PLT transfusion. FFP administration is indicated only after administration of PCC and fibrinogen concentrate, in case of MCF_{EXTEM} <35 mm and MCF_{FIBTEM}<6 mm [126].

10.6.3 The Effects of Heparin

TEG is extremely sensitive to heparin (both endogenous and exogenous), its effect being sometimes detected even prior to reperfusion. This is why during OLT, it is recommended to run a heparinase-modified TEG in parallel with the native TEG. This advice is even more important after reperfusion, when heparinase TEG or HEPTEM (heparinase-modified thromboelastometry) test is helpful to distinguish between a coagulation factor deficiency and a heparin-produced prolongation of the R or CT respectively. A significant heparin effect is not frequent using activated (Kaolin) TEG and INTEM (intrinsic ROTEM). Even if the HLE is detected in many liver transplanted patients both before and after reperfusion of the donor graft, its clinical significance still remains unclear. In case of HLE thromboelastographic tracing and active bleeding, an empirical dose of 50 mg of protamine is often administered if the decision to treat is made [86].

In accordance to recent clinical experiences and practice, it seems reasonable, before treating long r or CT with FFP or PCC, to consider the possibility of fibrinogen administration, which not only increases clot firmness but also shortens both parameters as described by Ranucci and associates [127] in the treatment of complex cardiac surgery.

10.7 Indications to Prothrombin Complex Concentrates (PCC) Administration TEG/ROTEM Guided

Transfusion of PRC, FFP, and PLTs has been shown to be associated with increased morbidity and mortality both in major liver surgery and transplantation [108]. With the diffusion of the thromboelastography/metry, newer hemostatic strategies based on a goal-directed therapy with fibrinogen and PCC have been developed.

These therapeutic strategies were effective in the bleeding management and in reducing transfusion requirements as well as safe, according to the low incidence of thrombotic or thromboembolic events in cardiovascular surgery and liver transplant setting [115, 128]. According to the most recent available literature, readdressing the OLT coagulation management from a FFP- and PLT-based strategy to a fibrinogen concentrate and PCC supplementation seems to be possible, well-tolerated, and not burdened by thrombotic complications. This offers the great advantage to manage coagulation imbalance without circulatory overload and worsening of portal hypertension. Studies on the impact on outcome and cost-effectiveness are ongoing.

10.7.1 TEG-Based Indications

According to a single-center experience, PCC are administered at a dosage of 25 IU/kg in case of (unfortunately still not well-defined) prolonged r-time when circulatory overload is to be avoided. Some authors suggest to check the antithrombin activity before administering PCC, to avoid thrombosis [129]. The recently marketed 4-factor PCC products are not reported to increase the occurrence of thrombosis and ischemic events in the OLT setting [126]. This result is in line with a recently published pharmacovigilance study showing that one marketed four-factor PCC is an effective hemostatic treatment without demonstrated risk of thrombosis [130].

10.7.2 ROTEM-Based Indications

A clinically relevant deficiency in vitamin K-dependent coagulation factors results in a prolongation of the coagulation time (CT) in EXTEM. In OLT setting, in case of a clinically relevant diffuse bleeding and a prolongation of the CT in EXTEM >80 s, 25 IU PCC per kg body weight (corresponding to 1 mL PCC per kg body v) administration is recommended [101, 115, 126, 131]. This strategy may avoid the risk of circulatory overload, acute lung injury, and infections, which can occur following a large amount of FFP administration [102].

10.8 Indications to TEG-/ROTEM-Guided Platelet (PLT) Transfusion

Although there is no consensus regarding the appropriate threshold for PLT transfusion, platelet concentrates are frequently administered during OLT to prevent or treat bleeding.

According to Pereboom and associates [88], patients and graft survivals were significantly reduced in patients who received PLTs transfusions when compared with those who did not. Acute lung injury and its major consequences were considered the main reason for the lower survival rate associated with the use of platelets [88]. Indeed, recent data clearly demonstrated that platelet transfusion during liver transplantation is associated with a significantly increased 1-year mortality (26 vs. 8 %) due to acute lung injury, independently from RBC transfusion [108]. In animal models of liver transplantation, studies have demonstrated that platelets are involved in the pathogenesis of reperfusion injury of the liver graft by inducing endothelial cell apoptosis [87].

In addition, platelet transfusions are associated to a risk of viral transmission, the potential for bacterial contamination especially for platelets stored at room temperature, and the risk of alloimmunization, graft-versus-host disease, and nonspecific immunosuppressive effects [108].

PLT transfusion should be avoided if a severe thrombocytopenia or platelet dysfunction is not associated to signs of clinically relevant bleeding [60, 84]. To decide if thrombocytopenia needs to be treated in OLT setting is a difficult task. It is a common experience that patients with a very low platelet level can show a dry surgical field. Therefore, a simple numeric cutoff value does not offer a real help.

The available evidence suggests that conventional laboratory tests (platelet count) are of little use in providing information on platelet function; TEG/ROTEM tracings may offer a help, even though both a dysfunctional and a functional platelet coagulation process may not be detected by VET methods when platelet count is significantly reduced [102].

In the liver transplant setting, the VET-based algorithms have shown to reduce platelet transfusions [115, 119].

10.8.1 TEG-Based Suggested Indications

Recommendations for correction of TEG parameters are often not standardized across transplant centers and commonly refer to kaolin-activated assay.

Wang and associates suggested to transfuse a single apheresis unit (corresponds to approximately 6–8 pooled units) of platelets when the maximum amplitude was less than 55 mm (kaolin-activated TEG assay) [99].

The same authors in a subsequent paper adopted a TEG-guided transfusion protocol using different threshold values to initiate transfusions:

Two units of FFP if the r-time was greater than 15 min and 1 unit of apheresis platelets if the MA was less than 40 mm and 6 units of cryoprecipitate (6 pooled units) for an alpha angle <45° [120]

Another transfusion algorithms proposed by Larsen [121] suggest to transfuse:

1 unit of apheresis platelets if MA is between 46 and 60 mm
2 units of apheresis platelets if MA is <46 mm (kaolin-activated TEG assay)

Although not standardized across transplantation centers, recommendations for correction of TEG parameters on native (without activators) TEG assay are often those suggested by Kang and associates [100] during OLT:

10 units (1 apheresis unit) of platelets for a maximum amplitude less than 40 mm, 2 units of plasma for an r-time longer than 15 min, and 6 units of cryoprecipitate for an α-angle less than 40°–45°

Unfortunately, these indications refer to 1985. Compared to this period very far in time, there have been numerous improvements in both the surgical and anesthetic management that led to a revision of the parameters to guide transfusions, originally proposed by Kang.

If TEG is performed on native blood, the available literature (but unfortunately without strong evidence) suggests to administer 1 unit of apheresis platelets if MA <30 mm.

Maximum amplitude (MA) reflects the contribution of fibrin and platelets to clot strength, approximately 80 % of the clot strength being related to platelet number and function. The functional fibrinogen (FF) assay (TEG) and FIBTEM (ROTEM) define the relative contribution of fibrinogen to clot strength. Hypofibrinogenemia (TEG or ROTEM) has to be ruled out before PLT transfusion. In case of contemporary reduction of MA and FF amplitude, the initial administration of fibrinogen concentrate, instead of PLT, might be the correct action. In presence of MA <30 mm (native blood without activator), a possible algorithm might be to run a FF-TEG test. In case of FFMA test >7 mm, the indication is to first transfuse PLT, while with FFFMa <7 mm fibrinogen correction is indicated (a single-center experiences). Should fibrinogen be unavailable, cryoprecipitate are to be transfused.

10.8.2 ROTEM-Based Indications

According to the ROTEM-guided transfusion protocol, 1 unit of apheresis platelets has to be transfused if EXTEM MCF is <35 mm and FIBTEM MCF >than 6 mm. On the contrary, in case of EXTEM and FIBTEM MCF values <35 and 6 mm, respectively, the administration of fibrinogen concentrate has to be considered, instead of PLTs [126].

As evident, both with TEM and ROTEM indications, fibrinogen supplementation has to be considered a priority to correct MA, when hypofibrinogenemia might be the most probable cause of reduced clot strength.

10.9 Indications to TEG-/ROTEM-Guided Fibrinogen and Cryoprecipitate Administration

Fibrinogen levels in cirrhotic patients are reduced, mainly due to a decreased synthesis and an increased turnover. The ESLD and the slow recovery of graft function after reperfusion make quite unlikely a spontaneous postoperative increase in fibrinogen blood levels. Several studies have shown that besides a decreased fibrinogen concentration, coagulation is also impaired by dysfibrinogenemia and disorders of fibrin polymerization due to fibrin-degrading products, increased circulating sialic acid, and/or infused artificial colloids [132, 133].

Because of its relatively high initial plasma concentration, fibrinogen is the first clotting factor to decrease to critically low levels in case of severe bleeding, while all other coagulation factors provide sufficient hemostatic power being as low as 30 % of their activity [134, 135]. Hypofibrinogenemia has a significant influence on blood product transfusions and is correlated to severe bleeding complications in cirrhotic patients.

There are three main approaches to fibrinogen supplementation: fresh frozen plasma, cryoprecipitate, or fibrinogen concentrate.

FFP contains approximately 2.0 g/L of fibrinogen: the great variability of fibrinogen concentrations between FFP units makes it difficult to predict the increase in patient plasma fibrinogen concentrations after transfusion.

Cryoprecipitate is a human plasma concentrate derived from FFP. Cryoprecipitate transfusion is the therapeutic option often used for fibrinogen supplementation in the United States and United Kingdom while has been withdrawn in some European countries (not in Italy), due to safety concerns (immunological reactions, transmission of infectious agents) [136].

Fibrinogen concentrate is derived from human plasma, and as a pasteurized, lyophilized powder significantly reduces the risk of viral infections and immunological reactions and allows a predictable increase in plasma fibrinogen levels.

In the liver transplant setting, fibrinogen concentrate has shown to be effective in reducing perioperative bleeding and transfusion needs and in optimizing coagulation profile [115, 119]. A fibrinogen concentration <1.5–2 g/L or ROTEM/TEG signs of functional fibrinogen deficit (see above) should trigger fibrinogen supplementation [102]. According to the viscoelastic tests, clot strength (MA/MCF) is the result of platelets-fibrinogen interaction: even in presence of a low platelet count, an adequate clot strength is achieved, provided that fibrinogen concentration is within the normal range or even above the upper limit [86]. The most recent ESA guidelines recommend the use of ROTEM/TEG for targeted management of perioperative coagulation management. However, while FIBTEM test is reported to possibly guide administration of fibrinogen concentrate or cryoprecipitate to reduce platelet and RBC transfusions, there is no formal recommendation for fibrinogen supplementation in OLT surgery. Instead, in a different setting (obstetric hemorrhagic emergencies), trigger levels for fibrinogen substitution were formally addressed, varying between 1 and 2 g/L, with a mean administered dose of 2–4 g.

The FIBTEM test and FF test to guide fibrinogen concentrate supplementation or cryoprecipitate transfusion are reported to reduce platelet and RBC transfusions [119].

10.9.1 TEG-Based Indications

As far as we are aware, there is no definite and shared definition of fibrinogen cutoff values to support a rationale supplementation during OLT when TEG is used to manage coagulation, apart from the correction of fibrinogen blood level below 100 mg/dL (Kang 1985). The functional fibrinogen test is relatively recent [137], and traditionally TEG parameters associated with fibrinogen activity were alpha angle and *K*: however the correlation with clinical fibrinogen levels is considered suboptimal. *K*-time and α-angle are poor predictors of fibrinogen function with fibrinogen levels <115 and >400 mg/dL [138]. The most recent (and unique) experience in the OLT was reported by Planinsic using rapid TEG and FF-TEG. Correlation between rapid TEG and k-TEG was reported as "strong" for MA and "moderate" for α-angle. Instead, in spite of good estimation of the plasma fibrinogen level, FF-TEG is to be interpreted with caution because of an overestimation after graft reperfusion (fibrinogen levels often decreased to less than 100 mg/dL). Changes in hematocrit, coagulation factors levels, the release of procoagulant and anticoagulant factor, and hemodilution due to the use of colloids and/or crystalloids were among the possible explanation [139]

Major points to be considered when using TEG to correct alpha angle are the absence of standardization across transplant centers and the frequent use of kaolin (activated) and not natural assays. In this context, Wang and associates suggest to transfuse cryoprecipitate (5–6 pooled units) when the alpha angle is less than 45° [99], while Larsen and associates [121] suggest to transfuse 2 units of FFP or fibrinogen concentrates when the alpha angle is less than 52°. It has to be underlined that even if not standardized across transplantation centers, recommendations to correct TEG parameters on native traces (without activators) are those (sometimes slightly modified) originally proposed by Kang and associates in 1985 [103]. Unfortunately, neither the use of FF test nor fibrinogen concentrates supplementation were available: this explains why cryoprecipitate transfusion is proposed to correct reduced amplitudes of the alpha angle (6 units of cryoprecipitate for an α-angle <40–45°) while 10 units of platelets were to be transfused to correct MA <40 mm [100].

The quite recent introduction of FF-TEG test (as for FIBTEM test) might provide a better interpretation of the reduced amplitude of MA/MCF (reduced PLT function/count vs. reduced fibrinogen concentration). FF-TEG test provides FLEV value (estimated fibrinogen level, mg/dL) and a fibrinogen-dependent MA amplitude on the TEG trace (FF-MA) using a GPIIb/IIIa platelet inhibitor. As above reported [139], concern exists on the available results. Poor agreement between conventional Clauss method and FLEV results were also reported by Agren and associates [140]: according to this study, raw TEG FF-MA values (mm) might be used instead of functional fibrinogen (g/L) to track changes in an individual patient only. According to the personal, unpublished experience of one of the authors of this chapter (LDP), in case of MA <30 mm (native blood without activator), an FF test is run: if FF-MA is <7 mm (normal range: 9–26 mm), fibrinogen concentrate (25–50 mg/kg) is administered.

10.9.2 ROTEM-Based Indications

Based on thromboelastometry measurements, according to Gorlinger and associates (127) if the EXTEM and FIBTEM MCF values are below 35 and 6 mm respectively, the administration of fibrinogen concentrate is recommended [126]: FIBTEM MCF below 6 mm is used as a trigger value for fibrinogen substitution in bleeding transplant patients [126]. ROTEM algorithms are able, when compared to TEG kaolin active tests, to reduce PLT transfusion in favor of fibrinogen substitution, thus reducing the risk associated with the use of PLT [141]. Even if this statement is frequently reported, very recently published studies challenge this consideration. In a large LDLT series, Seo and associates [142] reported a minor influence of fibrinogen (22 %) on MCF-FIB variability even in case of severe hypofibrinogenemia (fibrinogen <100 mg/dL). In their series, MCF-FIB was less reliable in predicting the fibrinogen concentration in cases of severe hypofibrinogenemia. On the contrary, platelet count was a constant primary determinant of the MCF-EXT and MCF-INT. In a recent comparative, prospective, without-versus-with study, the implementation of a ROTEM-based transfusion algorithm during OLT had no influence on bleeding and transfusion requirements: again, while the ROTEM-based algorithm was associated with an increased perioperative use of fibrinogen, this was not associated with a difference in bleeding and the transfusion needs [143].

According to the most recent experiences in massively bleeding patients, the required fibrinogen dosage can be calculated based on the targeted increase in MCF or A10 in FIBTEM and the body weight (Table 10.1). In the authors' opinion, one of the major concerns with these formulas is the more than probable fibrinogen over administration, leading to prohibitive costs

Table 10.1 Required fibrinogen dosage expressed in grams

Body weight (kg)	Targeted increase in MCF (A10) FIB TEM			
	4 mm	8 mm	12 mm	16 mm
20	0.5 g	1 g	1.5 g	2 g
40	1 g	2 g	3 g	4 g
60	1.5 g	3 g	4.5 g	6 g
80	2 g	4 g	6 g	8 g

Modified from Gorlinger [101]

without demonstrated utility. An alternative, more balanced approach might be a progressive correction with repeatable boluses of 2 g fibrinogen concentrate followed by a new TEG/ROTEM test to document the correction.

$$\text{Fibrinogen dosage (g)} = \text{targeted } \Delta \text{ MCF in FibTEM (mm)} \times \text{body weight (kg)} / 140$$

Cryoprecipitate source of fibrinogen is now only indicated when there is a lack of available fibrinogen concentrate. The risks of infection and immune reaction are reported by some as a contraindication for the treatment of bleeding and hypofibrinogenemia [102].

TEG monitoring can reduce transfusion requirements by 30 % [119]. TEG/ROTEM might improve patient outcomes: however, larger trials are required to investigate/demonstrate this hypothesis [144].

TEG/ROTEM can identify hyperfibrinolysis, indicating antifibrinolytic therapy in case of bleeding (Table 10.2).

Every therapeutic decision (FFP, PLT, fibrinogen administration) should be done in case of ongoing bleeding and should be verified by a new TEG test (Table 10.3).

10.10 TEG-/ROTEM-Based Pharmacological Management of Bleeding

The management of bleeding and coagulopathy varies greatly between different centers. Again, VET devices offer a rapid diagnostic point-of-care test to aid the clinician in orienting/directing pharmacological therapeutic interventions.

10.10.1 Antifibrinolytic Drugs

Hyperfibrinolysis may play a significant role in nonsurgical blood loss requiring massive transfusion during liver transplantation. Antifibrinolytic therapy has been shown to reduce blood loss and blood product transfusions [102, 146] and to be a good therapeutic option in cases of enhanced fibrinolysis. Such a therapy has to be guided by clinical judgment, TEG/ROTEM signs of lysis and "evident" bleeding, and not administered for routine prophylaxis [102] due to potential (albeit not demonstrated in a comprehensive meta-analysis) thrombotic risk [78, 147].

Except for VET, no commercial test evaluates global fibrinolysis. Measurement of individual components of the fibrinolytic pathway is unlikely to help in assessing and managing bleeding risk of cirrhosis [148].

Table 10.2 Simplified summary of three published TEG-based transfusion algorithm on kaolin blood

11 min ≤ r-time ≤ 15 min	*40 ≤ MA ≤ 46 mm and FF-MA 7–19 mm*	*40 ≤ MA ≤ 46 mm and FF-MA 7–19 mm*	*alpha angle <52°*	*Ly 30 min > 8 %*
10 mL/kg FFP or 2 U FFP	Apheresis platelets 1U	Fibrinogen 25–50 mg/kg or Cryoprecipitate 6U	2 UI FFP or fibrinogen concentrate	Tranexamic acid 1–2 g
r-time > 15 min	*MA < 40 mm and FF-MA 7–19 mm*	*MA < 40 mm and FF-MA ≤7 mm*	*alpha angle <45°*	*Ly 30 min >8 %*
20 mL/kg FFP or 4 U FFP	Apheresis platelets 2 U	Fibrinogen 25–50 mg/kg or Cryoprecipitate 6 U	Fibrinogen 25–50 mg/kg or Cryoprecipitate, 6 U	Tranexamic acid 1–2 g

Modified from Larsen and associates [121], Kang and associates [100], Wang and associates [120]
FF functional fibrinogen, *FFP* fresh frozen plasma, *r* time to initiation clot formation, *Ly30* lysis 30 min after the maximum amplitude, *MA* maximum amplitude of clot formation

Table 10.3 Simplified summary of ROTEM-based transfusion algorithm

EXTEMCT >80 s	*INTEM CT >240 s*	*EXTEM MCF <35 mm and FIBTEMMCF >6 mm*	*EXTEM MCF <35 mm and FIBTEMMCF <6 mm*	*EXTEM and INTEM decline after MCF APTEM normal CLI30EX <50 %*
PCC 25 UI/kg	15–20 mL/kg FFP[a]	Apheresis platelets,1 U	Fibrinogen 25–50 mg/kg	Tranexamic acid 1–2 g or 25 mg/kg

Modified from Kirkner and associates [126], Larsen and associates [121], and Coackley and associates [145]
APTEM tissue factor and aprotinin, *CLI30* clot lysis index at 30 min, *CT* clotting time, *EXTEM* tissue factor, *FIBTEM* tissue factor and cytochalasin D, *FFP* fresh frozen plasma, *INTEM* ellagic acid, *MCF* maximum clot firmness
[a]If patients continue to bleed after correction with factor concentrates and show signs of FV and/or FXI deficiency (indicated by prolonged INTEM clotting time, cutoff value of ≥240 s), FFP can be administered at a dose of 15–20 mL/kg

The timing and severity of fibrinolysis is relevant to decide whether to treat or not this complication. It is not unusual to see a spontaneous resolution of lesser degree of fibrinolysis in the post-reperfusion phase. In the liver transplant settings, hyperfibrinolysis may occur in up to 60 % of the cases, but it is self-limiting in one third of these cases [101]. Hyperfibrinolysis typically subsides within an hour but may persist with poorly functioning or marginal grafts. This scenario rarely occurs in acute liver failure due to a high PAI-1 [149].

The drugs usually administered during liver transplant to treat hyperfibrinolysis are:

- Aprotinin: associated with reduced blood loss and transfusion requirements. It is no longer available (withdrawn from the market for safety concerns) [146, 149].
- Lysine analogues (tranexamic acid (TA) and E-aminocaproic acid (EACA)). TA and EACA are associated with lower risk of death when compared to aprotinin. Overall, TA seems to be the agent of choice in liver transplantation, being equally efficacious as the currently unavailable aprotinin [150]. According to a recent Cochrane review, antifibrinolytic therapy helps reduce blood loss and perioperative allogeneic blood transfusion [146].

As opposed to a blind prophylaxis with antifibrinolytics in liver transplantation, a goal-directed therapy, using thrombelastometry/graphy to assess fibrinolysis and evaluating the response to antifibrinolytic therapy, has been suggested [102]. Optimal timing and dose of TA during OLT have not been established [151]. Currently, in many centers, tranexamic acid is usually given to treat ongoing bleeding in 1–2 g increments (20–25 mg/kg body weight bolus) [102]; a continuous infusion of 1–2 mg/kg/h is also used in some institutions.

10.10.1.1 TEG-Based Indications

Fibrinolysis is defined as present when whole blood clot lysis index is less than 80 % [152]. Manufacturer reference values define fibrinolysis when LY30 min is >8 % and LY60 min >15 %. Therefore, the antifibrinolytic therapy is suggested by TEG monitoring and by the presence of coexisting microvascular oozing in the surgical field.

10.10.1.2 ROTEM-Based Indication

The presence of clinically relevant fibrinolysis can be detected as increased maximum lysis (ML >15 % of MCF), early starting reduction in MCF (<45 min), and improved measurement values obtained from a test containing aprotinin (APTEM) [150].

If APTEM clotting time (CT) is shorter than EXTEM CT, or CLI60 in EXTEM is <85 % during preanhepatic or early anhepatic, a therapeutic administration of tranexamic acid may be suggested.

If fibrinolysis is observed during the late anhepatic phase (CLI30EXTEM) <50 % therapeutic administration of tranexamic acid (25 mg/kg) is a useful option to reduce blood loss. Tranexamic acid administration is indicated after reperfusion when CLIEXTEM <50 % is present and persistent bleeding occurs [101].

10.10.2 Recombinant Activated Factor VII (rFVIIa)

Recombinant factor VIIa (rFVIIa) is recombinant human coagulation factor initially developed for bleeding episodes in hemophilia A and B patients who developed inhibitors against standard-factor replacements. It promotes hemostasis by activating the extrinsic pathway of the coagulation cascade. rFVIIa, bypassing factors VIII and IX, initiates coagulation of blood. The FVIIa tissue factor complex catalyzes the conversion of factor IX and factor X into the active proteases, leading to thrombin generation.

The administration of this drug during liver transplantation, enthusiastically welcomed after the first reports, and associated with reduction of blood loss and transfusion needs, was quickly stopped after two multicenter studies that showed an increased number of thromboembolic-related events and no reduction in blood loss and transfusion requirements [84, 153, 154].

According to a recent retrospective review, intraoperative versus preemptive administration of rFVIIa during liver transplant was associated with higher blood product use, lower graft and patient survival rates, longer ICU stays, and higher overall costs compared with preemptive administration [155]. The implication for clinical practice was the absence of clear evidence to promote FVIIa use in OLT apart from rescue therapy for uncontrolled bleeding after having ruled out other possible alternative causes and interventions [102].

Even if more trials are needed to adequately evaluate the use of prophylactic rFVIIa in liver transplantation, room for a specific role does not seem to be likely: as commented on by Yank and associates, however, available evidence is of low strength and too limited to compare the harms and benefits of rFVIIa in OLT [156].

10.10.3 Desmopressin

Desmopressin, a derivative of the antidiuretic hormone, was used for the first time to treat patients with hemophilia A and von Willebrand disease (vWD). Its indications were quickly expanded to bleeding disorders not involving a deficiency or dysfunction of factor VIII or vWf, as it can happen in liver diseases. Despite a reduction in the bleeding time in cirrhotic patients, controlled clinical trials were not able to confirm a positive effect in the management of acute variceal bleeding in ESLD patients [157]. Arshad and associates [158] showed that desmopressin administration had minimal hemostatic effects in cirrhotic patients while could be more effective in patients with mild disease: further clinical studies are required to confirm this point.

Desmopressin has been shown to improve laboratory parameters of primary hemostasis (including the ex vivo bleeding time) [159], but there is very little evidence at the available dosage (0.3 μg/kg) for clinical efficacy in patients with ESLD undergoing liver transplantation [160, 161].

Conclusions

In the last 10 years, a sort of copernican revolution changed the interpretation of the hemostatic and coagulation profiles of the ESLD patients. Cirrhotic patients are not by definition auto-anticoagulated and then by default predisposed to bleeding: instead, they react, according to the different stimuli (e.g., endotoxemia) with a "rebalanced coagulation." It is now clear that cirrhotic patients might be considered in some settings at greater risk of thrombosis than bleeding, even if routine plasmatic coagulation tests suggest hypocoagulability: this is the reason to explain the negative effects often associated with "fixed" prophylactic correction of laboratory values (mainly INR and R) with blood products. According to the above concepts, the use of rapid and more dynamic tests, as the viscoelastic TEG and ROTEM, are on the rise, providing a rapid diagnostic (and now reliable) bedside tests to aid the clinician in directing therapeutic interventions. An easy to use, rapid, flexible, and reliable VET point of care should guide a "step-by-step" evaluation of the ongoing hemostatic phenomenon/bleeding event, allowing an in vitro simulation of the correction (if and when needed) and the timely and appropriate correction of the disorder(s). In the near future, endothelial cells seeded onto microbeads or microchips flow chamber technique will improve the in vitro coagulation assessment, adding to the available technology the two missing links, endothelium and flow rate [144]. Algorithms, in some cases, even quite complex, are now available: however a strong evidence of their effects on outcome, blood loss, and transfusion needs is still lacking, particularly according to the most recent available experiences [144]. As a matter of fact, still unmet needs are consensus on MBT definition and shared attitudes/consensus on each step of the algorithm designed to guide coagulation monitoring and substitution/transfusion management. While VET point-of-care devices are not under discussion as monitors, cutoff values of the single TEG/ROTEM parameters are at least as far as we are aware. Thus, we consider wise and mandatory to design large clinical trials to find a consensus on values below which fibrinogen or PCC is to be administered (the same is for tranexamic acid in hyperfibrinolysis) or to be considered for an appropriate correction: the actual ever-growing economic constraints and an appropriate use of resources mandate this step.

Finally yet importantly, in the absence of a clinically relevant bleeding, pathological laboratory results (VET tests or conventional laboratory tests) are not an indication for a hemostatic intervention: correction of bleeding and, perhaps before, of pH, calcium, and body temperature are the first targets of the anesthesiologist: "cosmetic correction" of numbers is indeed beyond the aim of this chapter.

References

1. Lisman T, Leebeek FW, de Groot PG (2002) Haemostatic abnormalities in patients with liver disease. J Hepatol 37:280–287
2. Rapaport SI (2000) Coagulation problems in liver disease. Blood Coagul Fibrinolysis 11(Suppl 1):S69–S74
3. Tripodi A, Salerno F, Chantarangkul V et al (2005) Evidence of normal thrombin generation in cirrhosis despite abnormal conventional coagulation tests. Hepatology 41:553–558
4. Lu SN, Wang JH, Liu SL et al (2006) Thrombocytopenia as a surrogate for cirrhosis and a marker for the identification of patients at high-risk for hepatocellular carcinoma. Cancer 107:2212–2222
5. Qamar AA, Grace ND, Groszmann RJ et al (2009) Incidence, prevalence, and clinical significance of abnormal hematologic indices in compensated cirrhosis. Clin Gastroenterol Hepatol 7:689–695
6. Ishikawa T, Ichida T, Matsuda Y et al (1998) Reduced expression of thrombopoietin is involved in thrombocytopenia in human and rat liver cirrhosis. J Gastroenterol Hepatol 13:907–913
7. Peck-Radosavljevic M, Wichlas M, Zacherl J et al (2000) Thrombopoietin induces rapid resolution of thrombocytopenia after orthotopic liver transplantation through increased platelet production. Blood 95:795–801
8. Aster RH (1966) Pooling of platelets in the spleen: role in the pathogenesis of "hypersplenic" thrombocytopenia. J Clin Invest 45:645–657
9. Wang CS, Yao WJ, Wang ST, Chang TT, Chou P (2004) Strong association of hepatitis C virus (HCV) infection and thrombocytopenia: implications from a survey of a community with hyperendemic HCV infection. Clin Infect Dis 39:790–796
10. Garcia-Suarez J, Burgaleta C, Hernanz N, Albarran F, Tobaruela P, Alvarez-Mon M (2000) HCV-associated thrombocytopenia: clinical characteristics and platelet response after recombinant alpha2b-interferon therapy. Br J Haematol 110:98–103
11. Bleibel W, Caldwell SH, Curry MP, Northup PG (2013) Peripheral platelet count correlates with liver atrophy and predicts long-term mortality on the liver transplant waiting list. Transpl Int 26:435–442
12. Ordinas A, Escolar G, Cirera I et al (1996) Existence of a platelet-adhesion defect in patients with cirrhosis independent of hematocrit: studies under flow conditions. Hepatology 24:1137–1142
13. Lisman T, Bongers TN, Adelmeijer J et al (2006) Elevated levels of von Willebrand Factor in cirrhosis support platelet adhesion despite reduced functional capacity. Hepatology 44:53–61
14. Hollestelle MJ, Geertzen HG, Straatsburg IH, van Gulik TM, van Mourik JA (2004) Factor VIII expression in liver disease. Thromb Haemost 91:267–275

15. Violi F, Leo R, Vezza E, Basili S, Cordova C, Balsano F (1994) Bleeding time in patients with cirrhosis: relation with degree of liver failure and clotting abnormalities. C.A.L.C. Group. Coagulation Abnormalities in Cirrhosis Study Group. J Hepatol 20:531–536
16. Amitrano L, Guardascione MA, Brancaccio V, Balzano A (2002) Coagulation disorders in liver disease. Semin Liver Dis 22:83–96
17. Lisman T, Leebeek FW, Mosnier LO et al (2001) Thrombin-activatable fibrinolysis inhibitor deficiency in cirrhosis is not associated with increased plasma fibrinolysis. Gastroenterology 121:131–139
18. Huber K, Kirchheimer JC, Korninger C, Binder BR (1991) Hepatic synthesis and clearance of components of the fibrinolytic system in healthy volunteers and in patients with different stages of liver cirrhosis. Thromb Res 62:491–500
19. vanDeWater L, Carr JM, Aronson D, McDonagh J (1986) Analysis of elevated fibrin(ogen) degradation product levels in patients with liver disease. Blood 67:1468–1473
20. Szczepanski M, Habior A, Szczepanik A, Soszka A, Grel K (1994) Thrombin clotting time and fibrin polymerization in liver cirrhosis. Mater Med Pol 26:87–90
21. Green G, Thomson JM, Dymock IW, Poller L (1976) Abnormal fibrin polymerization in liver disease. Br J Haematol 34:427–439
22. Rijken DC, Kock EL, Guimaraes AH et al (2012) Evidence for an enhanced fibrinolytic capacity in cirrhosis as measured with two different global fibrinolysis tests. J Thromb Haemost 10:2116–2122
23. Mammen EF (1994) Coagulopathies of liver disease. Clin Lab Med 14:769–780
24. Escolar G, Cases A, Bastida E et al (1990) Uremic platelets have a functional defect affecting the interaction of von Willebrand factor with glycoprotein IIb-IIIa. Blood 76:1336–1340
25. Piccinino F, Sagnelli E, Pasquale G, Giusti G (1986) Complications following percutaneous liver biopsy. A multicentre retrospective study on 68,276 biopsies. J Hepatol 2:165–173
26. Lisman T, Caldwell SH, Burroughs AK et al (2010) Hemostasis and thrombosis in patients with liver disease: the ups and downs. J Hepatol 53:362–371
27. Tripodi A, Mannucci PM (2007) Abnormalities of hemostasis in chronic liver disease: reappraisal of their clinical significance and need for clinical and laboratory research. J Hepatol 46:727–733
28. Giannini EG, Greco A, Marenco S, Andorno E, Valente U, Savarino V (2010) Incidence of bleeding following invasive procedures in patients with thrombocytopenia and advanced liver disease. Clin Gastroenterol Hepatol 8:899–902
29. Sharma P, McDonald GB, Banaji M (1982) The risk of bleeding after percutaneous liver biopsy: relation to platelet count. J Clin Gastroenterol 4:451–453
30. Janssen HL (2000) Changing perspectives in portal vein thrombosis. Scand J Gastroenterol Suppl 232:69–73
31. Tripodi A, Primignani M, Mannucci PM (2010) Abnormalities of hemostasis and bleeding in chronic liver disease: the paradigm is challenged. Intern Emerg Med 5:7–12
32. Tripodi A, Primignani M, Chantarangkul V et al (2006) Thrombin generation in patients with cirrhosis: the role of platelets. Hepatology 44:440–445
33. Pache I, Bilodeau M (2005) Severe haemorrhage following abdominal paracentesis for ascites in patients with liver disease. Aliment Pharmacol Ther 21:525–529
34. Grabau CM, Crago SF, Hoff LK et al (2004) Performance standards for therapeutic abdominal paracentesis. Hepatology 40:484–488
35. Perdigao JP, de Almeida PC, Rocha TD et al (2012) Postoperative bleeding after dental extraction in liver pretransplant patients. J Oral Maxillofac Surg 70:e177–e184
36. Segal JB, Dzik WH (2005) Paucity of studies to support that abnormal coagulation test results predict bleeding in the setting of invasive procedures: an evidence-based review. Transfusion 45:1413–1425
37. Fisher NC, Mutimer DJ (1999) Central venous cannulation in patients with liver disease and coagulopathy--a prospective audit. Intensive Care Med 25:481–485
38. Ewe K (1981) Bleeding after liver biopsy does not correlate with indices of peripheral coagulation. Dig Dis Sci 26:388–393
39. Grant A, Neuberger J (1999) Guidelines on the use of liver biopsy in clinical practice. British Society of Gastroenterology. Gut 45(Suppl 4):IV1–IV11
40. Gilmore IT, Burroughs A, Murray-Lyon IM, Williams R, Jenkins D, Hopkins A (1995) Indications, methods, and outcomes of percutaneous liver biopsy in England and Wales: an audit by the British Society of Gastroenterology and the Royal College of Physicians of London. Gut 36:437–441
41. Blake JC, Sprengers D, Grech P, McCormick PA, McIntyre N, Burroughs AK (1990) Bleeding time in patients with hepatic cirrhosis. BMJ 301:12–15
42. Suman A, Barnes DS, Zein NN, Levinthal GN, Connor JT, Carey WD (2004) Predicting outcome after cardiac surgery in patients with cirrhosis: a comparison of Child-Pugh and MELD scores. Clin Gastroenterol Hepatol 2:719–723
43. Farnsworth N, Fagan SP, Berger DH, Awad SS (2004) Child-Turcotte-Pugh versus MELD score as a predictor of outcome after elective and emergent surgery in cirrhotic patients. Am J Surg 188:580–583
44. de Goede B, Klitsie PJ, Lange JF, Metselaar HJ, Kazemier G (2012) Morbidity and mortality related to non-hepatic surgery in patients with liver cirrhosis: a systematic review. Best Pract Res Clin Gastroenterol 26:47–59

45. Shaikh AR, Muneer A (2009) Laparoscopic cholecystectomy in cirrhotic patients. JSLS 13:592–596
46. Ikeda Y, Kanda T, Kosugi S et al (2009) Gastric cancer surgery for patients with liver cirrhosis. World J Gastrointest Surg 1:49–55
47. Kao HK, Chang KP, Ching WC, Tsao CK, Cheng MH, Wei FC (2010) Postoperative morbidity and mortality of head and neck cancers in patients with liver cirrhosis undergoing surgical resection followed by microsurgical free tissue transfer. Ann Surg Oncol 17:536–543
48. Porte RJ (1993) Coagulation and fibrinolysis in orthotopic liver transplantation: current views and insights. Semin Thromb Hemost 19:191–196
49. Lu MS, Liu YH, Wu YC, Kao CL, Liu HP, Hsieh MJ (2005) Is it safe to perform esophagectomy in esophageal cancer patients combined with liver cirrhosis? Interact Cardiovasc Thorac Surg 4:423–425
50. Perkins L, Jeffries M, Patel T (2004) Utility of preoperative scores for predicting morbidity after cholecystectomy in patients with cirrhosis. Clin Gastroenterol Hepatol 2:1123–1128
51. Johnson PJ, Poon TC, Hjelm NM et al (1999) Glycan composition of serum alpha-fetoprotein in patients with hepatocellular carcinoma and non-seminomatous germ cell tumour. Br J Cancer 81:1188–1195
52. Friedman LS (1999) The risk of surgery in patients with liver disease. Hepatology 29:1617–1623
53. Garrison RN, Cryer HM, Howard DA, Polk HC Jr (1984) Clarification of risk factors for abdominal operations in patients with hepatic cirrhosis. Ann Surg 199:648–655
54. Chen CC, Hsu PW, Lee ST et al (2012) Brain surgery in patients with liver cirrhosis. J Neurosurg 117:348–353
55. An Y, Xiao YB, Zhong QJ (2007) Open-heart surgery in patients with liver cirrhosis: indications, risk factors, and clinical outcomes. Eur Surg Res 39:67–74
56. Murashita T, Komiya T, Tamura N et al (2009) Preoperative evaluation of patients with liver cirrhosis undergoing open heart surgery. Gen Thorac Cardiovasc Surg 57:293–297
57. Hayashida N, Shoujima T, Teshima H et al (2004) Clinical outcome after cardiac operations in patients with cirrhosis. Ann Thorac Surg 77:500–505
58. Tripodi A, Mannucci PM (2011) The coagulopathy of chronic liver disease. N Engl J Med 365:147–156
59. van Veen JJ, Spahn DR, Makris M (2011) Routine preoperative coagulation tests: an outdated practice? Br J Anaesth 106:1–3
60. Weeder PD, Porte RJ, Lisman T (2014) Hemostasis in liver disease: implications of new concepts for perioperative management. Transfus Med Rev 28:107–113
61. Lisman T, Porte RJ, Leebeek FW, Caldwell SH (2006) Methodological issues with coagulation testing in patients with liver disease. J Thromb Haemost 4:2061–2062
62. Tripodi A (2009) Tests of coagulation in liver disease. Clin Liver Dis 13:55–61
63. Lang T, von Depka M (2006) Possibilities and limitations of thrombelastometry/-graphy. Hamostaseologie 26:S20–S29
64. Stravitz RT (2012) Potential applications of thromboelastography in patients with acute and chronic liver disease. Gastroenterol Hepatol (N Y) 8:513–520
65. Fenger-Eriksen C, Moore GW, Rangarajan S, Ingerslev J, Sorensen B (2010) Fibrinogen estimates are influenced by methods of measurement and hemodilution with colloid plasma expanders. Transfusion 50:2571–2576
66. Molinaro RJ, Szlam F, Levy JH, Fantz CR, Tanaka KA (2008) Low plasma fibrinogen levels with the Clauss method during anticoagulation with bivalirudin. Anesthesiology 109:160–161
67. Kang Y, Gaisor TA (1999) Hematologic considerations in the transplant patient. In: Sharpe MA, Gelb AW (eds) Anesthesia and Transplantation. Butterworth Heinemann, Boston, pp 363–387
68. Niemann CU, Eilers H (2010) Abdominal organ transplantation. Minerva Anestesiol 76:266–275
69. Yost CS, Nieman CU (2010) Anesthesia for Organ transplantation. In: Miller RD (ed) Millers anaesthesia, 7th edn. Elsevier, Philadelphia 2155–2184
70. Hannaman MJ, Hevesi ZG (2011) Anesthesia care for liver transplantation. Transplant Rev (Orlando) 25:36–43
71. Mitra B, Cameron PA, Gruen RL, Mori A, Fitzgerald M, Street A (2011) The definition of massive transfusion in trauma: a critical variable in examining evidence for resuscitation. Eur J Emerg Med 18:137–142
72. Sharpe JP, Weinberg JA, Magnotti LJ, Croce MA, Fabian TC (2012) Toward a better definition of massive transfusion: focus on the interval of hemorrhage control. J Trauma Acute Care Surg 73: 1553–1557
73. Rossaint R, Bouillon B, Cerny V et al (2010) Management of bleeding following major trauma: an updated European guideline. Crit Care 14:R52
74. Hoyt DB (2004) A clinical review of bleeding dilemmas in trauma. Semin Hematol 41:40–43
75. McCluskey SA, Karkouti K, Wijeysundera DN et al (2006) Derivation of a risk index for the prediction of massive blood transfusion in liver transplantation. Liver Transpl 12:1584–1593
76. Kashuk JL, Moore EE, Johnson JL et al (2008) Postinjury life threatening coagulopathy: is 1:1 fresh frozen plasma:packed red blood cells the answer? J Trauma 65:261–270; discussion 270–261
77. Reichert B, Kaltenborn A, Becker T, Schiffer M, Klempnauer J, Schrem H (2014) Massive blood transfusion after the first cut in liver transplantation predicts renal outcome and survival. Langenbecks Arch Surg 399:429–440
78. Feltracco P, Brezzi M, Barbieri S et al (2013) Blood loss, predictors of bleeding, transfusion practice and strategies of blood cell salvaging during liver transplantation. World J Hepatol 5:1–15

79. de Boer MT, Molenaar IQ, Hendriks HG, Slooff MJ, Porte RJ (2005) Minimizing blood loss in liver transplantation: progress through research and evolution of techniques. Dig Surg 22:265–275
80. Massicotte L, Denault AY, Beaulieu D et al (2012) Transfusion rate for 500 consecutive liver transplantations: experience of one liver transplantation center. Transplantation 93:1276–1281
81. Massicotte L, Beaulieu D, Roy JD et al (2009) MELD score and blood product requirements during liver transplantation: no link. Transplantation 87:1689–1694
82. Cywinski JB, Alster JM, Miller C, Vogt DP, Parker BM (2014) Prediction of intraoperative transfusion requirements during orthotopic liver transplantation and the influence on postoperative patient survival. Anesth Analg 118:428–437
83. Martell M, Coll M, Ezkurdia N, Raurell I, Genesca J (2010) Physiopathology of splanchnic vasodilation in portal hypertension. World J Hepatol 2:208–220
84. Saner FH, Gieseler RK, Akiz H, Canbay A, Gorlinger K (2013) Delicate balance of bleeding and thrombosis in end-stage liver disease and liver transplantation. Digestion 88:135–144
85. Tripodi A, Fracanzani AL, Primignani M et al (2014) Procoagulant imbalance in patients with non-alcoholic fatty liver disease. J Hepatol 61:148–154
86. Clevenger B, Mallett SV (2014) Transfusion and coagulation management in liver transplantation. World J Gastroenterol 20:6146–6158
87. Cywes R, Packham MA, Tietze L et al (1993) Role of platelets in hepatic allograft preservation injury in the rat. Hepatology 18:635–647
88. Pereboom IT, Adelmeijer J, van Leeuwen Y, Hendriks HG, Porte RJ, Lisman T (2009) Development of a severe von Willebrand factor/ADAMTS13 dysbalance during orthotopic liver transplantation. Am J Transplant 9:1189–1196
89. Porte RJ, Bontempo FA, Knot EA, Lewis JH, Kang YG, Starzl TE (1989) Systemic effects of tissue plasminogen activator-associated fibrinolysis and its relation to thrombin generation in orthotopic liver transplantation. Transplantation 47:978–984
90. Molenaar IQ, Warnaar N, Groen H, Tenvergert EM, Slooff MJ, Porte RJ (2007) Efficacy and safety of antifibrinolytic drugs in liver transplantation: a systematic review and meta-analysis. Am J Transplant 7:185–194
91. Senzolo M, Burra P, Cholongitas E, Burroughs AK (2006) New insights into the coagulopathy of liver disease and liver transplantation. World J Gastroenterol 12:7725–7736
92. Bayly PJ, Thick M (1994) Reversal of post-reperfusion coagulopathy by protamine sulphate in orthotopic liver transplantation. Br J Anaesth 73:840–842
93. Agarwal S, Senzolo M, Melikian C, Burroughs A, Mallett SV (2008) The prevalence of a heparin-like effect shown on the thromboelastograph in patients undergoing liver transplantation. Liver Transpl 14:855–860
94. Findlay JY, Rettke SR (2000) Poor prediction of blood transfusion requirements in adult liver transplantations from preoperative variables. J Clin Anesth 12:319–323
95. Yeung MC, Tong SY, Tong PY, Cheung BH, Ng JY, Leung GK (2014) Use of viscoelastic haemostatic assay in emergency and elective surgery. Hong Kong Med J 21(1):45–51
96. Mallett SV, Chowdary P, Burroughs AK (2013) Clinical utility of viscoelastic tests of coagulation in patients with liver disease. Liver Int 33:961–974
97. Alamo JM, Leon A, Mellado P et al (2013) Is "intra-operating room" thromboelastometry useful in liver transplantation? A case–control study in 303 patients. Transplant Proc 45:3637–3639
98. Gurusamy KS, Pissanou T, Pikhart H, Vaughan J, Burroughs AK, Davidson BR (2011) Methods to decrease blood loss and transfusion requirements for liver transplantation. Cochrane Database Syst 1:1–127
99. Wang SC, Shieh JF, Chang KY et al (2010) Thromboelastography-guided transfusion decreases intraoperative blood transfusion during orthotopic liver transplantation: randomized clinical trial. Transplant Proc 42:2590–2593
100. Kang YG, Martin DJ, Marquez J et al (1985) Intraoperative changes in blood coagulation and thrombelastographic monitoring in liver transplantation. Anesth Analg 64:888–896
101. Gorlinger K (2006) Coagulation management during liver transplantation. Hamostaseologie 26:S64–S76
102. Kozek-Langenecker SA, Afshari A, Albaladejo P et al (2013) Management of severe perioperative bleeding: guidelines from the European Society of Anaesthesiology. Eur J Anaesthesiol 30:270–382
103. Peyrou V, Lormeau JC, Herault JP, Gaich C, Pfliegger AM, Herbert JM (1999) Contribution of erythrocytes to thrombin generation in whole blood. Thromb Haemost 81:400–406
104. Thachil J (2011) Anemia--the overlooked factor in bleeding related to liver disease. J Hepatol 54:593–594, author reply 594–595
105. Villanueva C, Colomo A, Bosch A et al (2013) Transfusion strategies for acute upper gastrointestinal bleeding. N Engl J Med 368:11–21
106. Carson JL, Noveck H, Berlin JA, Gould SA (2002) Mortality and morbidity in patients with very low postoperative Hb levels who decline blood transfusion. Transfusion 42:812–818
107. Massicotte L, Lenis S, Thibeault L, Sassine MP, Seal RF, Roy A (2006) Effect of low central venous pressure and phlebotomy on blood product transfusion requirements during liver transplantations. Liver Transpl 12:117–123
108. de Boer MT, Christensen MC, Asmussen M et al (2008) The impact of intraoperative transfusion of platelets and red blood cells on survival after liver transplantation. Anesth Analg 106:32–44, table of contents

109. Liu LL, Niemann CU (2011) Intraoperative management of liver transplant patients. Transplant Rev (Orlando) 25:124–129
110. Massicotte L, Denault AY, Beaulieu D, Thibeault L, Hevesi Z, Roy A (2011) Aprotinin versus tranexamic acid during liver transplantation: impact on blood product requirements and survival. Transplantation 91:1273–1278
111. Kato M, Sugawara Y, Orii R et al (2001) Lactate levels in cirrhotic patients undergoing liver resection. Hepatogastroenterology 48:1106–1109
112. Sarani B, Dunkman WJ, Dean L, Sonnad S, Rohrbach JI, Gracias VH (2008) Transfusion of fresh frozen plasma in critically ill surgical patients is associated with an increased risk of infection. Crit Care Med 36:1114–1118
113. Lisman T, Bakhtiari K, Pereboom IT, Hendriks HG, Meijers JC, Porte RJ (2010) Normal to increased thrombin generation in patients undergoing liver transplantation despite prolonged conventional coagulation tests. J Hepatol 52:355–361
114. Amarapurkar PD, Amarapurkar DN (2011) Management of coagulopathy in patients with decompensated liver cirrhosis. Int J Hepatol 2011:1–5
115. Gorlinger K, Fries D, Dirkmann D, Weber CF, Hanke AA, Schochl H (2012) Reduction of fresh frozen plasma requirements by perioperative point-of-care coagulation management with early calculated goal-directed therapy. Transfus Med Hemother 39:104–113
116. Al Dieri R, Peyvandi F, Santagostino E et al (2002) The thrombogram in rare inherited coagulation disorders: its relation to clinical bleeding. Thromb Haemost 88:576–582
117. Chowdary P, Saayman AG, Paulus U, Findlay GP, Collins PW (2004) Efficacy of standard dose and 30 ml/kg fresh frozen plasma in correcting laboratory parameters of haemostasis in critically ill patients. Br J Haematol 125:69–73
118. Ganter MT, Hofer CK (2008) Coagulation monitoring: current techniques and clinical use of viscoelastic point-of-care coagulation devices. Anesth Analg 106:1366–1375
119. Noval-Padillo JA, Leon-Justel A, Mellado-Miras P et al (2010) Introduction of fibrinogen in the treatment of hemostatic disorders during orthotopic liver transplantation: implications in the use of allogenic blood. Transplant Proc 42:2973–2974
120. Wang SC, Lin HT, Chang KY et al (2010) Use of higher thromboelastogram transfusion values is not associated with greater blood loss in liver transplant surgery. Liver Transpl 18:1254–1258
121. Larsen OH, Fenger-Eriksen C, Christiansen K, Ingerslev J, Sorensen B (2011) Diagnostic performance and therapeutic consequence of thromboelastometry activated by kaolin versus a panel of specific reagents. Anesthesiology 115:294–302
122. Roche AM, James MF, Grocott MP, Mythen MG (2003) Citrated blood does not reliably reflect fresh whole blood coagulability in trials of in vitro hemodilution. Anesth Analg 96:58–61, table of contents
123. Zambruni A, Thalheimer U, Leandro G, Perry D, Burroughs AK (2004) Thromboelastography with citrated blood: comparability with native blood, stability of citrate storage and effect of repeated sampling. Blood Coagul Fibrinolysis 15:103–107
124. Hardisty RM, Hutton RA (1965) The kaolin clotting time of platelet-rich plasma: a test of platelet factor-3 availability. Br J Haematol 11:258–268
125. Durila M (2011) Kaolin activated thromboelastography can result in false positive fibrinolytic trace. Anaesth Intensive Care 39:775–776
126. Kirchner C, Dirkmann D, Treckmann JW et al (2014) Coagulation management with factor concentrates in liver transplantation: a single-center experience. Transfusion 54((10 Pt 2)):2760–2768
127. Ranucci M, Baryshnikova E, Crapelli GB et al (2015) Randomized, double-blinded, placebo-controlled trial of fibrinogen concentrate supplementation after complex cardiac surgery. J Am Heart Assoc 4(6). pii: e002066. doi:10.1161/JAHA.115.002066
128. Gorlinger K, Dirkmann D, Hanke AA et al (2011) First-line therapy with coagulation factor concentrates combined with point-of-care coagulation testing is associated with decreased allogeneic blood transfusion in cardiovascular surgery: a retrospective, single-center cohort study. Anesthesiology 115:1179–1191
129. Dalmau A, Sabate A, Aparicio I (2009) Hemostasis and coagulation monitoring and management during liver transplantation. Curr Opin Organ Transplant 14:286–290
130. Hanke AA, Joch C, Gorlinger K (2013) Long-term safety and efficacy of a pasteurized nanofiltrated prothrombin complex concentrate (Beriplex P/N): a pharmacovigilance study. Br J Anaesth 110:764–772
131. Schochl H, Nienaber U, Hofer G et al (2010) Goal-directed coagulation management of major trauma patients using thromboelastometry (ROTEM)-guided administration of fibrinogen concentrate and prothrombin complex concentrate. Crit Care 14:R55
132. Fenger-Eriksen C, Tonnesen E, Ingerslev J, Sorensen B (2009) Mechanisms of hydroxyethyl starch-induced dilutional coagulopathy. J Thromb Haemost 7:1099–1105
133. Caldwell SH, Sanyal AJ (2009) Coagulation disorders and bleeding in liver disease: future directions. Clin Liver Dis 13:155–157
134. Tripodi A, Primignani M, Chantarangkul V et al (2009) The coagulopathy of cirrhosis assessed by thromboelastometry and its correlation with conventional coagulation parameters. Thromb Res 124:132–136

135. Hiippala ST, Myllyla GJ, Vahtera EM (1995) Hemostatic factors and replacement of major blood loss with plasma-poor red cell concentrates. Anesth Analg 81:360–365
136. Sorensen B, Bevan D (2010) A critical evaluation of cryoprecipitate for replacement of fibrinogen. Br J Haematol 149:834–843
137. TEG 5000 User Manual. Niles IH (1999–2007). 178–180
138. Jeger V1, Willi S, Liu T et al (2012) The Rapid TEG α-Angle may be a sensitive predictor of transfusion in moderately injured blunt trauma patients. Scientific World Journal 2012:821794. doi:10.1100/2012/821794. Epub 2012 Apr 1
139. Yang Lu S, Tanaka KA, Abuelkasem E, Planinsic RM, Sakai T (2014) Clinical applicability of rapid thrombelastography and functional fibrinogen thrombelastography to adult liver transplantation. Liver Transpl 20:1097–1105
140. Agren A, Wikman AT, Ostlund A, Edgren G (2014) TEG(R) functional fibrinogen analysis may overestimate fibrinogen levels. Anesth Analg 118:933–935
141. Pereboom IT, de Boer MT, Haagsma EB, Hendriks HG, Lisman T, Porte RJ (2009) Platelet transfusion during liver transplantation is associated with increased postoperative mortality due to acute lung injury. Anesth Analg 108:1083–1091
142. Seo H, Choi JH, Moon YJ, Jeong SM (2015) FIBTEM of thromboelastometry does not accurately represent fibrinogen concentration in patients with severe hypofibrinogenemia during liver transplantation. Ann Transplant 20:342–350
143. Roullet S, Freyburger G, Cruc M et al (2015) Management of bleeding and transfusion during liver transplantation before and after the introduction of a rotational thromboelastometry-based algorithm. Liver Transpl 21:169–179
144. Wikkelso A, Lunde J, Johansen M et al (2013) Fibrinogen concentrate in bleeding patients. Cochrane Database Syst
145. Coakley M, Reddy K, Mackie I, Mallett S (2006) Transfusion triggers in orthotopic liver transplantation: a comparison of the thromboelastometry analyzer, the thromboelastogram, and conventional coagulation tests. J Cardiothorac Vasc Anesth 20(4):548–553
146. Henry DA, Carless PA, Moxey AJ et al (2011) Antifibrinolytic use for minimising perioperative allogeneic blood transfusion. Cochrane Database Syst
147. Makwana J, Paranjape S, Goswami J (2010) Antifibrinolytics in liver surgery. Indian J Anaesth 54(6):489–495
148. Ferro D, Celestini A, Violi F (2009) Hyperfibrinolysis in liver disease. Clin Liver Dis 13:21–31
149. Warnaar N, Mallett SV, de Boer MT et al (2007) The impact of aprotinin on renal function after liver transplantation: an analysis of 1,043 patients. Am J Transplant 7:2378–2387
150. Trzebicki J, Flakiewicz E, Kosieradzki M et al (2010) The use of thromboelastometry in the assessment of hemostasis during orthotopic liver transplantation reduces the demand for blood products. Ann Transplant 15:19–24
151. Groenland TH, Porte RJ (2006) Antifibrinolytics in liver transplantation. Int Anesthesiol Clin 44: 83–97
152. Kang Y (1995) Thromboelastography in liver transplantation. Semin Thromb Hemost 21(Suppl 4):34–44
153. Lodge JP, Jonas S, Jones RM et al (2005) Efficacy and safety of repeated perioperative doses of recombinant factor VIIa in liver transplantation. Liver Transpl 11:973–979
154. Planinsic RM, van der Meer J, Testa G et al (2005) Safety and efficacy of a single bolus administration of recombinant factor VIIa in liver transplantation due to chronic liver disease. Liver Transpl 11:895–900
155. Scheffert JL, Taber DJ, Pilch NA, McGillicuddy JW, Baliga PK, Chavin KD (2013) Timing of factor VIIa in liver transplantation impacts cost and clinical outcomes. Pharmacotherapy 33:483–488
156. Yank V, Tuohy CV, Logan AC et al (2011) Systematic review: benefits and harms of in-hospital use of recombinant factor VIIa for off-label indications. Ann Intern Med 154:529–540
157. Mannucci PM (1997) Desmopressin (DDAVP) in the treatment of bleeding disorders: the first 20 years. Blood 90:2515–2521
158. Arshad F, Stoof SC, Leebeek FW et al (2015) Infusion of DDAVP does not improve primary hemostasis in patients with cirrhosis. Liver Int 35:1809–1815
159. Agnelli G, Parise P, Levi M, Cosmi B, Nenci GG (1995) Effects of desmopressin on hemostasis in patients with liver cirrhosis. Haemostasis 25:241–247
160. Pivalizza EG, Warters RD, Gebhard R (2003) Desmopressin before liver transplantation. Can J Anaesth 50:748–749
161. Wong AY, Irwin MG, Hui TW, Fung SK, Fan ST, Ma ES (2003) Desmopressin does not decrease blood loss and transfusion requirements in patients undergoing hepatectomy. Can J Anaesth 50:14–20

Disorders of Hemostasis in the Bleeding Intensive Care Unit Patient

11

Lucio Bucci, Luca Monastra, and Andrea De Gasperi

11.1 Overview

Hemostasis disorders (coagulopathies involving both prothrombotic states and bleeding due to several pathological mechanisms) are common clinical conditions in critically ill patients admitted in the intensive care unit (ICU) [1, 2]. Different hemorrhagic scenarios represent a challenging aspect of daily practical activity of anesthesiologists and intensivists facing perioperative bleeding in major surgery, trauma, burns, obstetrical hemorrhage and even in medical and septic patients, all of these conditions involving possible life-threatening coagulation disorders. The management of bleeding in these patients involves outstanding clinical aspects, requiring a pathophysiological and, possibly, a clinicopathological approach together with diagnostic tools. These include conventional laboratory coagulation tests or, more recently, point-of-care (POC) devices (thromboelastography/thromboelastometry: TEG®/TEM®; platelet aggregometry), to ensure a rapid, appropriate and correct diagnosis to activate a *theranostic approach* (a term derived from the fusion of two words: *thera*-peutic and diag-*nostic)*, in order to administer the appropriate and goal-directed treatment(s) [3, 4]. Coagulation disorders and severe bleeding conditions associated with postpartum hemorrhage (PPH), acute trauma with trauma-induced coagulopathy (TIC), and cardiac surgery-associated coagulopathy are treated in other chapters of this textbook. We will overview and summarize the pathophysiology of the coagulation disorders most frequently recorded in patients admitted to a general ICU after major surgery, polytrauma treated according to damage control surgery and "damage control resuscitation" with hemostatic control approach, burns, and severe sepsis/septic shock patients, looking at clinical and laboratory features of DIC (Disseminated Intravascular Coagulopathy). This chapter will focus on the more recent evidences regarding the costant relationships and cross talks between the coagulation and the inflammation systems, summarizing and outlining the importance of approaching these bleeding and unstable patients looking at a rapid, POC evaluation with viscoelastic hemostatic tests (VHT) such as TEG®/TEM®. Finally this chapter will report the principal therapeutically approaches, looking at the actual evidences, if

L. Bucci, MD (✉)
ICU "Bozza" – 1st Service Anesthesia and Intensive Care, Ospedale Niguarda Ca' Granda, Milan, Italy
e-mail: lucio.bucci@ospedaleniguarda.it; doclucio61@yahoo.it

L. Monastra, MD
UOC Anesthesia and Intensive Care, A.O. Ospedale dei Colli Presidio Monaldi, Naples, Italy

A. De Gasperi, MD
2nd Service Anesthesia Critical Care Medicine, Ospedale Niguarda Ca' Granda, Milan, Italy

M. Ranucci, P. Simioni (eds.), *Point-of-Care Tests for Severe Hemorrhage: A Manual for Diagnosis and Treatment*, DOI 10.1007/978-3-319-24795-3_11

any, to administer blood products and/or blood derivatives in a timely, goal-directed, and appropriated fashion.

11.2 Pathophysiology of the Most Common Coagulation Abnormalities in Critical Patients Admitted to the ICU

In critically ill patients admitted to the ICU due to major surgery, trauma, burns, obstetrical severe bleeding (PPH: postpartum hemorrhage), sepsis and in patients undergoing extracorporeal life support, the entire coagulation system may show several degrees of abnormalities at multiple levels [1, 2]. The risk of hemorrhage due to a coagulopathy in these settings and the administration of allogeneic blood products has been reported as independent risk factors of adverse and worse outcome, in terms of morbidity and mortality [5]. As a consequence, a rapid and correct diagnosis of the underlying main causes sustaining the coagulopathy is mandatory, since every different deranged and identified mechanism necessitates an appropriate and goal-directed therapeutic approach. Standard coagulation tests have shown several limitations, in terms of partial diagnostic informations and time of turnaround response from laboratory [6]. However, using conventional tests, important coagulopathy identification and pathophysiological mechanisms (like reduced clot firmness, hyperfibrinolysis or platelet dysfunction) remain undetected, therefore leading to no goal-directed management. Standard coagulation tests do not provide the right answers to clinical acute care requests, representing week *biomarkers* of abrupt coagulation derangements and poor predictors of bleeding and related mortality [4, 7, 8]. Therefore, in recent years, there has been a renewed and increasing interest for POC devices such as thromboelastography/thromboelastometry and platelet aggregometry tools, in order to obtain a rapid whole blood, near-patient analysis of the hemostatic function [7, 9]. Moreover, an increasing number of institutions worldwide have developed and adopted local protocols to manage hemorrhage, which include POC-based assessment, aiming at three main points: (1) a rapid diagnosis of the underlying coagulopathy, (2) an early goal-directed treatment approach, and (3) the potential for a timely and rapid clinical follow-up in terms of coagulation management [10]. The comprehensive goal seeks for blood loss containment, reduced allogeneic blood components requirements, favorable impact on the potentially severe or even life-threatening transfusion-related adverse effects, prevention of thromboembolic events and, finally, cost containment.

11.2.1 Diagnostic Approach to Coagulopathy in Intensive Care Patients

The main (but not exclusive) pathophysiological derangements at the basis of the ICU coagulopathies are the following [1]:

- Alterations of the physiological profile able to interfere with basic conditions for hemostating capabilities (pH, concentration of ionized calcium, temperature and hematocrit)
- Disturbances of primary hemostasis, e.g., pre-existing or perioperatively acquired alterations of platelet count and function due to antiplatelets medications, sepsis, disseminated intravascular coagulation (DIC), heparin-induced thrombocytopenia (HIT) and massive blood loss
- Abnormalities of the coagulation cascade due to preoperative anticoagulation medications such as vitamin K antagonists (VKA) and/or the novel oral anticoagulants (NOAC: dabigatran, rivaroxaban, apixaban) as well as isolated or global clotting-factor deficits (impaired synthesis, massive loss, consumption)
- Complex systemic hemostatic derangements (DIC or hyperfibrinolysis)

In Fig. 11.1, a schematic representation of the main aspects of the most relevant coagulopathies observed in the ICU patients is represented.

In patients with extracorporeal life support such as ECMO, the risk of coagulopathy is

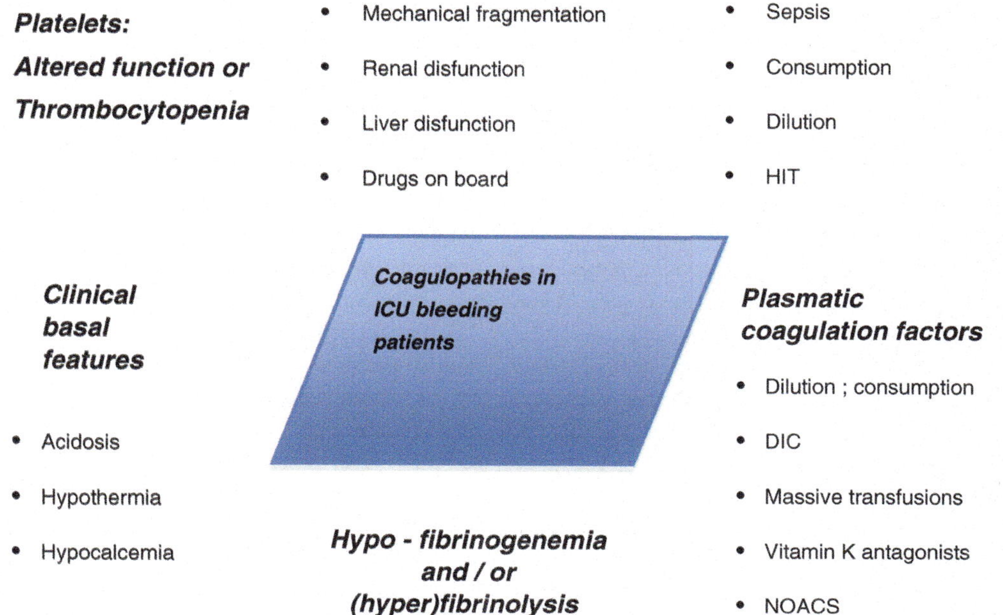

Fig. 11.1 A schematic overview of the main principal coagulopathies in ICU critical patients. *DIC* disseminated intravascular coagulopathy, *HIT* heparin-induced thrombocytopenia, *NOAC* novel oral anticoagulant (Modified from Levi and van der Poll [11])

further increased by therapeutic anticoagulation using unfractionated heparin (UFH) to prevent blood clotting and by hemodilution, both resulting in the activation and consumption of coagulation factors and platelets [12, 13].

11.2.2 Limitations of Conventional Laboratory Coagulation Tests

Standard laboratory coagulation tests (prothrombin time, PT; activated partial thromboplastin time, aPTT; platelet count; fibrinogen plasmatic concentration; D-dimer) appear to be of limited value for the precise assessment and the timely monitoring of ICU coagulopathies and for their treatment strategies, in particular in patients with critical and ongoing bleeding [4, 8, 14]. Hypothermia-induced coagulopathy might be masked by the usual sample analysis at a standardized temperature of 37 °C. The conventional "static" tests (PT and aPTT) only partially reflect the initial thrombin generation; platelet count is merely quantitative and does not detect preexisting, drug-induced or perioperatively acquired platelet dysfunction. Moreover, conventional coagulation tests do not provide information about clot stability over time, giving a limited information regarding (hyper)fibrinolysis. It is therefore of paramount importance to acknowledge the intrinsic limitations of routine coagulation tests in detecting clinically significant conditions which may influence bleeding.

11.3 Point-of-Care Devices

For an appropriate and clinically useful hemostatic evaluation of the critically ill patient, the analysis of a rapid, reproducible and reliable hemostatic profile is mandatory. Differently from the standard tests, POC techniques, including whole blood platelet function tests (impedance or turbidimetric aggregometry) and particularly viscoelastic tests (thromboelastography/thromboelastometry: TEG®/TEM®) might provide detailed results, including the correction for the core temperature of the patient. When compared to conventional laboratory test, viscoelastic assay results are available much earlier (analysis time of 20–25 min vs. laboratory turnaround time of 40–90 min) and might identify in a large part of the cases the underlying hemostatic derangement (i.e. factor deficiency, low fibrinogen, altered platelet function, increased fibrinolysis). Therefore, they can provide the indication for a targeted drug therapy or the appropriate blood component administration [6, 15]. More importantly, the results of the hemostatic interventions are real-time available, an opportunity which might become critical in this setting (rapid display of the *in vitro* drug effect and of the *in vivo* results early after the therapeutic intervention). Viscoelastic POC techniques (ROTEM®, TEG®) are based on thromboelastography, which was described several decades ago by Hartert [16]. These tests are used to measure the time until clot formation begins, the dynamics of clot formation and the firmness and stability of clots over time. A special and unique advantage provided by the viscoelastic techniques is the direct detection of hyperfibrinolysis [17]. Platelet aggregation tests combined with viscoelastic methods yield a far broader diagnostic spectrum than conventional laboratory testing of coagulation may offer [15]. However, none of the currently available POC techniques can provide adequate information about all aspects of the complex process of blood clotting. For more detailed informations regarding the techniques, the points of strengths and limitations of POC devices, see elsewhere in Chaps. 2 and 3.

11.4 Coagulation and Inflammation: Relationships and Cross talk Pathways between the Two Systems

In recent years, evidences from basic researches and clinical studies focused on the profound relationships and the costantly cross talks between the coagulation system and the inflammatory cascade. This involves the cellular elements of the immune response, the released substances (i.e. cytokines, PAMPs and DAMPs, and more recently microparticles and histones; see below) [18], the endothelium with its complex system of signals' mechano-transducers such as glycocalyx and receptors [19] and the inflammatory response to tissue damages, due to invading pathogens or sterile injuries [20]. Blood coagulation and inflammation represent the two main ancient human host defense systems, aiming to recognize, contain and kill invaders, trying to limit tissue injury and to start repair mechanisms [21, 22]. The interplay of the coagulation and inflammatory pathways shows a formidable complexity, in which laboratory researches and animal model studies offer even more elements to clinical queries to reach (possibly) solid evidences. The need is for *biomarkers* and rapid diagnostic POC tools. The ultimate goal is to define precise targets for appropriate drug delivery to guide a goal-directed treatment; the final result should be to modulate both coagulation and inflammatory systems' responses and, definitively, to counteract possible impending bleeding situations.

11.4.1 Inflammatory Response in ICU Patients due to Surgery, Trauma, and Burns: Lessons Learned from Sepsis

Tissue injury following major surgery, trauma and burns represents a formidable boost of inflammatory response, with the host immune system involved both in protection from infection (a major factor of increased morbidity, mortality and overall costs) and in the initiation and guidance of the repair mechanisms aiming at the final "*restitutio ad integrum*". Immunological variations following surgery and trauma are only partially understood. They appear as characterized by an increase of expression of T-helper 2 (Th2) lymphocytes with impaired cell-mediated immunity. Moreover, an imbalance between the pro- and the anti-inflammatory pathways of Th1/Th2 occurs, with changes over time, following activation of hypothalamic-pituitary-adrenal (HPA) axis and sympathetic adrenal system activation, with the release of cortisol and catecholamines [23]. In trauma patients, the host's immune response is widely believed to follow a bimodal sequential organized forms, represented by the systemic inflammatory response syndrome (SIRS, a pro-inflammatory activated condition) followed by a series of mechanisms of compensatory anti-inflammatory response syndrome (CARS) to counteract, balance and dump the overwhelming and possibly dangerous inflammatory reaction. However, recent data in severely injured patients with blunt trauma and burns seem to suggest a different view and this paradigm may not be correct [24]. This proposed new model accounts for a simultaneous and rapid boost of innate immunity (with activation of both pro- and anti-inflammatory genes) and suppression of those genes involved in adaptive immune response. In this paradigmatic shift of view, those complicated recoveries are delayed, resulting in a prolonged and dysregulated immune-inflammatory state.

11.5 Clinical Scenarios of Critical ICU Patients with Coagulopathy

11.5.1 Perioperative Coagulation Management in Major Surgery and Trauma Bleeding Patients

By definition, the intraoperative and the postoperative phases are summarized together as "perioperative" period. "Surgical bleeding" from an uncontrolled source, with no clinical and laboratory evidence of coagulopathy, may present as an early pathomechanism of perioperative hemorrhage in ICU. During ongoing major bleeding requiring a massive transfusion approach, coagulopathy may develop in a high percentage of cases. Depending on the patient's compensatory capability, bleeding situations with a blood loss exceeding 20 % of the blood volume may represent an emergency as well as a risk factor for postoperative anemia, tissue hypoperfusion, transfusion requirements and associated adverse events and, ultimate, coagulopathy [4]. All these factors are independent predictors for survival outcome in postoperative critical care patients and are major drivers for resource application and costs [4, 9, 14]. Moreover, as surgery and trauma injuries are not limited to previously healthy people, the increasing number of patients treated with oral anticoagulants and antiplatelet drugs poses an additional problem to clinicians. Diagnosis of perioperative coagulation derangements in major bleeding necessitating massive transfusion needs to be addressed by appropriate coagulation tests. Repeated coagulation monitoring is the rational basis for the introduction of prothrombotic and/or antithrombotic interventions. In the last decade, there has been a paradigmatic shift in the management of these patients, with an increased awareness for the limitations of routine coagulation tests to guide coagulopathy treatment in massive bleeding, pointing out that predominant pathomechanism(s) of bleeding in the complex scenario of perioperative coagulopathy cannot be differentiated. A prolonged activated partial thromboplastin time (aPTT) may be due to "intrinsic coagulation factor" deficiency requiring specific substitution, fibrinogen deficiency requiring fibrinogen substitution, hypothermia necessitating rewarming, residual heparinization requiring protamine reversal or hyperfibrinolysis requiring antifibrinolytic drugs. Normal viscoelastic assay results and normal platelet count/function are unlikely to coincide with bleeding (high negative predictive value), which should trigger a requirement of surgical re-exploration. In major trauma patients, coagulopathy is recorded in approximately 25–30 % of patients admitted to the emergency room, being involved in up to 40 % of all trauma-related deaths [25]. Although fresh frozen plasma (FFP) transfusion is often a routine part of transfusion protocols, its efficacy is uncertain. Most notably, FFP administration is also associated with acute lung injury (TRALI), transfusion-associated cardiac overload (TACO) and nosocomial infections [26, 27]. Additionally, trauma-associated coagulopathy is a very complex biological process; for the updated informations of early trauma-induced coagulopathy (TIC) and its detection and treatment approach, see Chap. 7. However, care of the most injured trauma patients does not end in the trauma resuscitation bay and/or in the operating room. ICU physicians must be skilled to receive patients at any point along the continuum of care, both with an assessment of the patient's physiologic status and addressing ongoing needs in a prompt and rapid fashion [28]. Once the patient is more stable, the ICU physician must begin the mainstays of care focusing on clinical issues such as organ function support, potential for infectious, thromboembolic events and the need for planned re-exploration (e.g. in case of open abdomen strategy) and staged definitive repair.

The resuscitation strategies from surgery or trauma injury are based on the prerequisite of stopping hemorrhage. Life-threatening coagulopathy is one of the most dangerous complications of patients in severe hemorrhagic shock and increased transfusion requirements are generally predictive of subsequent organ dysfunction; moreover, there are data showing that persistent bleeding with ongoing coagulopathy of patients admitted to the ICU is independently associated with increasing in morbidity and mortality [29, 30]. In these critical care settings, there are more and more urgent needs for the ICU physicians for reliable POC hemostatic monitoring devices, with clinical relevance in conditions of severe coagulopathy due to massive hemorrhage. There is increasing evidence that viscoelastic monitoring systems such as TEG (Haemonetics Corp., Niles, IL, USA) and ROTEM (Tem Innovations GmbH, Munich, Germany) are useful for detecting clinically relevant hemostatic alterations in surgical and trauma patients with critical bleeding and diffuse coagulopathy [31, 32]. Viscoelastic monitoring has been much more widely used in Europe than in the United States, both for perioperative and ICU management of the hemorrhagic patients [3, 33, 34]. In the recent published ESA Guidelines on Perioperative Bleeding Management, the authors suggest the use of viscoelastic tests (ROTEM/TEG) for monitoring perioperative hemostatic function in major orthopedic surgery and neurosurgery (Grade of Evidence: 2C), as well as a recommendation in visceral and transplant surgery for a targeted coagulation disorders management (Grade of Evidence: 1C) [7].

11.5.2 Burn Injury

Severe burn injury (burned body surface area >15 % in adult and >10 % in children) triggers a SIRS with serious metabolic derangements. One of the best known systemic manifestations evidenced in the first hours after a major burn trauma is related to systemic microcirculation damage with increased capillary permeability and protein leakage into the interstitial space, with clinical evidence of huge generalized edema and hemodynamic features of hypovolemic shock. Adequate fluid replacement is mandatory in the first hours after a traumatic burn. However, in burn patients other systemic disorders are also accompanied by SIRS such as cardiac dysfunction, acute respiratory distress syndrome, acute renal failure, increased intestinal permeability resulting in bacterial translocation, hypermetabolism, hypercatabolism and sepsis [35]. These severe alterations in homeostatic balance may escalate in multiple organ failure (MOF) and death. Therefore, research seeking new mechanisms by which to attenuate inflammation after severe burn injury is urgently needed. The goal for early excision of burns is the reduction in release of inflammatory mediators and bacterial colonization of wounds. This currently worldwide adopted strategy can attenuate SIRS phenomena and reduce the incidence of metabolic derangements, sepsis and multiorgan failure. Once performed as early as possible, excisions and immediate wound closure have shown an improvement in survival, with a decrease in ICU and hospital length of stay [36]. Once activated, inflammation and coagulation systems in septic burn patients can definitively lead to increased mortality [37]. Coagulation system derangements during the early phases of burn injury are characterized by activation of procoagulation pathways, enhanced fibrinolysis and consumption of natural anticoagulant factors. Both the thrombotic and fibrinolytic pathways are triggered proportionally to the degree and the extent of the burn [38–40]. Conflicting results about a possible, early acute burn-induced coagulopathy with similarities to TIC are reported. Sherren and associates showed that, in major burns, the dysfunction of the procoagulant, anticoagulant and fibrinolytic pathways may occur early [41], arguing that, to date, the existent trials were focused on the incidence and the time course of DIC and a hypercoagulable state. The initial coagulation test reported values referred to the first 24–36 h; therefore, if any laboratory evidence of the coagulation derangements was observed, it was often delayed [42, 43]. Lu and associates found in their single-center, retrospective study that the screening hematologic profile of burn patients at admission was normal and the standard screening assays did not suggest the existence of an admission coagulopathy analogous to TIC [44]. The current trend for increased survival in burn patients has been attributed to various improvements in care, including early total burn wound excision and grafting, both with dedicated intensive care units and an improved infection control due to a more coordinated multidisciplinary approach [45, 46]. A major challenge for the anesthesiologists regards blood loss and transfusion management during early burn wound excision. The surgical approach is often associated with severe bleeding [47]. Despite multiple attempts to reduce blood losses, patients still need large amounts of allogeneic blood products both with blood derivatives (red blood cells, FFP, platelet concentrates and coagulation factor concentrates) [48–50]. Schaden and associates reported data from a prospective, single-center, randomized study focused on the management of coagulation disorders through a treatment algorithm centered on POC (ROTEM) evaluation, aiming at reduction of allogeneic blood products transfusions during surgical burn wound excisions [51]. The primary endpoint was the evaluation of the cumulative transfused number of allogeneic blood units on the day of surgery. Given the limitations due to the power of the study, a significant decrease in blood product transfusions was observed in the ROTEM-based algorithm group. No FFP was administered in the algorithm group. Low fibrinogen levels or hyperfibrinolysis was not significant pathomechanisms requiring goal-directed treatment.

11.5.3 Severe Sepsis

Hemostatic derangements represent a common early event in patients with severe sepsis. Sepsis is characterized by a procoagulant state and the resultant hypercoagulability may lead in the most severe cases to DIC. An excessive activation of the coagulation system involves platelets and coagulation factor consumption, which may shift the hypercoagulant state into a hypocoagulant state, ultimately leading to the hemorrhagic complications [52].

For the diagnosis of DIC, a simple scoring system has been developed from the International Society of Thrombosis and Haemostasis, which can be adopted and repeated daily for the management of these patients [11].

In clinical practice, it is well known that commonly used biomarkers of sepsis such as procalcitonin and interleukin-6 (IL-6) may also increase in patients with trauma or surgery even without infection. However, thromboelastometry variables may play a potential role as early coagulopathy biomarkers in critical septic patients [53]. Adamzik and associates [54] reported in their observational cohort study (56 patients with severe sepsis and 52 patients after major surgery) that the thromboelastometry-derived lysis index was a more reliable biomarker of severe sepsis compared with procalcitonin, IL-6 and C-reactive protein. More interestingly, a multivariate analysis of another cohort study of 98 septic patients evidenced that the absence or presence of at least one pathological thromboelastometry variable allowed better prediction of 30-day survival in severe sepsis, compared with the simplified acute physiology system (SAPS) II and sequential organ failure assessment (SOFA) scores [55]. This again highlights the relevance of the coagulation system and the possible role in the next future of POC techniques in critical septic patients. In a very recent multicenter prospective observational study, Haase and associates investigated the outcome in patients with severe sepsis evaluated with repeated TEG measurements (standard TEG and functional fibrinogen) [56]. This was a subgroup of the 6S Trial, comparing hydroxyethyl starch (HES) vs. Ringer's acetate as fluid resuscitation in severe septic patients [57]. Two hundred sixty patients were assessed consecutively for 5 days, and data including death and bleeding were retrieved from the original databases. For all TEG variables, a hypocoagulability state was significantly associated with an increased risk of death. Patients treated with HES had lower values of functional fibrinogen maximum amplitude compared with patients who received Ringer's acetate with a consistent increased risk of bleeding (hazard ratio 2.43, 95 % CI 1.16–5.07). However, to date, a clear relationship between viscoelastic test variables and clinically relevant outcomes such as hemorrhage and mortality has not yet been demonstrated in patients with sepsis, because previous published studies were relatively low powered and only few made sequential measurements [58].

11.6 Therapeutical Options in Managing Coagulopathies in ICU Patients

The cornerstone of the therapeutical strategies in managing coagulopathy in the critical patients is that transfusional decisions should not be based only on coagulation test results, rather being guided by global clinical evaluation and possibly through an individualized approach. In a stable patient with no clinical signs of an ongoing bleeding, an unexpected abnormal coagulation test result must be repeated, in order to exclude possible sampling and/or laboratory errors.

The need to transfuse allogeneic blood products and/or blood derivatives is indicated for patients who are actively bleeding; actually, limited data exist regarding a prophylactic use of blood products in order to prevent a possible hemorrhage [2, 15]. Moreover, the very recent Practice Guidelines for Perioperative Blood Management by the ASA Task Force on Perioperative Blood Management emphasized new evidences including preoperative evaluation, assessment for transfusion risk and the use of adjunctive therapies to prevent and/or to treat bleeding [59]. These updated ASA guidelines promote the use of transfusion algorithms, in particular those based on thromboelastographic evaluations, blood ordering schedules and restrictive transfusion regimens. They advocate for implementing the adoption of pharmacologic therapies aiming to reduce allogeneic blood transfusions, using alternatives like coagulation factors concentrates (e.g. prothrombin complex concentrate) for rapid reversal of vitamin K antagonists or antifibrinolytic drugs during selected cardiac and noncardiac procedures with a high risk of bleeding.

A brief overview on the principal therapeutical options as blood components and blood derivates used in treating coagulopathy in the bleeding ICU patients is presented.

11.6.1 Fresh Frozen Plasma (FFP)

Transfusions with FFP are increased in recent years, with a usage up to 39 % of all patients admitted in the ICU [60, 61]. The most common clinical indications for FFP transfusion are prolonged PT or aPTT coagulation tests, meaning a decrease in coagulation factors with a major contribution and an increased risk for bleeding. FFP transfusion is able to increase the levels of coagulation factors normalizing coagulation tests and decreasing bleeding [62]. However, several observations should be applied to these rationales. A reduction in coagulation factor levels can increase the risk of bleeding but only when coagulation factors activity decreases below the minimum hemostatic threshold of 30 %, which correlates with an INR >1.7 [63]. FFP transfusions increase coagulation factor levels, but the effect on the laboratory tests (INR and aPTT) depends on two factors: the amount of transfused FFP (which is quite large to reach an effective result) and the degree of the coagulopathy [60]. Finally, a recent systematic review of 80 randomized trials failed to identify any evidence of effectiveness for FFP [64].

For the use of FFP in critical ill patients see indications, mode of uses and possible adverse events in published guidelines [7, 9, 59], reviews on this topic [2, 4] and in Chap. 6 of this manual.

11.6.2 Thrombocytopenia and Platelet Dysfunction

For thrombocytopenia, the main trigger for transfusion occurs in approximately 35–45 % of the ICU patients; approximately, 15–30 % of patients who develop thrombocytopenia in the ICU will receive platelet concentrates [65, 66].

The rationales for transfusion of platelets in the critically ill patient are (1) a therapeutic intervention to stop bleeding, (2) prophylactically prior to a surgical intervention or (3) for patients at a high suspicion of bleeding risk including those with combined coagulation deficits, platelet dysfunction due to treatment with antiplatelet agents or renal disease.

However, other concomitant factors may increase the bleeding risk in the critical patients due to the presence of other coagulation abnormalities or DIC, uremia, continuous renal replacement therapy in case of renal failure, as well as medications like antiplatelet drugs that may interfere with platelet function [67].

A failure to increase platelet count after platelet concentrate transfusions may be due to the presence of antiplatelet antibodies; however, these are unlikely in patients who have not been previously transfused. In the critically ill, the commonest reason for the platelet count not to increase is due to the ongoing consumption either by hemorrhage or thrombosis. Heparin-induced thrombocytopenia (HIT) is a rare, adverse drug reaction caused by heparin. It is a prothrombotic disorder which can lead to a worse outcome when a delay in diagnosis occurs. The treating team and hematologist must have a high index of suspicion to facilitate diagnosis and treatment. The pathophysiology of HIT centers on the development of pathological antibodies to the combination of heparin and platelet factor 4 (PF4). These antibodies activate platelets, triggering the release of their procoagulant substances and precipitating the development of pathological thrombus [15]. The timing of onset of the thrombocytopenia is of key importance, with classical onset HIT occurring between 5 and 10 days after heparin has been initiated. The treatment consists in stopping heparin and start an alternative anticoagulation (e.g. fondaparinux or a direct thrombin inhibitor).

Desmopressin (DDAVP, 1-deamino-8-D-arginine vasopressin) enhances platelet adherence and platelet aggregation on human subendothelium and is the first choice in the treatment of bleeding in patients with von Willebrand disease. Its use at a dose of 0.3 μg/kg has been recommended in patients treated with antiplatelet drugs, suffering from intracerebral bleeding and in trauma patients with von Willebrand disease (Grade 2C) [9].

11.6.3 Fibrinogen Supplementation

In some countries (the United States and United Kingdom among others) cryoprecipitate is the first-line product to supplement fibrinogen. Cryoprecipitate is rich in fibrinogen factor VIII, vWF (von Willebrand Factor), fibronectin and factor XIII. A standard transfusion of two bags of cryoprecipitate is expected to increase the fibrinogen concentration by 0.5–1 g/l. The transfusion of cryoprecipitate is appropriate when a patient is bleeding and the fibrinogen level is below 1.5 g/l [68]. There are no randomized controlled trials on the use of cryoprecipitate and the recommendations are based on expert opinion. Fibrinogen concentrate is produced from pooled donor plasma, and during manufacturing, it undergoes several steps designed to produce viral inactivation [69]. Its usage appears appealing in several clinical settings with critical bleeding like severe trauma and postpartum hemorrhage (PPH) (see Chaps. 7 and 9).

11.6.4 Prothrombin Complex Concentrate (PCC)

If coagulopathy persists even after fibrinogen supplementation and if the INR is >1.4 or if viscoelastic measures reveal a deficiency of coagulation factors, then substitution of these is indicated. A dosage of FFP 15–30 ml/kg is necessary to increase their concentration. However, the use of a prothrombin complex concentrate, depending on different production techniques (as a three-factor or four-factor) marketed forms. In the four-factor form, PCC contains factors II, VII, IX and X, proteins C and S, heparin and antithrombin; it represents an attractive alternative to FFP because of the smaller volumes required to supplement the deficiency [70].

Moreover, the use of PCC as a rapid reversal of vitamin K antagonist in case of ongoing bleeding when an urgent surgery or an interventional procedure is indicated has been claimed. Its use has been advocated also in case of bleeding as rapid reversal of the novel anticoagulant drugs [71–73], however with limited evidence of efficacy.

11.6.5 Recombinant Activated Factor VII (rFVIIa) and Factor XIII (FXIII)

If the coagulopathy persists with an ongoing bleeding and surgical causes have been ruled out, *off-label* use of two additional coagulation factor concentrates such as human recombinant activated factor VII (rFVIIa) and factor XIII (FXIII) may represent an "extrema ratio" therapeutic approach. As an additional pro-hemostatic agent, rFVIIa has undergone an ever-increasing *off-label* use within the first 10 years of its approval for treatment of hemophilia patients with inhibitors. Administration of recombinant factor VIIa (90 μg/kg) induces a so-called thrombin burst. As a "last-ditch" attempt of the therapy algorithm, this approach may potentially reverse life-threatening coagulopathy. However, several conditions, such as pH ≥7.2, fibrinogen concentration >150 mg/dl, platelet count >50,000/μl, hematocrit ≥25 %, ionized calcium concentration >1 mmol/l and body temperature >36 °C should be reached, before factor VIIa be administered. Moreover, as highlighted in a recent systematic review, the effectiveness of recombinant factor VIIa in reducing perioperative bleeding and the transfusion rate of blood products remains controversial [74].

Factor XIII (FXIII) enhances blood clot stability by cross-linking fibrin monomers and integrating alpha 2-antiplasmin into developing clots. There is no routinely available test parameter for factor XIII deficiency. In addition, there are currently no standardized reference values. However, especially in diffuse bleeding, factor XIII substitution (15–30 IU/kg) may be indicated as a "last ditch" to achieve a factor XIII activity above 60–70 % [75].

Conclusion

Coagulopathy is very common in the critically ill patients once admitted in ICU in several clinical settings. Blood product support is frequently required, but there are very limited evidence-based data to support their use. Clinicians should try to collect all the possibly available data at the bedside, aiming to approach these bleeding patients in goal-directed fashion guided by a rapid viscoelastic analysis through POC devices. In many cases, as the so-called magic bullet does not exist to date, no specific product support is required and the core management approach is the treatment of the underlying condition(s) triggering and sustaining the coagulopathy itself. Further basic researches and well-built clinical studies are urgently warranted to assure the best diagnostic approaches (e.g. POC techniques) and the optimal goal-directed treatment(s) for these patients. POC tests themselves are an integral part of a Patient Blood Management program [76] and the future studies should aim to demonstrate that hemostatic therapies, based on POC algorithms, are beneficial in improving the outcome of the critical care patients.

References

1. Levi M, Opal SM (2006) Coagulation abnormalities in critically ill patients. Crit Care 10:222
2. Hunt BJ (2014) Bleeding and coagulopathies in critical care. N Engl J Med 370:847–859

3. Levy JH, Faraoni D, Sniecinski RM (2013) Perioperative coagulation management in the intensive care unit. Curr Opin Anaesthesiol 26:65–70
4. Kozek-Langenecker SA (2014) Coagulation and transfusion in the postoperative bleeding patient. Curr Opin Crit Care 20:460–466
5. Glance LG, Dick AW, Mukamel DB et al (2011) Association between intraoperative blood transfusion and mortality and morbidity in patients undergoing noncardiac surgery. Anesthesiology 114:283–292
6. Toulon P, Ozier Y, Ankri A, Fléron MH, Leroux G, Samama CM (2009) Point-of-care versus central laboratory coagulation testing during haemorrhagic surgery. A multicenter study. Thromb Haemost 101:394–401
7. Kozek-Langenecker SA, Afshari A, Albaladejo P et al (2013) Management of severe perioperative bleeding: guidelines from the European Society of Anaesthesiology. Eur J Anaesthesiol 30:270–382
8. Haas T, Fries D, Tanaka KA, Asmis L, Curry NS, Schöchl H (2015) Usefulness of standard plasma coagulation tests in the management of perioperative coagulopathic bleeding: is there any evidence? Br J Anaesth 114:217–224
9. Spahn D, Bouillon B, Cerny V et al (2013) Management of bleeding and coagulopathy following major trauma: an updated European guideline. Crit Care 17:R76
10. Schochl H, Schlimp CJ, Voelckel W (2013) Potential value of pharmacological protocols in trauma. Curr Opin Anaesthesiol 26:221–229
11. Levi M, van der Poll T (2013) Disseminated intravascular coagulation: a review for the internist. Intern Emerg Med 8:23–32
12. Gorlinger K, Bergmann L, Dirkmann D (2012) Coagulation management in patients undergoing mechanical circulatory support. Best Pract Res Clin Anaesthesiol 26:179–198
13. Esper SA, Levy JH, Waters JH, Welsby IJ (2014) Extracorporeal membrane oxygenation in the adult: a review of anticoagulation monitoring and transfusion. Anesth Analg 118:731–743
14. Kozek-Langenecker S (2007) Management of massive operative blood loss. Minerva Anestesiol 73:401–415
15. Retter A, Barrett NA (2015) The management of abnormal haemostasis in the ICU. Anaesthesia 70(S1):121–127
16. Hartert H (1951) Thrombelastography, a method for physical analysis of blood coagulation. Z Gesamte Exp Med 117:189–203
17. Bolliger D, Seeberger MD, Tanaka KA (2012) Principles and practice of thromboelastography in clinical coagulation management and transfusion practice. Transfus Med Rev 26:1–13
18. Esmon CT, Xu J, Lupu F (2011) Innate immunity and coagulation. J Thromb Haemost 9(Suppl 1):182–188
19. Fu BM, Tarbell JM (2013) Mechano-sensing and transduction by endothelial surface glycocalyx: composition, structure, and function. WIREs Syst Biol Med. doi:10.1002/wsbm.1211
20. Bianchi ME (2007) DAMPs, PAMPs and alarmins: all we need to know about danger. J Leukoc Biol 81:1–5
21. Levi M, van der Poll T (2010) Inflammation and coagulation. Crit Care Med 38(Suppl 2):S26–S34
22. Petaja J (2011) Inflammation and coagulation. An overview. Thromb Res 127(Suppl 2):S34–S37
23. Marik PE, Flemmer M (2012) The immune response to surgery and trauma: implications for treatment. J Trauma Acute Care Surg 73:801–808
24. Xiao W, Mindrinos MN, Seok J et al (2011) A genomic storm in critically injured humans. J Exp Med 208:2581–2590
25. Maegele M, Lefering R, Yucel N et al (2007) Early coagulopathy in multiple injury: an analysis from the German Trauma Registry on 8724 patients. Injury 38:298–304
26. Sarani B, Dunkman WJ, Dean L, Sonnad S, Rohrbach JI, Gracias VH (2008) Transfusion of fresh frozen plasma in critically ill surgical patients is associated with an increased risk of infection. Crit Care Med 36:1114–1118
27. Watson GA, Sperry JL, Rosengart MR et al (2009) Inflammation and Host Response to Injury Investigators: fresh frozen plasma is independently associated with a higher risk of multiple organ failure and acute respiratory distress syndrome. J Trauma 67:221–227
28. Shere-Wolfe RF, Galvagno SM Jr, Grissom TE (2012) Critical care considerations in the management of the trauma patient following initial resuscitation. Scand J Trauma Resusc Emerg Med 20:68–83
29. Moore FA, Moore EE, Sauaia A (1997) Blood transfusion. An independent risk factor for postinjury multiple organ failure. Arch Surg 132:620–624
30. Johansson PI, Stensballe J, Vindelov N, Perner A, Espersen K (2010) Hypocoagulability, as evaluated by thrombelastography, at admission to the ICU is associated with increased 30-day mortality. Blood Coagul Fibrinolysis 21:168–174
31. Johansson PI, Stissing T, Bochsen L, Ostrowski SR (2009) Thrombelastography and tromboelastometry in assessing coagulopathy in trauma. Scand J Trauma Resusc Emerg Med 17:45
32. Levi M, Fries D, Gombotz H et al (2011) Prevention and treatment of coagulopathy in patient receiving massive transfusions. Vox Sang 101:154–174
33. Teodoro da Luz L, Nascimento B, Rizoli S (2013) Thrombelastography (TEG): practical considerations on its clinical use in trauma resuscitation. Scand J Trauma Resusc Emerg Med 21:29–36
34. Jakoi A, Kumar N, Vaccaro A, Radcliff K (2014) Perioperative coagulopathy monitoring. Musculoskelet Surg 98:1–8
35. Farina JA Jr, Rosique MJ, Rosique RG (2013) Curbing inflammation in burn patients. Int J Inflam; Article ID 715645, http://dx.doi.org/10.1155/2013/715645
36. Ong YS, Samuel M, Song C (2006) Meta-analysis of early excision of burns. Burns 32:145–150

37. Lavrentieva A, Kontakiotis T, Bitzani M et al (2008) Early coagulation disorders after severe burn injury: impact on mortality. Intensive Care Med 34:700–706
38. Lippi G, Ippolito L, Cervellin G (2010) Disseminated intravascular coagulation in burn injury. Semin Thromb Hemost 36:429–436
39. Niedermayr M, Schramm W, Kamolz L et al (2007) Antithrombin deficiency and its relationship to severe burns. Burns 33:173–178
40. Kowal-Vern A, Gamelli RL, Walenga JM, Hoppensteadt D, Sharp-Pucci M, Schumacher HR (1992) The effect of burn wound size on hemostasis: a correlation of the hemostatic changes to the clinical state. J Trauma 33:50–56
41. Sherren PB, Hussey J, Martin R, Kundishora T, Parker M, Emerson B (2013) Acute burn induced coagulopathy. Burns 39:1157–1161
42. King DR, Namias N, Andrews DM (2010) Coagulation abnormalities following thermal injury. Blood Coagul Fibrinolysis 21:666–669
43. Garcia-Avello A, Lorente JA, Cesar-Perez J et al (1998) Degree of hypercoagulability and hyperfibrinolysis is related to organ failure and prognosis after burn trauma. Thromb Res 89:59–64
44. Lu RP, Ni A, Lin FC et al (2013) Major burn injury is not associated with acute traumatic coagulopathy. J Trauma Acute Care Surg 74:1474–1479
45. Latenser BA (2009) Critical care of the burn patient: the first 48 h. Crit Care Med 37:2819–2826
46. Hendon DN (2003) Total burn care, vol 3. Saunders, London
47. Sterling JP, Heimbach DM (2011) Hemostasis in burn surgery: a review. Burns 37:559–565
48. Cartotto R, Musgrave MA, Beveridge M, Fish J, Gomez M (2000) Minimizing blood loss in burn surgery. J Trauma 49:1034–1049
49. O'Mara MS, Hayetian F, Slater H, Goldfarb IW, Tolchin E, Caushaj PF (2005) Results of a protocol of transfusion threshold and surgical technique on transfusion requirements in burn patients. Burns 13:558–561
50. Johansson PI, Eriksen K, Nielsen SL, Rojkjaer R, Alsbjørn B (2007) Recombinant FVIIa decreases perioperative blood transfusion requirement in burn patient undergoing excision and skin grafting—results of a single centre pilot study. Burns 33:435–440
51. Schaden E, Kimberger O, Kraincuk P, Baron DM, Metnitz PG, Kozek-Langenecker S (2012) Perioperative treatment algorithm for bleeding burn patients reduces allogeneic blood product requirements. Br J Anaesth 109:376–381
52. Levi M (2008) The coagulant response in sepsis. Clin Chest Med 29:627–642
53. Meybohm P, Zacharowski K, Weber CF (2013) Point-of-care coagulation management in intensive care medicine. Crit Care 17:218, http://ccforum.com/content/17/2/218
54. Adamzik M, Eggmann M, Frey UH et al (2010) Comparison of thromboelastometry with procalcitonin, interleukin 6, and C-reactive protein as diagnostic tests for severe sepsis in critically ill adults. Crit Care 14:R178
55. Adamzik M, Langemeier T, Frey UH et al (2011) Comparison of thrombelastometry with simplified acute physiology score II and sequential organ failure assessment scores for the prediction of 30-day survival: a cohort study. Shock 35:339–342
56. Haase N, Ostrowski SR, Wetterslev J et al (2015) Thromboelastography in patients with severe sepsis: a prospective cohort study. Intensive Care Med 41:77–85
57. Perner A, Haase N, Guttormsen AB et al (2012) Hydroxyethyl starch 130/0.42 versus Ringer's acetate in severe sepsis. N Engl J Med 367:124–134
58. Muller MC, Meijers JC, Vroom MB, Juffermans NP (2014) Utility of thromboelastography and/or thromboelastometry in adults with sepsis: a systematic review. Crit Care 18:R30
59. American Society of Anesthesiologists Task Force on Perioperative Blood Management Practice Guidelines for Perioperative Blood Management (2015) An Updated Report by the American Society of Anesthesiologists Task Force on Perioperative Blood Management. Anesthesiology 122:241–275
60. Stanworth SJ, Walsh TS, Prescott RJ et al (2011) A national study of plasma use in critical care: clinical indications, dose and effect on prothrombin time. Crit Care 15:R108
61. Vlaar AP, in der Maur AL, Binnekade JM, Schultz MJ, Juffermans NP (2009) A survey of physicians' reasons to transfuse plasma and platelets in the critically ill: a prospective single-centre cohort study. Transfus Med 19:207–212
62. McIntyre L, Tinmouth AT, Fergusson DA (2013) Blood component transfusion in critically ill patients. Curr Opin Crit Care 19:326–333
63. Callum JL, Dzik WH (2010) The use of blood components prior to invasive bedside procedures: a critical appraisal. In: Mintz PD (ed) Transfusion therapy: clinical principles and practice, 3rd edn. AABB Press, Bethesda, pp 1–36
64. Yang L, Stanworth S, Hopewell S, Doree C, Murphy M (2012) Is fresh-frozen plasma clinically and effective? An update of a systematic review of randomized controlled trials. Transfusion 52:1673–1686
65. Arnold DM, Crowther MA, Cook RJ et al (2006) Utilization of platelet transfusions in the intensive care unit: indications, transfusion triggers, and platelet count responses. Transfusion 46:1286–1291
66. Nydam TL, Kashuk JL, Moore EE et al (2011) Refractory postinjury thrombocytopenia is associated with multiple organ failure and adverse outcomes. J Trauma 70:401–406
67. Gajic O, Dzik WH, Toy P (2006) Fresh frozen plasma and platelet transfusion for nonbleeding patients in the intensive care unit: benefit or harm? Crit Care Med 34:S170–S173

68. Nascimento B, Rizoli S, Rubenfeld G et al (2011) Cryoprecipitate transfusion: assessing appropriateness and dosing in trauma. Transfus Med 21:394–401
69. Franchini M, Lippi G (2012) Fibrinogen replacement therapy: a critical review of the literature. Blood Transfus 10:23–27
70. Sorensen B, Spahn DR, Innerhofer P, Spannagl M, Rossaint R (2011) Clinical review: prothrombin complex concentrates – evaluation of safety and thrombogenicity. Crit Care 15:201
71. Patanwala AE, Acquisto NM, Erstad BL (2011) Prothrombin complex concentrate for critical bleeding. Ann Pharmacother 45:990–999
72. Levy JH, Levi M (2014) New oral anticoagulant–induced bleeding. Clinical presentation and management. Clin Lab Med 34:575–586
73. Moorman ML, Nash JE, Stabi KL (2014) Emergency surgery and trauma in patients treated with the new oral anticoagulants: dabigatran, rivaroxaban, and apixaban. J Trauma Acute Care Surg 77:486–494
74. Yank V, Tuohy CV, Logan AC et al (2011) Systematic review: benefits and harms of in-hospital use of recombinant factor VIIa for off-label indications. Ann Intern Med 154:529–540
75. Korte W (2010) FXIII in perioperative coagulation management. Best Pract Res Clin Anaesthesiol 24:85–93
76. Shander A, Van Aken H, Colomina MJ et al (2012) Patient blood management in Europe. Br J Anaesth 109:55–68

Assessment of the Effects of Antithrombotic Drugs

12

Blanca Martinez, Ekaterina Baryshnikova, Maria Lucia Bindi, and Domenico Prisco

12.1 Introduction

One of the main causes involved in acquired hemorrhagic disturbs are the side effects of antithrombotic drugs that can lead to bleeding complications due to overdosage or accumulation or contribute to worsening a bleeding status triggered by other causes like surgery or trauma. Bleeding is the major adverse reaction to anticoagulants, leading to significant morbidity and even mortality [1]. Moreover, one of the most challenging aspects of antithrombotic drugs management is their capability to be monitored in order to establish their adequate anticoagulant effect protecting versus thrombosis and to be able to modulate their dosage quickly in case of overdosage or to reverse their action in case of life-threatening bleeding or schedule for an emergency procedure.

Recently, several efforts have been made to create point-of-care versions of the main laboratory test routinely used to monitor antithrombotic drugs. Furthermore, viscoelastic tests (VET) (i.e., TEG® and ROTEM®) that are currently widely used to detect global coagulation changes and guide blood product replacement in cardiac and liver surgery perioperative context, trauma, and peripartum settings have been increasingly tested to monitor the effect of anticoagulants bedside.

Actually, there are not many evidences regarding the monitoring of the majority of the antithrombotic drugs supported by large clinical randomized trials involving patients assuming these drugs and affected by bleeding complications. Therefore, to date, the current available recommendations are given from small in vitro studies and experts' opinion.

In the following sections the authors will expose the point-of-care tests to monitor the anticoagulant action of the main antithrombotic drugs currently available on the market. The laboratory POC monitoring of the effect of antiplatelet drugs has been study in deep in previous chapters.

B. Martinez, MD (✉)
Department of Anesthesiology and Intensive Care Medicine, Santa Maria della Misericordia University Hospital, Udine, Italy
e-mail: martinez.blanca@aoud.sanita.fvg.it

E. Baryshnikova, PhD
Department of Cardiothoracic-Vascular Anesthesia and ICU, IRCCS Policlinico San Donato, San Donato Milanese, Milan, Italy

M.L. Bindi, MD
Liver Transplant Anaesthesia and Critical Care, Azienda Ospedaliera Universitaria Pisana, Pisa, Italy

D. Prisco, MD, PhD
Department of Experimental and Clinical Medicine, University of Florence; Careggi University Hospital, Florence, Italy

M. Ranucci, P. Simioni (eds.), *Point-of-Care Tests for Severe Hemorrhage: A Manual for Diagnosis and Treatment*, DOI 10.1007/978-3-319-24795-3_12

12.2 Heparin

Unfractionated heparin (UFH) is a heterogeneous mixture of branched glycosaminoglycans that acts as antithrombotic drug by means of an endogenous cofactor named antithrombin (AT). Heparin exerts its anticoagulant effect by binding to lysine sites on AT, modifying AT from a slow to a very rapid and powerful thrombin inhibitor [2].

The heparin-AT complex inactivates thrombin factor (IIa), factors Xa, IXa, XIa, and XIIa. Thrombin is about tenfold more sensitive to inhibition than factor Xa. Moreover, by inhibiting thrombin, heparin also inhibits thrombin-induced activation of factor V and factor VIII. Heparin presents other AT-independent anticoagulants effects. It induces secretion of tissue factor pathway inhibitor (TFPI) by vascular endothelial cells that reduce procoagulant activity of TF-fVIIa complex and release of tPA from endothelial cells, triggering hyperfibrinolysis.

Heparin is heterogeneous with respect to molecular size, anticoagulant activity, and pharmacokinetic properties, and its clearance is influenced by the chain length of the molecules. This differential clearance (the rapid plasmatic saturable route versus the slow non-saturable renal route) results in accumulation in vivo of the lower-molecular-weight species, which have a higher ratio of antifactor Xa to antifactor IIa activity [3].

Despite its imperfect profile due to its heterogeneous molecular size, anticoagulant activity, and pharmacokinetic profile [2, 4, 5], heparin still remains the gold standard for systemic anticoagulation in different settings such as cardiac surgery due to several advantages. First, it presents a short onset time and half-life, and secondly, its neutralization is possible by protamine. The main drawbacks of heparin are its high interindividual variability and the potential heparin rebound after adequate antagonization with protamine due to heparin release from certain tissues and due to shorter half-life of protamine than heparin [2].

Its pharmacokinetic characteristics and its dependency on the presence of antithrombin cause a high interindividual variability of heparin anticoagulant effect leading to numerous modification of heparin velocity of infusion with a risk of under- and overdosage that could produce dangerous thrombotic and bleeding complications, respectively.

Several assays are today available to monitor the UFH anticoagulant effect in laboratories and bedside. Point-of-care tests (POCT) are able to shorten the time to have a result leading to clinical decisions. They are mainly used in cardiac angiography laboratories, during cardiopulmonary bypass, and in critically ill patients admitted to intensive care units.

The POC tests to monitor UFH are based on activated partial thromboplastin time (aPTT), activated clotting time (ACT), and heparin concentration measurement.

12.2.1 Activated Partial Thromboplastin Time

The aPTT is a laboratory coagulation test that explores the intrinsic and common pathway. It is a modification of the partial thromboplastin time (PTT) that was first described in 1953 to detect clotting factors deficiencies in hemophiliacs [6]. Phospholipids without tissue factor associated to a particular matter such as kaolin, celite, and others are added to recalcified plasma to trigger a clot formation that is detected using an electromechanical or photo-optical device. It represents the in vitro analysis of coagulation factors of the intrinsic and common pathways. The aPTT is the suggested test to monitor the effect of heparin therapy in low ranges [2, 7].

Prolongation of the aPTT by 1.5–2.5 times the upper limit of the normal reference range is generally considered therapeutic, and the aim is to reach an aPTT of 1.5 times the upper limit of the normal range within 24 h [8]. It also exists in point-of-care versions.

Notwithstanding, several limits of heparin monitoring by aPTT have been described. Firstly, aPTT has a lack of specificity for heparin effects. Falsely prolonged aPTT due to short draw and in polycythemic patients (hematocrit >60 %) can be observed. Besides, concomitant deficiencies or presence of inhibitors of the intrinsic and common pathways factors and congenital disorders (lupus-like antibodies, antiphospholipid syndrome, etc.) can prolong aPTT. Acute phase high levels of fVIII can shorten the aPTT, despite the presence of heparin [8]. Secondly, the aPTT is a highly variable test that produces inconsistent results for several reasons. Significantly different aPTT results have been observed with different instruments, reagents, and different lots of the same reagent implying difficulties in standardization. To overcome this problem, some authors have suggested to express the aPTT result as a ratio of the aPTT. This issue still remains controversial because therapeutic heparin concentrations determined by factor Xa inhibition (0.3–0.7 antifactor Xa units) correspond to different aPTT ratio ranges. Consequently, the use of a standard aPTT therapeutic range of 1.5–2.5 for all reagents and instruments leads to the systematic administration of subtherapeutic doses of heparin [2, 9]. According to other authors, the therapeutic range for each aPTT reagent should be reported in seconds and calibrated to correspond with heparin serum concentrations of 0.2–0.4 units/mL by protamine titration or antifactor Xa activity of 0.3–0.7 units/mL [10]. It should be recommended that every clinical laboratory calibrate its therapeutic range using a minimum of 30–40 samples from patients receiving heparin [8, 11]. Finally, the aPTT is insensitive to heparin concentrations higher than 1.0 units/mL, so it is not useful to monitor large doses of heparin, such as during cardiopulmonary bypass (CPB) [8, 11].

Several aPTT POC devices are available today on the market. The main devices are GEM Portable Coagulation Laboratory (Instrumentation Laboratory, Lexington, MA), Hemochron 401 (International Technidyne, Edison, NJ), Hemochron Jr. Signature+ (International Technidyne, Edison, NJ), Hemochron Response (International Technidyne, Edison, NJ), and ACT II (Medtronic, Minneapolis, MN). The technical characteristics of each device have been described elsewhere [9].

Spinler and associates [9] analyzed the studies regarding the aPTT POCT, underscoring the inconsistencies between trials even if the same method of measurement was considered. The authors concluded that the aPTT test was associated with significant inherent inaccuracy, and POC testing of the aPTT may heighten this inaccuracy. Performing routine heparin concentrations may be useful albeit complex, to establish a reagent-specific therapeutic range for aPTT. Cuker and associates compared the interlaboratory agreement of the anti-FXa-correlated aPTT with that of the traditional 1.5–2.5 times normal method and concluded that the anti-FXa–correlation method does not seem to improve the interlaboratory agreement in UFH monitoring compared with the traditional 1.5–2.5 times method [12].

Another important aspect is that POC aPTT should not be used interchangeably with standard laboratory assays [13]. Discrepancies between POC aPTT and laboratory assays are due to the nonstandardized nature of aPTT assay itself [9]. In conclusion, clinical application of POC aPTT seems limited at the moment.

12.2.2 Activated Clotting Time

The ACT was first described in 1966 [14] and widely diffused for clinical UFH monitoring in 1980. It measures the antithrombotic (anti-IIa) action of heparin in a whole-blood sample containing an activator of contact phase (kaolin, celite, or glass particles). ACT is the laboratory test most frequently used to measure the anticoagulant effect of high doses of heparin or bivalirudin [15, 16]. It is a point-of-care whole-blood clotting test, performed bedside and expressed in seconds.

ACT and aPTT are not equivalent tests and can lead to discordant clinical decisions [17].

Different technologies according to magnetic, optical, or viscoelastic detection of fibrin are currently available to measure ACT. Generally, whole blood is collected into a tube containing a coagulation activator and a magnetic stir bar. The clot formation interrupts a magnetic field and stops the timer [18].

ACT is typically used to monitor heparin activity during cardiac surgery. However, its use presents several limits. First, during CPB the ACT has been shown to be highly susceptible to variation. It does not correlate well with anti-Xa measures and heparin concentration especially in case of hemodilution, hypothermia and severe thrombocytopenia. Secondly, the type of activator can modify the result of ACT. Celite prolongs ACT in the presence of aprotinin or anti-GPIIb/IIIa drugs [19, 20].

Some authors have observed a good correlation between ACT and plasma heparin concentration after the initial bolus of UFH in cardiac surgery patients population [20]. Nevertheless, after the beginning of cardiopulmonary bypass, this correlation is lost due to the effects of hemodilution, hypothermia, and platelet dysfunction [21, 22]. Besides that, warfarin, aprotinin, and glycoprotein IIb/IIIa receptor inhibitors prolong ACT independently of the heparin presence and amount [23, 24].

Regarding ACT accuracy, correlations between the ACT and heparin concentrations have ranged from 0.24 to 0.98 in different studies. The more significant variability was observed in case of low-range heparin concentrations (0–0.7 IU/mL by antifactor Xa assay) [9]. On the contrary, ACT offers interpretable results in case of high plasma levels of heparin [25].

The main ACT devices currently available on the market are Hemochron Jr. Signature (International Technidyne, Edison, NJ), Hemochron Response and Hemochron 401 (International Technidyne, Edison, NJ), Actalyke XL and Actalyke Mini (Helena Laboratories, Beaumont, TX), ACT Plus Automated Coagulation Timer (Medtronic Biologic Therapeutics and Diagnostic, Minneapolis), Hepcon HMS Plus (Medtronic Perfusion Systems, Minneapolis), and ACT from viscoelastic global test of hemostasis such as ACT RapidTEG (Haemoscope Thrombelastograph® Haemostasis Analyzer TEG®) and kaolin-based ACT test from the Sonoclot® Analyzer (SkACT, Sienco Inc, Arvada, CO). Technical characteristics of each device have been described elsewhere [9, 18, 19, 26].

A main issue is that ACT which results from different instruments may not be interchangeable [9] and, as a consequence, the target ACT range can vary according to the device used [27, 28].

12.2.3 Heparin Concentration Monitoring

The multiple limitations of ACT and the fact that ACT does not correlate well with heparin levels in specific situations like hypothermia or hemodilution during cardiopulmonary bypass have led to develop an alternative strategy to anticoagulation management during cardiac surgery. A combination of ACT with heparin plasmatic levels measurement has been proposed. The most widely available POC systems for measuring heparin levels are the Hepcon HMS Plus (Medtronic Inc., Minneapolis, MN, USA) and the Hemochron Response RxDx System (International Technidyne Corporation) which allow a tailored management of anticoagulation by heparin and protamine titration creating an individualized heparin dose-response curve [29]. The Hepcon HMS Plus uses the protamine titration method to establish the heparin plasma concentration and correlates well with the laboratory anti-Xa values [30]. A strong association ($r=0.74$) between the Hepcon HMS and the anti-Xa plasma heparin has been found [31]. Despotis and associates compared the conventional management of anticoagulation during CPB using ACT or the maintenance of a target heparin plasma concentration as determined by the Hepcon HMS. The heparin concentration method resulted in both larger doses of administered UFH and a lower hemostatic blood products administration because higher concentrations of heparin more effectively suppress coagulation activation and thrombin formation, leading to less consumption of coagulation factors [32]. Noui and associates compared the standard coagulation management during CPB using ACT and the antagonization of heparin dose/dose by protamine with Hepcon HMS. The authors demonstrated that heparin and protamine titration using Hepcon HMS device predicted a lower protamine dose, decreased postoperative bleeding and perioperative red blood cell transfusion rate, and shortened chest closure time [29]. As the protamine/heparin ratio has been described as one of the main factors associated with the postoperative bleeding and transfusion requirements in cardiac surgery [33], this strategy could influence the outcome. On the contrary, other authors have found opposite results with HMS management leading to higher postoperative bleeding, but these studies included small numbers of patients and heterogeneous populations [34, 35]. At the current time, further studies are necessary to establish if these devices can really influence the clinical outcome and are cost-effective [9, 36].

12.2.4 Viscoelastic Hemostatic Assays

In cardiac surgery setting, excessive postoperative bleeding has been frequently associated to insufficient reversal of heparin by protamine after the weaning from CPB, in part due to the routine monitoring of heparin anticoagulation with ACT, which does not differentiate between coagulopathy caused by heparinization, hemodilution, platelet dysfunction, and others [33, 37].

The TEG is the best predictor of trace amounts of heparin [38]. Heparin causes a dose-dependent inhibition of TEG clotting of normal blood [39]. As heparin inhibits thrombin formation, in the presence of heparin the reaction time and the *K*-time of TEG and the CT and CFT of ROTEM are expected to be prolonged. In a study from Coppell and associates [40], UFH prolonged *R*-time at blood concentrations ≥0.25 IU/mL and *K*-time at concentrations ≥0.1 IU/mL. Besides, UFH reduced the α-angle at concentrations ≥0.1 IU/mL and the MA at any concentration. The *R*-time and α-angle were the least sensitive of the TEG parameters to UFH in this study. Overall, TEG has a higher sensitivity than standard laboratory tests as concentrations of heparin of less than 0.1 IU/mL had no effect on PT, aPTT, or thrombin time (TT) assays [40].

In order to discriminate the prolongation of *R*-time due to heparin rebound or insufficient reversal from prolonged *R*-time due to other causes such as lack of coagulation factors, a modified viscoelastic test has been developed. Adding heparinase I to the TEG/ROTEM cuvettes, heparin becomes neutralized allowing to assess the global coagulation status independently of heparin activity [40, 41] (see Fig. 12.1). Inhibition of TEG clotting by heparin is reversed in vitro by both protamine sulfate and heparinase, but heparinase is more effective than protamine sulfate [39, 42].

In the presence of heparin, TEG parameters return within reference ranges if the tests are performed in heparinase-coated cuvettes, suggesting that the enzyme is able to successfully neutralize the anticoagulant effect of UFH [40]. Heparinase-modified TEG is useful to monitor heparin reversal in special clinical settings such as cardiac surgery [43].

Heparinase I is an enzyme derived from the bacterium *Flavobacterium heparinum* that neutralizes heparin by enzymatic cleavage of alpha-glycosidic linkages at the antithrombin-binding site [44, 45]. If heparin activity is identified as the cause of bleeding, reversal with protamine can be performed avoiding unnecessary and potentially harmful blood transfusions.

In addition, heparinase is able to antagonize up to 6 IU/mL of heparin, so during cardiopulmonary bypass, the heparinase-modified thromboelastogram and the HEPTEM test of ROTEM are feasible despite anticoagulation with heparin in doses of 300 IU/kg, giving the chance to early understand the potential hemostatic deficiency regardless of heparin before CBP weaning [45, 46].

Therapeutic UFH affects TEG parameters at lower concentrations than those that affect the PT, aPTT, TT, and ACT and in a dose-dependent fashion. For example, the aPTT is only slightly prolonged at doses of heparin that will completely inhibit TEG clotting. The standard TEG is more sensitive to UFH and low-molecular-weight heparin (LMWH) than most conventional coagulation tests, except the anti-FXa activity. The difference between standard and heparinase-modified TEG parameters increases the sensitivity of the

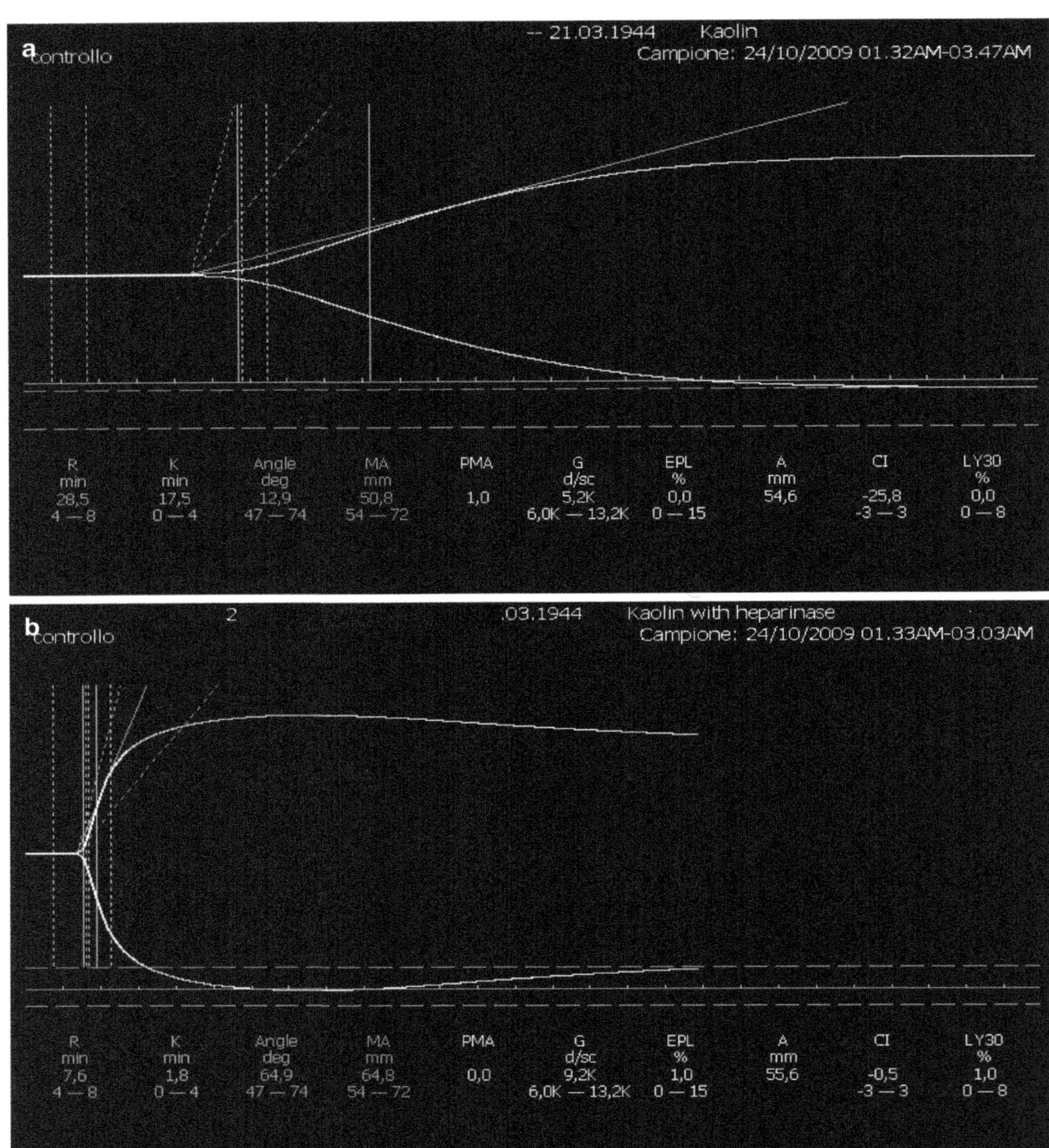

Fig. 12.1 Heparin rebound. Postoperative bleeding in aortic valve replacement. (**a**) Kaolin-TEG trace without heparinase. (**b**) Kaolin-TEG trace with heparinase. The presence of heparinase reduces *R*-time and *K*-time and normalizes alpha angle and MA

assay for the effects of heparins and is more sensitive to very low doses of UFH than anti-FXa activity [40].

The influence of unfractionated heparin on thromboelastometry parameters is markedly stronger than that of the LMWHs [47].

12.2.5 Low-Molecular-Weight Heparin Antithrombotic Effect Monitoring

LMWHs are derived from UFH by chemical or enzymatic depolymerization and have higher antifactor Xa and reduced antifactor IIa activity (in an antifactor Xa/antifactor IIa ratios between 2:1 and 4:1 depending on the type of LMWH). LMWHs present superior pharmacokinetic properties with a more predictable dose-response with respect to UFH due to their reduced binding to plasma proteins, endothelial cells, and macrophages [2]. As a rule, laboratory monitoring is needed when the variation in the individual response to a given drug is so variable that a correlation between dose and standard effect is difficult to predict [48]. The good bioavailability and long half-life of subcutaneous LMWHs provide a predictable anticoagulation effect and consequently routine monitoring of their action is not necessary. However, in special populations prone to overdosing such as pediatric, obese, and pregnant patients and in case of renal insufficiency (creatinine clearance <30 mL/min) LMWH anticoagulant effect is not foreseeable and laboratory measurements are recommended [2], LMWHs do not prolong the assays used to monitor UFH (aPTT and ACT) [49]. The antifactor Xa activity monitored by chromogenic assay is the test currently recommended by the College of American Pathologist [50]. However, this assay is neither standardized nor routinely available universally and around the clock. To overcome this drawback, a point-of-care qualitative test called enoxaparin clotting time has been developed, but currently it is withdrawn from the market [9].

In case of bleeding complications during LMWH therapy a quick bedside qualitative/semiquantitative monitoring able to discriminate the effect of the LMWHs as a major contributor to the hemostatic disturbance could be useful [51]. In this clinical setting, viscoelastic assays have been tested. Coppell and associates have investigated the correlation between the variables of the standard and heparinase-modified TEG with conventional clotting tests (aPTT, TT and antifactor Xa activity) obtained from in vitro citrated samples spiked with increasing amounts of UFH, LMWH, and danaparoid from 0.025 to 1.0 U/mL. The results of this study pointed out that UFH and LMWH (dalteparin) are able to modify the following TEG parameters: the *R*-time, the *K*-time, the α-angle and the MA. In Coppell's study, LMWH prolongs *R*-time at blood concentrations ≥0.5 IU/mL and *K*-time at concentrations ≥0.0025 IU/mL, and reduces α-angle at concentrations ≥0.25 IU/mL and the MA at any concentration. Furthermore, the addition of heparinase neutralizes LMWH and normalizes TEG parameters [40] (see Fig. 12.2).

In case of bleeding due to multiple and dynamic factors, VETs are able not only to establish the contribution of anticoagulants to the coagulation disorder but also to monitor the normalization of hemostasis after a reversal of the drug has been administered [1]. Regarding different LMWH agents, Zmuda and associates showed that enoxaparin caused a dose-dependent inhibition of TEG clotting of normal blood. Abnormal TEG clotting was observed in patients receiving enoxaparin whose plasma level of the drug was more than 0.1 anti-Xa U/mL. However, the degree of TEG abnormality did not always coincide with plasma levels of the agent. The inhibition of TEG clotting by enoxaparin was reversed by protamine sulfate and heparinase [39]. TEG is able to detect the presence of enoxaparin but does not seem an appropriate assay for monitoring adequate enoxaparin antithrombotic therapy. This statement is based on the inconsistent findings for the TEG parameters (reaction time, *K*-time and alpha angle) for plasma levels of anti-Xa activity [39]. Similar results have been pointed out by other authors. White and associates showed that there was no evidence of association between *R* and anti-Xa in patients treated with 1 mg/kg of enoxaparin. In addition, TEG was unable to predict anti-Xa activity. However, TEG *R* was prolonged in more than 90 % patients and showed a correlation with the dose of enoxaparin [52]. These conclusions are not share by other authors. Klien and associates underlined that the *R*-time from thromboelastogram correlates with serum anti-Xa in an orthopedic population treated with enoxaparin [53]. Therefore, the correlation between *R*-time and antifactor Xa in patients treated with LMWH remains still controversial. In order to optimized the thromboelastometric capability to monitor the anticoagulant effects

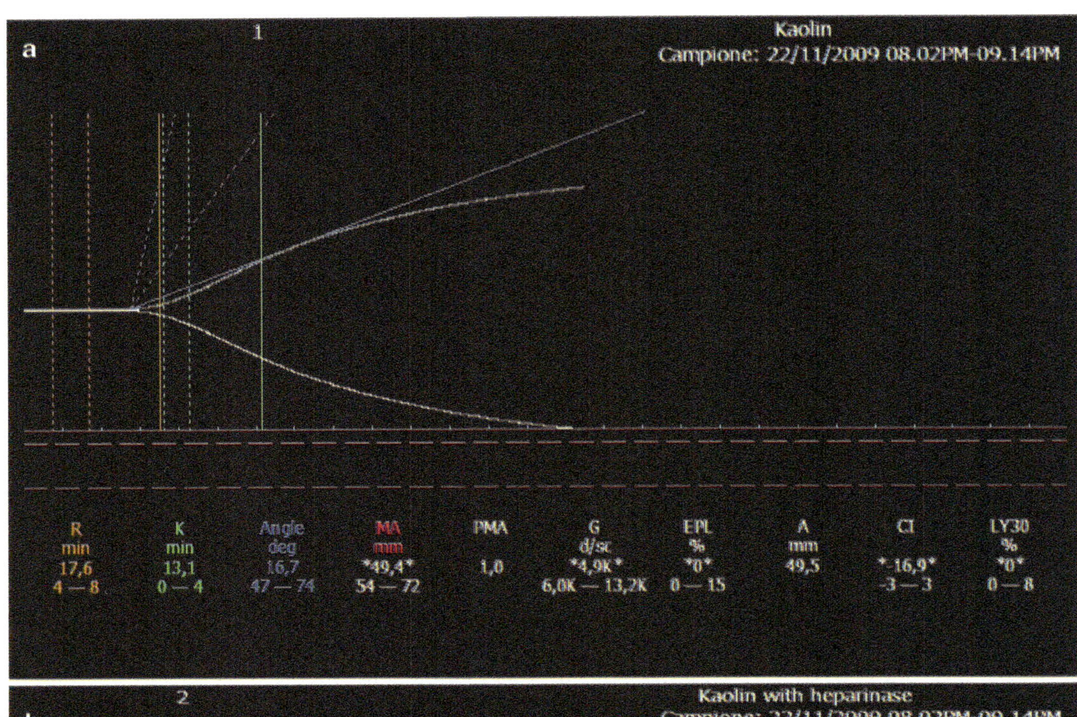

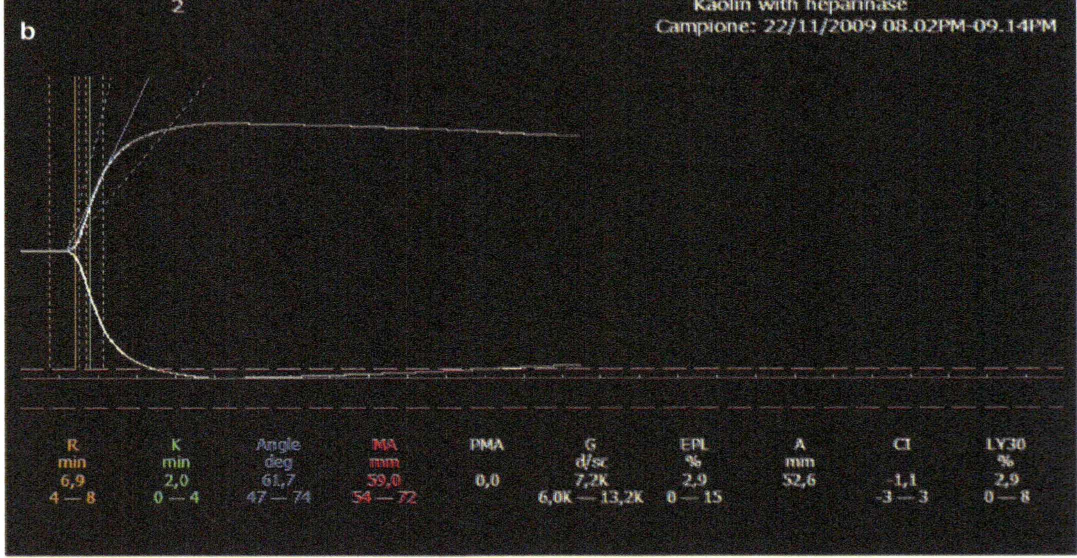

Fig. 12.2 Effects of therapeutic doses of enoxaparin (80 IU/kg twice a day) in a patient with thrombosis of right jugular subclavian axis. (**a**) Plain kaolin-TEG trace. (**b**) Kaolin-TEG trace with heparinase. In the presence of low-molecular-weight heparin, heparinase normalized the prolonged *R*- and *K*-times and the reduced alpha angle and maximum amplitude

of LMWH, new reagents like prothrombinase-induced clotting time reagent are currently under investigation [54].

Regarding the possibility of preventing bleeding associated to LMWH administration in surgical populations, the use of thromboelastography has been also proposed preoperatively to establish an adequate window of anticoagulant effect leading to a decreased risk of perioperative bleeding complications [55].

12.3 Fondaparinux

Fondaparinux is a synthetic factor Xa inhibitor analog of the active pentasaccharide present in UFH and LMWHs that involves the antithrombin-binding site [56–58]. It is approved for thromboprophylaxis in medical and orthopedic patients, for treatment of venous thromboembolism, and for NSTEMI-acute coronary syndromes in Europe after the results of the OASIS-5 trial [59, 60].

Due to its 100 % bioavailability after subcutaneous administration, fondaparinux elimination is completely dependent on renal clearance; therefore, it is contraindicated in patients with severe renal insufficiency (creatinine clearance <30 mL/min). In patients with moderate renal insufficiency (creatinine clearance 30–50 mL/min), the dose should be reduced by 50 %.

Routine anticoagulant monitoring is not recommended, but, considering that fondaparinux activity is not reversed by a specific antidote, in special situations such as renal insufficiency, extremes of body weight, and bleeding complications, it is useful to determine its real anticoagulant effect [48, 58, 61]. Fondaparinux slightly (but without clinical significance) prolongs the PT and the aPTT [62] and has no effect on the ACT. Therefore, these assays are not adequate to monitor the anticoagulant effect of fondaparinux [63]. A standard curve taking fondaparinux as a calibrator should be used for reporting fondaparinux levels using an antifactor Xa assay [62]. Patients with Non-ST segment elevation-Acute Coronary Syndrome (NSTE-ACS) often require urgent percutaneous coronary interventions (PCI) or aortocoronary bypass surgery, so a point-of-care test able to monitor quickly the anticoagulant effect of this agent should be useful. The main limitation of antifactor Xa assay calibrated for fondaparinux is the same that happens for LMWHs. It is not available in every laboratory at every time. In order to try to overcome this drawback, clinicians have analyzed the possibility of monitoring the fondaparinux anticoagulant activity using the point-of-care tests of hemostasis usually present in the intensive care units and operating theaters.

Gerotziafas and associates analyzed in vitro the influence of clinically relevant concentrations (prophylactic and therapeutic) of fondaparinux on thromboelastographic profiles of citrated whole blood of 12 healthy volunteers after triggering TF pathway with a minimal amount of thromboplastin. Diluted thromboplastin was added to samples supplemented with fondaparinux (0.25; 0.5; 1 μg/mL). At concentrations used in prophylaxis regimen (0.25 μg/mL equivalent to 0.27 anti-Xa IU/mL), fondaparinux significantly prolonged the *R*- and *K*-times but did not significantly modify the alpha angle as compared to the control. At concentrations observed after administration of therapeutic doses for the treatment of deep venous thrombosis (≥0.5 μg/mL for fondaparinux), fondaparinux induced a significant prolongation of *R*- and *K*-times and a significant decrease of the alpha angle ($p<0.05$). Fondaparinux did not induce modifications of MA at any concentration. In this study, *R*- and *K*-times were the most sensitive parameters of the modified TF-TEG assay to reveal the anticoagulant effect of prophylactic concentrations of fondaparinux. A ceiling effect of the inhibitory effect of fondaparinux was observed at the concentration of 0.55 anti-Xa IU/mL. This study provides evidence that the whole-blood TF-triggered TEG assay is sensitive to the presence of clinically relevant concentrations of fondaparinux. Moreover, the alpha angle may be used in order to distinguish the effect of prophylactic and therapeutic concentrations [64].

However, these results have been not confirmed by other authors. Eller and associates spiked blood samples from healthy volunteers with therapeutic and supra-therapeutic concentrations of fondaparinux and other direct antifactor Xa and antifactor IIa drugs. Only supra-therapeutic concentrations of fondaparinux significantly influenced the clotting time (CT) of INTEM assay of ROTEM. No significant modifications were observed at therapeutic and prophylactic doses. Moreover, no modifications of EXTEM-CT were observed at any concentration.

Again, in another study, the authors prospectively measured the antifactor Xa levels and analyzed the thromboelastographic profile triggered by kaolin of whole-blood samples of orthopedic patients treated with prophylactic doses of fondaparinux (2.5 mg once a day). Samples were taken at baseline (before first postoperative injection of fondaparinux), 2 h after administration, 17 h after administration (half-life of fondaparinux), and 24 h after administration of the drug. The *R*-time was into the normal range at any phase of the study, and there were not significant differences between the *R* mean value at the different phases. Moreover, the reaction time did not correlate with antifactor Xa levels at any phase. Only the parameter MA had a significant variation over time [66].

In conclusion, further studies are necessary to establish the real capability of viscoelastic point-of-care assays to monitor the anticoagulant effect of pentasaccharides.

Regarding the fondaparinux anticoagulant effect reversal, recombinant factor VIIa is able to reverse in vitro the TEG modifications caused by fondaparinux [1], so if uncontrollable bleeding occurs with fondaparinux, recombinant factor VIIa may be effective [67].

12.4 Parenteral Direct Thrombin Inhibitors

As well known, heparin is far to be the ideal anticoagulant. Its main drawbacks are that heparin can inhibit only fluid-phase thrombin as opposed to other thrombin inhibitors (e.g., bivalirudin) that can inhibit clot-bound thrombin. Heparin is not a direct thrombin inhibitor and requires antithrombin (AT) as a cofactor, thus heparin efficacy is susceptible to pharmacodynamic differences based on AT level and activity (heparin resistance). Finally, heparin binds to endothelial surfaces and has high affinity to platelets (platelet factor 4), potentially leading to heparin-induced thrombocytopenia [4, 5].

In order to overcome these limitations, parenteral direct thrombin inhibitors (DTI) have been developed. The current marketed parenteral DTIs are bivalirudin, argatroban, and danaparoid. The FDA-approved indications of bivalirudin are anticoagulation during percutaneous transluminal coronary angioplasty (PTCA), percutaneous coronary intervention (PCI) with use of glycoprotein IIb/IIIa inhibitors, and for patients with or at risk of heparin-induced thrombocytopenia (HIT) and HIT with thrombosis (HITT) undergoing PCI. In Canada, bivalirudin is also approved for patients with or at risk of HIT undergoing cardiac surgery [68]. Moreover, bivalirudin has been proposed as an off-label alternative to UFH during on-pump and off-pump cardiac surgery in patients affected by HIT [69–72].

Bivalirudin is a potent reversible bivalent direct inhibitor of free and clot-bounded thrombin. It inhibits the activation of fibrinogen and the thrombin-mediated activation of factors V, VIII, and XIII and platelets. One of its main advantages is its low immunogenic potential. Bivalirudin has a unique pharmacologic profile: it undergoes predominant non-organ elimination by plasmatic proteolysis with only a 20 % of renal elimination that imposes, in any case, a dose reduction in case of renal insufficiency. Bivalirudin is the parenteral DTI with the shortest half-life (25 min) [73]. Bleeding is the major adverse effect, more commonly found in patients with renal impairment.

Regarding laboratory monitoring, PT, ACT, aPTT, and TT are all prolonged in a linear fashion with increased doses of bivalirudin, but this linearity is lost at high doses [74].

Bivalirudin is usually monitored by aPTT in case of anticoagulation for HIT/HITT [68] maintaining a therapeutic range from 1.5 to 2.5 times the upper limit of normal range.

INR rises in the presence of bivalirudin, so attention must be paid during DTI shift to vitamin K antagonist (VKA) when concomitant administration of both drugs occurs, as thrombosis risk exits with premature discontinuation of DTI due to wrong INR interpretation [75].

ACT is generally used to monitor bivalirudin during interventional cardiology and in cardiac surgery (with and without CPB) [69–72]. However, the ecarin thrombin time would be the preferred assay, if available [75].

Monitoring bivalirudin with a point-of-care ecarin clotting time (ECT) during cardiac surgery has been anedoctically proposed too [76].

Argatroban is the second parenteral DTI currently on the market. It is a synthetic DTI that reversibly binds to activated thrombin. It exerts its anticoagulant effects by inhibiting thrombin-induced reactions including fibrin formation and activation of factors V, VIII, and XIII and platelet aggregation. Its half-life is longer than that of bivalirudin (45 min). It has a hepatic clearance, so no dose modification is necessary in case of renal impairment [77]. It has been approved for prophylaxis and treatment of thrombosis complicating HIT and in patients with or at risk of HIT undergoing PCI.

As bivalirudin, argatroban dose dependently increases aPTT/ACT/PT/INR and TT. The aPTT is the recommended assay for monitoring the anticoagulant effect of argatroban in patients with HIT. The suggested aPTT target is 1.5–3 times the baseline value and it should never exceed 100 s. aPTT loses its linear relationship with argatroban plasma concentrations if aPTT is higher than 60 s. In this case, shift to ECT is necessary. ACT is the suggested test in patients undergoing PCI with a therapeutic target of 300–450 s [77].

Regarding the capacity of viscoelastic point-of-care tests to monitor parenteral DTI, an in vitro study has demonstrated that argatroban at supratherapeutic and therapeutic concentrations prolongs the INTEM-CT and the EXTEM-CT [65]. In a clinical study involving patients undergoing PCI the *R*-time of a modified thromboelastograph, ecarin clotting time had a better correlation ($r^2=0.746$) with bivalirudin level than the standard ACT ($r^2=0.306$) [78]. Again, ecarin modified rotational thromboelastometry (EMT) has been proposed as a point-of-care monitor of argatroban. Ecarin acts as a direct thrombin activator. It is a metalloprotease isolated from the venom of the saw-scaled viper that activates prothrombin without affecting other coagulation factors and independently of the calcium, phospholipids, factor V, and heparin. In this study, the correlation between argatroban concentration and EMT-CT was high ($r^2=0.94$) and statistically significant [79].

Definitely, the development of a reliable point-of-care monitoring of DTIs still remains a challenging issue because a strict control of the level of anticoagulation is necessary as specific antidotes are not available. Unlike that for argatroban, in case of bleeding due to overdose of bivalirudin, hemodialysis, hemofiltration, and plasmapheresis can be helpful because they are able to remove significant amount of the drug [68].

12.5 Vitamin K Antagonists

Arterial and venous thromboses are common causes of morbidity and mortality for the surgical and medical patients and increase with age. The thrombosis risk stays for about a year after the triggering event [80], and among the drugs used for the long-term anticoagulation in the risk patients, the vitamin K antagonists (VKA), which are used for those up to 60 years, symbolize the cornerstone of the treatment. They are approved for the prevention and/or treatment of venous thrombosis, pulmonary embolism, and thromboembolic complication [81]. These drugs are prothrombin synthesis inhibitors, and they can be divided in two categories: the coumarins and the indandiones [82].

Those belonging to the first class work with the same mechanism of action: they interfere with the carboxylation of glutamate residues on the N-terminal regions of vitamin k-dependent proteins as II, VII, IX, and X. The principal action develops through the cyclic interconversion of vitamin K, so the vitamin K-dependent coagulation factors are produced by the liver partially carboxylated and decarboxylated with reduced coagulation activity. These drugs inhibit also the synthesis of endogenous anticoagulant proteins such as protein C and S [82].

However, the coumarins have a different pharmacokinetic and pharmacodynamic mechanism.

The molecules differ primarily for half-lives 9 h for acenocoumarol, 30–40 h for warfarin, and up 120 h for phenprocoumon [81]. Their use is influenced by pharmacological interactions, particularly the drugs which work through the hepatic P450 cytochrome. Moreover vegetables and also some other food can alter the pharmacokinetics and the pharmacodynamics of these drugs.

Warfarin is the most common used in clinical situations, it is given orally and it is rapidly adsorbed from the gastrointestinal tract. Its mechanism is influenced by metabolic clearance and vitamin K intake.

Acenocoumarol is derivate from coumarin, and the age and its dosage is established by two parameter, body mass index and international normalized ratio (INR). The therapeutic effects are faster than warfarin that gives more steady hematic concentration.

The use of VKA is increasing, but bleeding is a frequent and important complication affecting between 10 and 16 % of the treated patients. The reasons are due to incorrect treatment in 20–40 % of them and to spontaneous bleeding which has a frequency of 14 % in the emergency department's admissions due to drug-related adverse effects, while during hospitalization is 25 % [83].

Monitoring of VKA therapy is the tool for the effectiveness of these drugs and INR is the only parameter used until now: the typical target of INR range for the anticoagulation is 2–3 [84]. INR (international normalized ratio = patient PT/mean normal PT) is the standardization of the PT based on ISI values derived from the plasma of patients who had received stable anticoagulant doses for at least 6 weeks [82]. It explores the extrinsic or vitamin K-dependent factors of the coagulation cascade. In some settings, such as surgery and trauma, INR is not reliable to predict the coagulopathy and has a relatively long turnaround time [85].

A still open question is if the POCT could result useful to manage or to understand the variations on hemostatic balance induced by VKA.

The POCT can rapidly assess global hemostasis and give information to treat patients at bedside [18], to manage bleeding, and to measure the anticoagulation level in order to prevent thrombotic events.

Among POCT, the coagulometers perform a valuable aid to measure INR. Several devices are available: the CoaguChek XS, INRatio Time, ProTime, and SmartCheck. All start the clotting process by a recombinant thromboplastin, except SmartCheck which uses thromboplastin from rabbit brain. These coagulometers differ in the methodology of clotting detection: respectively, electrochemical detection of thrombin activity, electrochemical detection of changes in impedance of blood, and cessation of blood flow through capillary channel and a magnetic field. These tests are assessed by their accuracy and precision, and the imprecision is expressed by means of coefficient of variation, which should be less than 3 % [86]. Furthermore, the coagulometers are not subject to control and standardization as laboratory measurements: only CoaguChek presents a calibration process of each lot with the corresponding code chip.

The coagulometers are tools to self-monitoring the INR: the frequent control confirms the clinical efficacy and safety of VKA treatment also if the choice of coagulation monitor had no effect on clinical outcome of a large patients' cohort [87].

Regarding VET POCT, there is not an agreement about indications to the use of TEG or ROTEM for monitoring the VKA effect.

The TEG assesses the global process of hemostasis, analyzing the viscoelastic properties of blood during the clotting process. The role of the activator is very important. The reagents can quicken the coagulation and the kaolin spur the intrinsic via. So clotting times measured by aPTT correspond to coagulation time (*R*-time) in TEG.

The patients treated with VKA and showing a therapeutic INR presented a TEG signature typically normal, and the literature described several case reports where there is no agreement between the variation of INR and the TEG parameter [88].

The kaolin-TEG is insensitive to warfarin effects and also, when triggered by both kaolin and tissue factor, is not able to show the alteration of hemostasis induced by coumarins, maybe due to that the intrinsic pathway activation may mitigate detection of an extrinsic pathway coagulopathy [88]. Again, Nascimento and associates conclude that in trauma patients, the reaction time of RapidTEG® is not superior to INR to identify vitamin K factors deficiency [85]. A recent analysis [89] confirmed this result, even if the markers of thrombus generation [reaction time (*R*), maximum rate of thrombus generation (MRTG), and time to maximum range thrombus generation (TMRTG)] correlated with INR in a series of 104 patients.

With regard to the ROTEM, performed in patients treated with VKA and triggered by calcium chlorides and tissue factor, a marked significant increase in clotting time (CT) [4] and higher levels of maximum clot firmness (MCF) and area under curve (AUC) even if their values were in range were obtained. Of special interest is the MCF in FIBTEM, which was significantly higher in VKA patients than in the control group: this feature probably describes a hypercoagulable paradox of the patients anticoagulated, being MCF in FIBTEM a parameter influenced by fibrinogen concentration and fibrin polymerization [90].

In conclusion, among POCTs the coagulometers are safe and adequate for clinical use, even if they need quality control and calibration. Although several papers were published during the last years about the use of the TEG and ROTEM to identify and manage the coagulopathy and antithrombotic therapy, at present these techniques are puzzling to understand the hemostatic alteration induced by VKA and data from literature are few and lacking. Despite all its criticisms, to date the INR remains the gold standard laboratory test for warfarin monitoring.

12.6 Novel Oral Anticoagulants

Agents directly inhibiting thrombin (dabigatran) and activated factor X (rivaroxaban and apixaban) are now increasingly employed in preventing and treating venous thromboembolism in orthopedic surgery and preventing arterial thromboembolism in non-valvular atrial fibrillation [91]. Thrombin and factor Xa have a central role in the coagulation cascade, being the converging point of the extrinsic and the intrinsic pathways. Activated factor X is the enzyme that triggers the prothrombinase to thrombin activation. Thrombin catalyzes the conversion of fibrinogen to fibrin, activates positive feedback signals for coagulation amplification, and is a strong platelet activator, being the final and the most important contributor to clot formation and stability. The development of these novel drugs was aimed at increasing the efficacy and overcome variable dosing and safety issues of the traditional anticoagulants. Indeed, these inhibitors show a faster onset of action, reduced half-lives, a wider therapeutic window, fewer drug interactions, and more predictable pharmacokinetics allowing to get over the routine coagulation monitoring required in patients administered with traditional drugs, such as warfarin and heparin. Noteworthy, the anticoagulant effect of these inhibitors cannot be reversed specifically and antidotes are still to undergo definitive clinical testing and approval [92, 93]. Interindividual variability of patient response to anticoagulant administration and thus a particular need for drug activity monitoring, especially in patients with changing renal function and in the elderly, still remains a not fully clarified matter [94]. Till then, rapidly recognizing and monitoring the extent of the coagulation suppression in settings where bleeding could put the patient in danger of life is of fundamental importance.

Emergency situations, such as urgent invasive surgery, hemorrhage, or overdose, may require a rapid and reliable assessment of the extent of the anticoagulant effect. Monitoring is also required in assessing the patient compliance to the treatment or tracking the anticoagulation reversal in critical settings [95]. To date there are no commercially available antidotes towards these novel anticoagulant agents. Until the promising specific antibodies will be available, prothrombin complex concentrate (PCC), activated prothrombin complex concentrate (aPCC), factor VIII inhibitor bypassing activity (FEIBA), and recombinant activated factor VII (rFVIIa) have been proposed for managing bleeding complications in patients under active treatment [95, 96].

Dabigatran etexilate is an oral prodrug that is rapidly converted to active dabigatran that competitively inhibits thrombin through binding to its active site. Dabigatran is excreted almost completely by the kidney, so this is why renal failure is a major issue for the management of anticoagulation effect and dialysis has been shown to be efficient for drug removal but poorly applicable in most cases [97].

Apixaban and rivaroxaban are not prodrugs and competitively bind to the active site of both free factor Xa and factor Xa bound in the prothrombinase complex. The major part of circulating rivaroxaban (67 %) is metabolized to inactive metabolites in liver, but a part of unmodified rivaroxaban is eliminated through renal route (33 %). Apixaban undergoes excretion mainly through hepatobiliary route (75 %) and only 25 % in excreted through kidneys [98, 99]. These drugs circulate mainly in protein-bound form, and dialysis is not efficient in removing them from circulation [95].

12.6.1 Traditional Laboratory Testing

Standard laboratory methods have shown important limitations in quantitative assessment of novel oral anticoagulants (NOACs) activity that have not been overcome yet. Different reagents, classical and modified analytical methods, and a wide range of laboratory instruments have been described with results still requiring further clinical validation and standardization. However, despite its limitations, laboratory testing could provide important qualitative information regarding the presence of drug of interest.

For dabigatran, the PT shows a low sensitivity and is not recommended. Nevertheless, a prolonged PT is reliable in predicting the presence of dabigatran in amounts sufficient to produce an anticoagulant effect. The aPTT time is suitable for the purpose but values seem variable depending on the reagent used; a prolonged aPTT may indicate the presence of dabigatran but does not accurately reflect plasma drug concentration. Thrombin clotting time is linearly correlated to drug concentration in plasma but is too sensitive even at therapeutic dosages and not routinely available in most laboratories. Ecarin thrombin time needs standardization and is poorly available in most laboratories as well. Hemoclot, a commercial dabigatran calibrator, where a diluted TT test has been coupled with a dabigatran calibration curve, has been developed recently and is now more and more widely applied in clinical setting [100, 101].

For factor Xa inhibitors, PT is more sensitive than aPTT, but the results are depending on the reagents used, and apixaban seems to have less effect on PT than rivaroxaban. However, the degree of PT prolongation is not reliable for assessing the amount of circulating drug because it is influenced by reagents used for the assay. The dilute PT test (or modified PT test) offers a better sensitivity for apixaban detection. Commercially available antifactor Xa chromogenic assays with appropriate calibration curves may provide sensitive and specific measurement of drug concentration [101].

12.6.2 Point-of-Care Tests

Multiple studies pointed out that point-of-care tests were applicable for qualitatively monitoring the anticoagulant effect of novel oral anticoagulants and the eventual reversibility of their activity with the most commonly available prothrombotic drugs as well.

In an in vitro experiment employing blood samples from healthy volunteers, Xu and associates showed that dabigatran significantly affected both TEG and thrombin generation assay (TGA) parameters in a concentration-dependent manner [102]. In particular, *R*-time of TEG and the lag time of TGA were prolonged, whereas the maximum amplitude of the TEG curve and the endogenous thrombotic potential (ETP) and the peak height on the TGA curve were significantly depressed.

Eller and associates spiked blood samples from healthy volunteers with therapeutic and supratherapeutic concentrations of direct thrombin inhibitors (including dabigatran) and factor Xa inhibitors (rivaroxaban and apixaban) [65]. They showed that therapeutic concentrations of dabigatran prolonged ACT in a concentration-dependent manner and that only ROTEM CT parameter was affected when therapeutic concentrations of dabigatran, rivaroxaban, and apixaban were tested. Interestingly, they found that platelet function tests (except for the α-thrombin-induced aggregation on the light transmission aggregometer) were not affected by the tested inhibitors, speculating that their validity is not questioned when both anticoagulant and antiplatelet therapy are administered.

Dinkelaar and associates explored the in vitro reversal of dabigatran and apixaban with PCC as monitored by the most available laboratory and point-of-care technologies [103]. They pointed out that the reversal of NOACs anticoagulation by PCC will be primarily due to an increase of plasma levels of vitamin K-dependent coagulation factors rather than to the interference between the NOAC agent and its ligand. Assays based on the measurement of residual thrombin or factor Xa activity (TT, ECT, or chromogenic anti-Xa assays) are inappropriate for the purpose. Moreover, assays based on contact activation of the coagulation cascade (aPTT or ROTEM INTEM test) were not sensitive to inhibitor reversal by PCC as well. It was confirmed that thrombin generation was depressed when plasma samples from healthy volunteers were added with apixaban or dabigatran and found that PCC administration could achieve a significant but not full reversal (only ETP normalized) of the anticoagulation. TEG was sensitive as well to the NOAC activity showing a *R*-time prolongation and the angle reduction with dabigatran achieving a stronger effect than apixaban (being the only able to reduce the curve maximum amplitude of the TEG curve).

In another study, Dinkelaar and associates analogously explored the reversal of rivaroxaban with PCC as assessed by PT and thrombin generation tests [104]. They found that PCC only partially reverted the lengthening of PT and thrombin lag time due to rivaroxaban anticoagulation in vitro; however, the total thrombin potential could be neutralized. Noteworthy, they found that the results were somehow dependent of the assay conditions, pointing out the need for standardization and further studies to identify the best assay protocol for this scope. Future prospective studies in clinical setting are also strongly required.

Animal models have been used to observe the effect of NOACs and their reversal with point-of-care devices.

In a porcine trauma model, animals were orally administered with dabigatran, and the blood samples were ex vivo spiked with different prohemostatic agents, including a specific antidote to dabigatran [105, 106]. Dabigatran prolonged all the analyzed coagulation parameters, including PT, aPTT, and ROTEM EXTEM-CT; clot strength (MCF), platelet number, and fibrinogen concentration were not influenced. Additional intravenous infusion of dabigatran, further impairing thrombin bioavailability, finally reduced the maximum clot firmness, readily restored once sufficient thrombin is provided through prothrombin complex concentrate [105]. Therapeutic concentrations of PCC and activated PCC were able to reduce the extent of dabigatran-induced anticoagulation, but only the specific antidote fully neutralized the dabigatran activity [105, 106] without an associated thrombin overcorrection [106]. No significant correction was achieved using rFVIIa [105].

Herrman and colleagues analyzed samples of 17 patients on 150 mg dabigatran twice daily (for non-valvular atrial fibrillation therapy) and of 17 patients on 10 mg rivaroxaban daily (for DVT prevention after orthopedic surgery) for thrombin generation (using calibrated automatic thrombogram, CAT) and for thromboelastic parameters using TEG and ROTEM devices [108]. Dabigatran and rivaroxaban both significantly increased thrombin generation lag time and decreased the endogenous thrombotic potential (ETP) and the peak height of the curve. Dabigatran prolonged the *R*-time on TEG, whereas rivaroxaban administration kept the parameters within the normal range. On ROTEM dabigatran induced a significant increase in the clotting formation time for both INTEM and EXTEM tests, whereas rivaroxaban produced only a nonsignificant increase of CFT beyond the normal range on EXTEM CFT. Spiking the blood samples with therapeutic concentration of procoagulative agents, they observed prothrombin complex concentrate (PCC), factor VII inhibitor bypassing activity (FEIBA), and to a lesser extent recombinant activated factor VII (rFVIIa) significantly correcting all the abnormal parameters.

Kyriakou and associates focused on the comparison between the impact of dabigatran versus acenocoumarol using the nonactivated TEM test and thrombin generation assay [100]. Blood samples were drawn from patients undergoing active treatment, and Hemoclot assay was used to assess specific dabigatran concentration. They found that all the parameters of ROTEM were affected with greater effect of dabigatran as compared to acenocoumarol. Interestingly they noted a significant reduction of the lysis index in samples of patients on dabigatran. At thrombin generation assay, it was acenocoumarol to show a larger impact on all the observed parameters. However, they were able to verify the strong association between dabigatran concentration in plasma and the ETP parameters speculating that such a finding might account for a safer profile of dabigatran [100].

In conclusion, a wide range of clinical cases could require a rapid and sensitive assessment of NOACs anticoagulation activity or of the extent of its reversal. The most widely used point-of-care devices (TEG, ROTEM, and thrombin generation assay) seem to be sensitive enough to allow monitoring and help decision making. However, available research is still very limited and needs further deepening and investigation in order to clear the partially contradictory knowledge obtained so far.

Conclusions

Bleeding is the most severe side effect of antithrombotic drugs and one of the main causes of acquire hemorrhagic disorders. Strict control of dosages particularly in special populations by means of laboratory monitoring of plasma drug concentrations and/or anticoagulant activity is one of the pillars in order to improve the management of anticoagulated patients and to reduce bleeding complications. To date, there is quite an agreement regarding the most adequate laboratory assay to monitor the anticoagulant effect of the different drugs, but consensus regarding the capability of point-of-care tests to assess the effect of antithrombotic drugs is still lacking and remains a matter of debate, especially due to the fact that the current evidence is given only by small in vitro studies. Further clinical studies involving patients that really assume anticoagulants are necessary in order to create shared recommendations between clinicians and pathologists.

References

1. Young G, Yonekawa KE, Nakagawa PA et al (2007) Recombinant activated factor VII effectively reverses the anticoagulant effects of heparin, enoxaparin, fondaparinux, argatroban and bivalirudin ex vivo as measured using thromboelastography. Blood Coagul Fibrinolysis 18:547–553
2. Hirsh J, Raschke R (2004) Heparin and low-molecular-weight heparin: the Seventh ACCP Conference on Antithrombotic and Thombolytic Therapy. Chest 123:188S–203S
3. Hirsh J, Warkentin TE, Shaughnessy SG et al (2001) Heparin and low-molecular-weight heparin: mechanism of action, pharmacokinetics, monitoring, efficacy, and safety. Chest 119(1 Suppl):64S–94S
4. Ranucci M, Ballotta A, Kandil H et al (2011) Bivalirudin-based versus conventional heparin anticoagulation for postcardiotomy extracorporeal membrane oxygenation. Crit Care 15:R275
5. Kelton JG, Arnold DM, Bates SM (2013) Nonheparin anticoagulants for heparin-induced thrombocytopenia. N Engl J Med 368:737–744
6. Langdell RD, Wagner RH, Brinkhous KM (1953) Effect of antihemophilic factor on one-stage clotting tests; a presumptive test for hemophilia and a simple test one-stage antihemophilic factor assay procedure. J Lab Clin Med 41:637–647
7. Baglin T, Barrowcliffe W, Cohen A, Greaves M, British Committee for Standards in Haematology (2006) Guidelines on the use and monitoring of heparin. Br J Haematol 133:19–34
8. Winkler AM, Sheppard CA, Fantz CR (2007) Laboratory monitoring of heparin: challenges and opportunities. Lab Med 38:499–502
9. Spinler SA, Wittkowsky AK, Nutescu EA et al (2005) Anticoagulation monitoring part 2: unfractionated heparin and low-molecular-weight-heparin. Ann Pharmacother 39:1275–1285
10. Olson JD, Arkin CF, Brandt JT et al (1998) College of American Pathologists Conference XXXI on laboratory monitoring of anticoagulant therapy. Arch Pathol Lab Med 122:782–798

11. Bates SM, Weitz JI (2005) Coagulation assays. Circulation 112:e53–e60
12. Cuker A, Ptashkin B, Konkle BA et al (2009) Interlaboratory agreement in the monitoring of unfractionated heparin using the anti-factor Xa-correlated activated partial thromboplastin time. J Thromb Haemost 7:80–85
13. Reiss RA, HAAS CE, Griffis DL, Porter B, Tara MA (2002) Point-of-care versus laboratory monitoring of patients receiving different anticoagulant therapies. Pharmacotheray 22:677–685
14. Hattersley PG (1996) Activated coagulation time. JAMA 196:436–440
15. Jude B, Lasne D, Mouton C et al (2004) Monitoring of heparin therapy during extracorporeal bypass: what are the remaining questions? Ann Fr Anesth Reanim 23:589–596
16. Bull BS, Korpman RA, Huse WM, Briggs BD (1975) Heparin therapy during extracorporeal circulation: I. Problems inherent in existing heparin protocols. J Thorac Cardiovasc Surg 69:674–684
17. Smythe MA, Koerber JM, Nowak SN et al (2002) Correlation between activated clotting time and activated partial thromboplastin time. Ann Pharmacother 36:7–11
18. Prisco D, Paniccia R (2003) Point of care testing of hemostasis in cardiac surgery. Thrombosis J 1:1–10
19. Shore-Lesserson L (2005) Evidence based coagulation monitors: heparin monitoring, thromboelastography, and platelet function. Semin Cardiothorac Vasc Anesth 9:41–52
20. Despotis GJ, Summerfield AL, Joist JH et al (1994) Comparison of activated coagulation time and whole blood heparin measurements with laboratory plasma anti-Xa heparin concentration in patients having cardiac operations. J Thorac Cardiovasc Surg 108:1076–1082
21. Koster A, Despotis G, Gruendel M et al (2002) The plasma supplemented modified activated clotting time for monitoring of heparinization during cardiopulmonary bypass: a pilot investigation. Anesth Analg 95:26–30
22. Sniecinski RM, Levy JH (2015) Anticoagulation management associated with extracorporeal circulation. Best Practice Res Clin Anaesthesiol 29:189–202
23. Ammar T, Scudder LE, Coller BS (1997) In vitro effects of platelet glycoprotein IIb/IIIa receptor antagonist c7E3 Fab on the activated clotting time. Circulation 95:614–617
24. Wang JS, Lin CY, Hung WT, Thisted RA, Karp RB (1992) In vitro effects of aprotinin on activated clotting time measured with different activators. J Thorac Cardiovasc Surg 104:1135–1140
25. Simko RJ, Tsung FW, Stanck EJ (1995) Activated clotting time versus activated partial thromboplastin time for therapeutic monitoring of heparin. Ann Pharmacother 29:1015–1021
26. Ganter MT, Monn A, Tavakoli R, Klaghofer R, Zollinger A, Hofer CK (2007) Kaolin-based activated coagulation time measured by sonoclot in patients undergoing cardiopulmonary bypass. J Cardiothorac Vasc Anesth 21:524–528
27. Smith SC Jr, Dove JT, Jacobs AK et al (2001) ACC/AHA guidelines of percutaneous coronary interventions (revision of the 1993 PTCA guidelines)-executive summary. A report of the American College of Cardiology/American Heart Association Task Force on Practice Guidelines (committee to revise the 1993 guidelines for percutaneous transluminal coronary angioplasty). J Am Coll Cardiol 37:2215–2239
28. Popma JJ, Berger P, Ohman EM, Harrington RA, Grines C, Weitz JL (2004) Antithrombotic therapy during percutaneous coronary intervention. The Seventh ACCP Conference on Antithrombotic and Thrombolytic Therapy. Chest 126:576S–599S
29. Noui N, Zogheib E, Walczak K et al (2012) Anticoagulation monitoring during extracorporeal circulation with the Hepcon/HMS device. Perfusion 27:214–220
30. Despotis G, Joist JH, Goodnough LT et al (1997) Whole blood heparin concentration measurements by automated protamine titration agrees with plasma anti-Xa measurements. J Thorac Cardiovasc Surg 113:611–613
31. Raymond PD, Ray MJ, Callen SN, Marsh NA (2003) Heparin monitoring during cardiac surgery. Part 1: validation of whole-blood heparin concentration and activated clotting time. Perfusion 18:269–276
32. Despotis GJ, Joist JH, Hogue CW Jr et al (1995) The impact of heparin concentration and activated clotting time monitoring on blood conservation. A prospective, randomized evaluation in patients undergoing cardiac operation. J Thorac Cardiovasc Surg 110:46–54
33. Despotis GJ, Filos KS, Zoys TN et al (1996) Factors associated with excessive postoperative blood loss and hemostatic transfusion requirements: a multivariate analysis in cardiac surgical patients. Anesth Analg 82:13–21
34. Koster A, Fischer T, Praus M et al (2002) Hemostatic activation and inflammatory response during cardiopulmonary bypass: impact of heparin management. Anesthesiology 97:837–841
35. Beholz S, Grubitzsach H, Bergamann B, Wollert HG, Eckel L (1999) Hemostasis management by use of Hepcon/HMS: increasing bleeding without increased need for blood transfusion. Thorac Cardiovasc Surg 47:322–327
36. Shore-Lesserson L (2002) Point of care coagulation monitoring for cardiovascular patients: past and present. J Cardiothorac Vasc Anesth 16:99–106
37. Johansson PI, Solbeck S, Genet G, Stensballe J, Ostrwski SR (2012) Coagulopathy and hemostatic monitoring in cardiac surgery: an update. Scand Cardiovasc J 46:194–202
38. Shore-Lesserson L, Spiess BD (2006) Perioperative coagulation monitoring. In: Ed Spiess BD, Spence RK, Shander A (eds) Perioperative transfusion

medicine, 2nd edn. Lippincott Williams and Wilkins, Philadelphia
39. Zmuda K, Neofotistos D, Ts'ao CH (2000) Effects of unfractionated heparin, low-molecular-weight heparin, and heparinoid on thromboelastograhic assay of blood coagulation. Am J Clin Pathol 113:725–731
40. Coppell JA, Thalheimer U, Zambruni A et al (2006) The effects of unfractionated heparin, low molecular weight heparin and danaparoid on the thromboelastogram (TEG): an in-vitro comparison of standard and heparinase-modified TEGs with conventional coagulation assays. Blood Coagul Fibrinolysis 17:97–104
41. Salooja N, Perry DJ (2001) Thrombelastography. Blood Coagul Fibrinolysis 12:327–337
42. Spiess BD, Wall MH, Gillies BS et al (1997) A comparison of thromboelastography with heparinase or protamine sulfate added in vitro during heparinized cardiopulmonary bypass. Thromb Haemost 78:820–826
43. Levin AI, Hein AM, Coetzee JF, Coetzee A (2014) Heparinase thromboelastography compared with activated coagulation time for protamine titration after cardiopulmonary bypass. J Cardiothorac Vasc Anesth 28:224–229
44. Hutt ED, Kingdon HS (1972) Use of heparinase to eliminate heparin inhibition in routine coagulation assays. J Lab Clin Med 79:1027–1034
45. Tuman KJ, McCarthy RJ, Djuric M, Rizzo V, Ivankovich AD (1994) Evaluation of coagulation during cardiopulmonary bypass with heparinase-modified thromboelastographic assay. J Cardiothorac Vasc Anesth 8:144–149
46. Gronchi F, Perret A, Ferrari E et al (2014) Validation of rotational thromboelastometry during cardiopulmonary bypass: a prospective, observational in vivo study. Eur J Anaesthesiol 31:68–75
47. Cvim G, Wagner T, Juergens G, Koestenberger M (2009) Effects of nadroparin, enoxaparin, and unfractionated heparin on endogenous factor Xa and IIa formation and on thromboelastometry profiles. Blood Coagul Fibrinolysis 20:71–77
48. Tripodi A, van den Besselaar A (2009) Laboratory monitoring of anticoagulation: where do we stand? Semin Thromb Hemost 35:34–41
49. Hery TD, Satran D, Knox LL, Iacarella CL, Laxson DD, Antman EM (2001) Are activated clotting times helpful in the management of anticoagulation with subcutaneous low-molecular-weight heparin? Am Heart J 142:590–593
50. Laposata M, Green K, Elisabeth MVC et al (1998) College of American Pathologist Conference XXXI on laboratory monitoring of low-molecular-weight heparin, danaparoid, hirudin and related compounds, and argatroban. Arch Pathol Lab Med 122:799–807
51. Pittalis A, Tuccillo ML, Savron F, Schember C, Morri D, Dell'Oste C (2013) Pediatric enoxaparin overdose: more attention to thromboelastography monitoring. Minerva Anestesiol 79:1203–1204
52. White H, Sosonowski K, Bird R, Jones M, Solano C (2012) The utility of thromboelastography in monitoring low molecular weight heparin therapy in the coronary care unit. Blood Coagul Fibrinolysis 23:304–310
53. Klein SM, Slaughter TF, Vail PT et al (2000) Thromboelastography as a perioperative measure of anticoagulation resulting from low molecular weight heparin: a comparison with anti-Xa concentration. Anesth Analg 91:1091–1095
54. Schade E, Schober A, Hacker S, Spiss C, Chiari A, Kozek-Langenecker S (2010) Determination of enoxaparin with rotational thromboelastometry using the prothrombinase-induced clotting time reagent. Blood Coagul Fibrinolysis 21:256–261
55. Simons R, Mallett SV (2007) Use of thromboelastography to demonstrate persistent anticoagulation after stopping enoxaparin. Anaesthesia 62:1173–1178
56. Bauer KA (2004) Fondaparinux: a new synthetic and selective inhibitor of Factor Xa. Best Pract Res Clin Haematol 17:89–104
57. Sharma T, Mehta P, Gajra A (2010) Update on fondaparinux: role in management of thromboembolic and acute coronary events. Cardiovasc Hematol Agents Med Chem 8:96–103
58. Garcia DA, Baglin TP, Weitz JI, Samama MM (2012) Parenteral anticoagulants. Antithrombotic Therapy and Prevention of Thrombosis, 9th ed: American College of Chest Physicians Evidence-Based Clinical Practice Guidelines. Chest 141(2):e24S–e43S
59. Mehta SR, Granger CB, Eikelboom JW et al (2007) Efficacy and safety of fondaparinux versus enoxaparin in patients with acute coronary syndromes undergoing percutaneous coronary intervention: results from the OASIS-5 trial. J Am Coll Cardiol 50:1742–1751
60. De Caterina R, Husted S, Wallentin L et al (2013) Parenteral anticoagulants in heart disease: current status and perspectives (Section II). Position paper of the ESC Working Group on Thrombosis-Task Force on Anticoagulants in Heart Disease. Thromb Haemost 109:769–786
61. Nagler M, Haslauer M, Wuillemin WA (2011) Fondaparinux-data on efficacy and safety in special situations. Thromb Res 129:407–417
62. Smogorzewska A, Brandt JT, Chandler WL et al (2006) Effect of fondaparinux on coagulation assay. Arch Pathol Lab Med 130:1605–1611
63. Linkins LA, Julian JA, Rischke J, Hirsh J, Weitz JI (2002) In vitro comparison of the effect of heparin, enoxaparin and fondaparinux on tests of coagulation. Thromb Res 107:241–244
64. Gerotziafas GT, Chakroun T, Samama MM, Elalamy I (2004) In vitro comparison of the effect of fondaparinux and enoxaparin on whole blood tissue factor-triggered thromboelastography profile. Thromb Haemost 92:1296–1302
65. Eller T, Busse J, Dittrich M et al (2014) Dabigatran, rivaroxaban, apixaban, argatroban and fondaparinux

and their effects on coagulation POC and platelet function tests. Clin Chem Lab Med 52:835–844
66. Martinez B, Giacomello R, Paniccia R (2013) Thromboelastographic monitoring of fondaparinux in surgical patients. Crit Care 17(Suppl 2):P356
67. Bijsterveld NR, Moons AH, BoeKholdt SM et al (2002) Ability of recombinant factor VIIa to reverse the anticoagulant effect of the pentasaccharide fondaparinux in healthy volunteers. Circulation 106:2550–2554
68. Warkentin TE, Greinacher A, Koster A (2008) Bivalirudin. Thromb Haemost 99:830–839
69. Smedira NG, Dyke CM, Koster A et al (2006) Anticoagulation with bivalirudin for off-pump coronary artery bypass grafting: the results of the EVOLUTION-OFF study. J Thorac Cardiovasc Surg 131:686–692
70. Dyke CM, Smedira NG, Koster A et al (2006) A comparison of bivalirudin to heparin with protamine reversal in patients undergoing cardiac surgery with cardiopulmonary bypass: the EVOLUTION-ON study. J Thorac Cardiovasc Surg 131:533–539
71. Dyke CM, Aldea G, Koster A et al (2007) Off-pump coronary artery bypass with bivalirudin for patients with heparin-induced thrombocytopenia or antiplatelet factor four/heparin antibodies. Ann Thorac Surg 84:836–839
72. Koster A, Dyke CM, Aldea G et al (2007) Bivalirudin during cardiopulmonary bypass in patients with previous or acute heparin-induced thrombocytopenia and heparin antibodies: results of the CHOOSE-ON trial. Ann Thorac Surg 83:572–577
73. Robson R (2000) The use of bivalirudin in patients with renal impairment. J Invasive Cardiol 12:33F–36F
74. Fox I, Dawson A, Loynds P et al (1993) Anticoagulant activity of Hirulog, a direct thrombin inhibitor, in humans. Thromb Haemost 69:157–163
75. Linkins LA, Dans AL, Moores LK et al (2012) Treatment and prevention of heparin-induced thrombocytopenia: Antithrombotic Therapy and Prevention of Thrombosis, 9th ed: American College of Chest Physicians Evidence-Based Clinical Practice Guidelines. Chest 141(2 Suppl):e495S–e530S
76. Koster A, Chew D, Gründel M, Bauer M, Kuppe H, Spiess BD (2003) Bivalirudin monitored with the ecarin clotting time for anticoagulation during cardiopulmonary bypass. Anesth Analg 96:383–386
77. Babuin L, Pengo V (2010) Argatroban in the management of heparin-induced thrombocytopenia. Vasc Health Risk Manag 6:813–819
78. Carroll RC, Chavez JJ, Simmons JW et al (2006) Measurement of patients' bivalirudin plasma levels by a thromboelastograph ecarin clotting time assay: a comparison to a standard activated clotting time. Anesth Analg 102:1316–1319
79. Schaden E, Schober A, Hacker S, Kozek-Langenecker S (2013) Ecarin modified rotational thromboelastometry: a point-of-care applicable alternative to monitor the direct thrombin inhibitor argatroban. Wien Klin Wochenschr 125:156–159
80. Previtali E, Bucciarelli P, Passamonti SM, Martinelli I (2011) Risk factors for venous and arterial thrombosis. Blood Transfus 9:120–138
81. Steffel J, Luscher TF (2012) Vitamin K antagonists. Ready to be replaced? Hamostaseologie 32:249–257
82. Ansell J, Hirsh J, Hylek E, Jacobson A, Crowther M, Palareti G (2008) Pharmacology and management of Vitamin K antagonists. Chest 133:160S–198S
83. Wysowski DK, Nouriah P, Swartz L (2007) Bleeding complications with warfarin use. A prevalent adverse effect resulting in regulatory action. Arch Intern Med 167:1414–1419
84. Schitt A, Jambor C, Spannagi M, Gogarten W, Schilling T, Zwisler B (2013) The perioperative management of treatment with anticoagulations and platelet aggregation inhibitors. Dtsch Arztebl Int 110:525–532
85. Nascimento B, Al Mahoos M, Callum J et al (2012) Vitamin K-dependent coagulation factor deficiency in trauma: a comparative analysis between international normalized ratio and thromboelastography. Transfusion 52:7–13
86. Christensen TD, Larsen TB (2012) Precision and accuracy of point of care testing coagulometers used for self-testing and self-management of oral anticoagulation therapy. J Thromb Haemost 10:251–260
87. Brouwer JLP, Stoevelaar H, Sucker C (2014) The clinical impact of different coagulometers on patient outcome. Adv Ther 31:639–656
88. Dunham CM, Rabel C, Hileman BM et al (2014) TEG® and RapidTEG® are unreliable for detecting warfarin-coagulopathy: a prospective cohort study. Thromb J 12:4
89. Franchi F, Hammad JS, Rollini F et al (2015) Role of thromboelastography and rapid thromboelastography to assess the pharmacodynamics effects of vitamin K antagonists. J Thromb Thrombolysis 40:118–125
90. Spiezia L, Bertini D, Simioni P, Salmaso L (2008) Whole blood rotation thromboelastometry in subjects undergoing vitamin k antagonist treatment: hypo- or hypercoagulant profiles? Thromb Res 122:568–569
91. Levy JH, Spyropoulos AC, Samama CM, Douketis J (2014) Direct oral anticoagulants: new drugs and new concepts. JACC Cardiovasc Interv 7:1333–1351
92. Bauer KA (2013) Pros and cons of new oral anticoagulants. Hematology Am Soc Hematol Educ Program 2013:464–470
93. Gomez-Outes A, Suarez-Gea ML, Lecumberri R, Terleira-Fernandez AI, Vargas-Castrillon E (2014) Specific antidotes in development for reversal of novel anticoagulants: a review. Recent Pat Cardiovasc Drug Discov 9:2–10
94. Charlton B, Redberg R (2014) The trouble with dabigatran. BMJ 349:g4681
95. Baglin T, Hillarp A, Tripodi A, Elalamy I, Buller H, Ageno W (2013) Measuring oral direct inhibitors (ODIs) of thrombin and factor Xa: a recommendation from the Subcommittee on Control Anticoagulation of the Scientific and Standardisation

Committee of the International Society on Thrombosis and Haemostasis. J Thromb Haemost 11:756–760
96. Siegal DM (2015) Managing target-specific oral anticoagulant associated bleeding including an update on pharmacological reversal agents. J Thromb Thrombolysis 39:395–402
97. Siegal DM, Crowther MA (2013) Acute management of bleeding in patients on novel oral anticoagulants. Eur Heart J 34:489–498b
98. Stangier J, Rathgen K, Stahle H, Mazur D (2010) Influence of renal impairment on the pharmacokinetics and pharmacodynamics of oral dabigatran etexilate: an open- label, parallel-group, single-centre study. Clin Pharmacokinet 49:259–268
99. Wang Y, Bajorek B (2014) New oral anticoagulants in practice: pharmacological and practical considerations. Am J Cardiovasc Drugs 14:175–189
100. Bhanwra S, Ahluwalia K (2014) The new factor Xa inhibitor: Apixaban. J Pharmacol Pharmacother 5:12–14
101. Kyriakou E, Ikonomidis I, Stylos D et al (2015) Laboratory assessment of the anticoagulant activity of dabigatran. Clin Appl Thromb Hemost 21:434–445
102. Cuker A, Siegal DM, Crowther MA, Garcia DA (2014) Laboratory measurement of the anticoagulant activity of the non-vitamin K oral anticoagulants. J Am Coll Cardiol 64:1128–1139
103. Xu Y, Wu W, Wang L et al (2013) Differential profiles of thrombin inhibitors (heparin, hirudin, bivalirudin, and dabigatran) in the thrombin generation assay and thromboelastography in vitro. Blood Coagul Fibrinolysis 24:332–338
104. Dinkelaar J, Patiwael S, Harenberg J, Leyte A, Brinkman HJ (2014) Global coagulation tests: their applicability for measuring direct factor Xa and thrombin inhibition and reversal of anticoagulation by prothrombin complex concentrate. Clin Chem Lab Med 52:1615–1623
105. Dinkelaar J, Molenaar PJ, Ninivaggi M, de Laat B, Brinkman HJ, Leyte A (2013) In vitro assessment, using thrombin generation, of the applicability of prothrombin complex concentrate as an antidote for Rivaroxaban. J Thromb Haemost 11:1111–1118
106. Grottke O, van Ryn J, Spronk HM, Rossaint R (2014) Prothrombin complex concentrates and a specific antidote to dabigatran are effective ex-vivo in reversing the effects of dabigatran in an anticoagulation/liver trauma experimental model. Crit Care 18:R27
107. Honickel M, Treutler S, van Ryn J, Tillman S, Rossaint R, Grottke O (2015) Reversal of dabigatran anticoagulation ex vivo: Porcine study comparing prothrombin complex concentrates and idarucizumab. Thromb Haemost 113:728–740
108. Herrmann R, Thom J, Wood A, Phillips M, Muhammad S, Baker R (2014) Thrombin generation using the calibrated automated thrombinoscope to assess reversibility of dabigatran and rivaroxaban. Thromb Haemost 111:989–995

Practical Issues in POCT

13

Vanessa Agostini

Viscoelastic tests favor the detection of hemostatic disorders and the implementation of a goal-directed strategy for the management of perioperative and traumatic bleeding [1].

In hospitals using this kind of approach, multidisciplinarity is mandatory. In fact, anesthetists, traumatologists, intensive care specialists, hematologists, and clinical pathologists have to cooperate in the management of critical bleeding.

Several issues merit a discussion before implementing a multimodal and point-of-care test (POCT)-based approach.

This chapter approaches the best location for viscoelastic testing and how to guarantee quality assurance.

13.1 The Best Location for Point-of-Care Testing Devices

To date there are insufficient data to decide where is the best location for the POCT devices. This in fact depends on hospital factors such as local infrastructures and human resources.

The viscoelastic tests can be used either as point-of-care tests at the bedside or as central laboratory-based tests [2, 3]. Both models have advantages and disadvantages.

In any case, a hospital using POCT devices should guarantee a POCT testing service, led by an expert management team with a good training program.

The management team should include, at the bare minimum, a director and a coordinator in order to guarantee that POCT users receive the same information regarding the test to ensure the consistency of practice through the procedure manual.

The procedure manual should describe the scope, the principle of tests, the specimen requirements, reagent and kit storage conditions, procedure for performing the test, safety precautions, test limitations and interferences, documentation of results, and procedure for performing quality controls.

In the manual it should be mentioned that a diagnostic test can be divided into three stages: pre-analytical, analytical, and post-analytical.

Each step is susceptible to errors that can affect the result.

The most common sources of errors in the pre-analytical stage are patient identification, specimen collection, inadequate sample, specimen identification, fasting versus nonfasting, wrong anticoagulant, contamination with intravenous fluids, and hemolysis.

As for standard coagulation tests, incorrect blood collection techniques and sampling result

V. Agostini, MD
Transfusion Medicine Cesena/Forlì and Blood Establishment, Clinical Pathology Department-Cesena Azienda U.S.L Romagna, Romagna, Italy
e-mail: vani.agostini@gmail.com

M. Ranucci, P. Simioni (eds.), *Point-of-Care Tests for Severe Hemorrhage: A Manual for Diagnosis and Treatment*, DOI 10.1007/978-3-319-24795-3_13

in activation of coagulation leading to erroneous results.

Recently the International Society for Thrombosis and Haemostasis Working Party (ISTH-WP) on standardization of thromboelastography tried [4] to determine the methodology for performing viscoelastic test in patients suffering from congenital bleeding disorders, such as hemophilia, at baseline and after treatment with coagulation factor concentrates.

During the analytical phase, sources of errors are inadequate mixing of samples with reagents, usage of expired reagents, and instrument failure.

In the post-analytical phase, the most common sources of errors are the incorrect reading of results and the nonrecognition of interferences.

13.1.1 Point-of-Care Testing at the Bedside

The devices could be located in the emergency department, in the operating room, in the intensive care unit, and in the delivery room or could be used in a mobile way, if the number of devices is limited. In these cases the turnaround time and the time to treatment can be very quick if coagulation factor concentrates are immediately available at the bedside.

To support this kind of choice, an extensive staff education and training is essential together with a rigorous quality control management [5]. Good communication between clinicians who are in charge of the patients and a consultant in hematology or an expert in hemostasis to share specific algorithms to support coagulation during critical bleeding is also very important.

13.1.2 Central Laboratory-Based Tests

If POCT is located in the central laboratory, an effective transportation system for blood samples is essential, as well as an immediate way to get results back to clinicians who are treating the patient.

For the first issue, there are no data to support the use of pneumatic tube transportation for blood samples for coagulation tests, so to overcome the problem, one possibility is to identify, in the standard operational procedure, the person in charge for the transport of blood samples in emergency situation.

Regarding the way to communicate the results to physicians who are in charge of the bleeding patient, an electronic connection could be the best option if a local multidisciplinary algorithm for the management of critical bleeding has been shared and coagulation factor concentrates are immediately available at the bedside.

Either in case of point-of-care testing at the bedside or in a central laboratory test model, a good communication with the blood bank or transfusion medicine specialists is important in order to reduce the time to receive blood component therapy such as fresh frozen plasma, cryoprecipitate, or platelet concentrates.

13.2 Other Models

Depending on local factors and human resources, other possibilities can be adopted.

An interesting initiative was started at the Department of Pathology and Laboratory Medicine of the University of Texas-Houston where a coagulation-based hemotherapy (CBH) service was created to support coagulation in bleeding patients undergoing cardiopulmonary bypass (CPB) [6].

The CBH service is managed by clinical pathologists and includes preoperative, intraoperative, and postoperative consultations through the monitoring of coagulation variables at defined times during surgery with either standard coagulation tests or thromboelastography or platelet function testing.

The devices are located close to the operating room, samples are hand delivered to reduce the turnaround time, the tests are immediately started on arrival of blood samples, and blood products are delivered to the operation room from a satellite blood bank located inside the operating room.

13.2.1 An Italian Experience: The Cesena Model

Viscoelastic tests were initially introduced at the Bufalini Hospital in Cesena for the management of trauma-induced coagulopathy.

Three integrated trauma care systems (SIAT) are present in Emilia-Romagna, Italy (Figs. 13.1 and 13.2).

The SIAT works according to hub and spoke model: severe and resource-consuming patients are centralized in first-level hubs to guarantee high-quality and efficient care. Every SIAT has a trauma center (hub) connected with a net of peripheral hospitals (spokes).

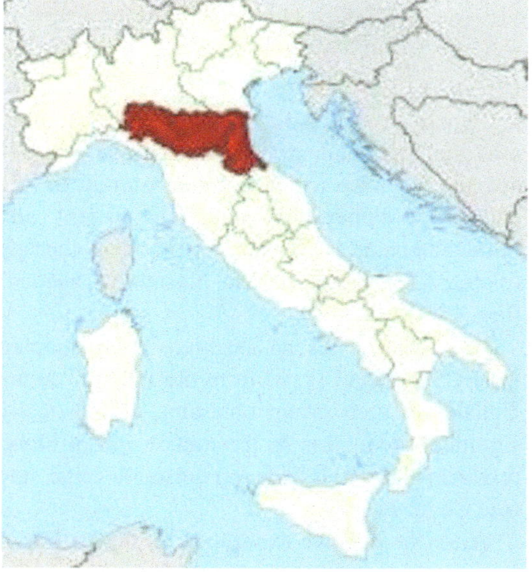

Fig. 13.1 Emilia-Romagna, Italy

The main goal of a SIAT is to organize and manage trauma care pathways, to enable quick and adequate treatments in the same way everywhere.

Bufalini Hospital in Cesena is the hub for the Area Vasta SIAT and serves a catchment area of about 1 million people doubling during summertime because of its geographical position on the Adriatic coast.

Moreover, at the Bufalini Hospital a hemophilia center and a thrombosis and hemostasis center inside the transfusion medicine ward are present in order to guarantee consultation on congenital and acquired bleeding disorders.

In 2001 the regional healthcare plan was published, and for the accreditation of the emergency department, a specific protocol and standard operative procedure for the management of major blood loss were required.

A multidisciplinary team for the implementation of the transfusion policy was created involving traumatologists, emergency physicians, and transfusion medicine specialists with expertise in hemostasis.

A first formula-driven protocol for the management of trauma-induced coagulopathy was adopted for the prompt release of the blood component therapy.

In 2012 the protocol was implemented with the introduction of the thromboelastometry

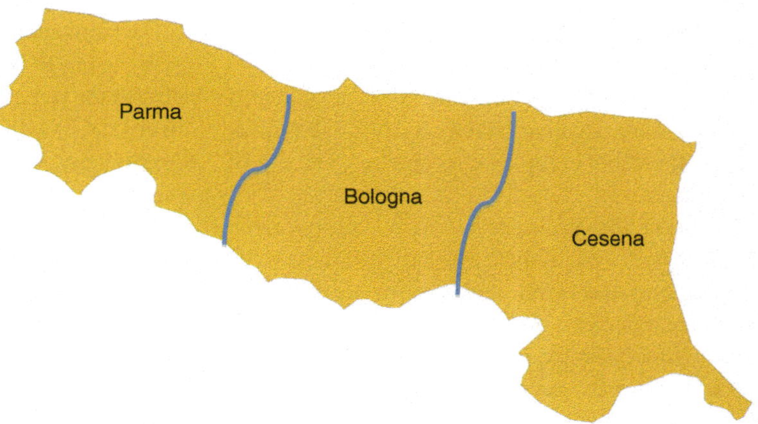

Fig. 13.2 Emilia-Romagna integrated trauma care system (SIAT)

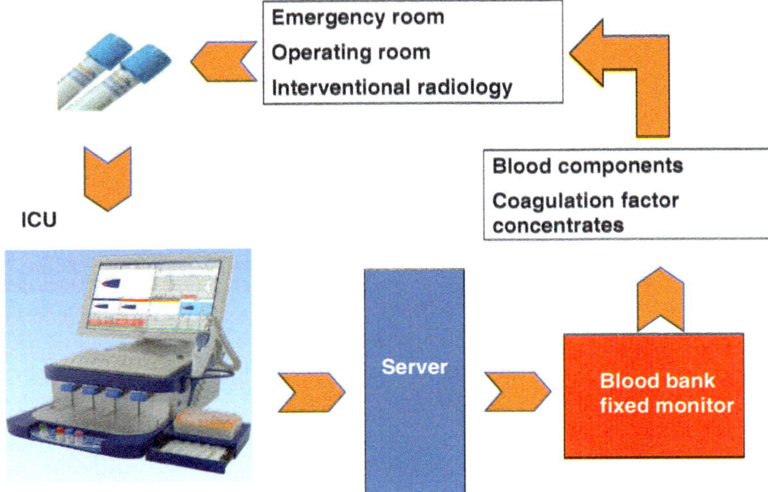

Fig. 13.3 Cesena organization

(ROTEM) device. The instrument was located in the intensive care unit (ICU), and an intensive training course was started. All the anesthetists and transfusion medicine specialists were trained by classroom lessons with a ratio of one tutor to three students. Every lesson lasted 4 h: two hours of theory and two practical hours of hands-on ROTEM using blood samples from patients in the ICU. Every year a refresh course is organized.

Before introducing the device in the clinical practice, a verification of ROTEM reference ranges was conducted performing assays on blood samples from 20 healthy blood donors with normal coagulation, and results were compared with the reference ranges provided by the manufacturer.

A specific algorithm was defined for the coagulation support to the trauma bleeding patients, and a laminated poster with the algorithm is present in the ICU and in the blood bank.

In the emergency department are available 6 units of zero negative red blood cells, 3,000 units of prothrombin complex concentrates, and 2 g of fibrinogen.

During the management of a major trauma patient with coagulopathy, in order to reduce the turnaround time and the time to treatment, a nurse or a porter is dedicated to the transportation of the blood sample to the ICU where the testing is immediately started. The ROTEM device is electronically connected to the blood bank monitor, where a transfusion medicine specialist oversees the trace and orders the administration of coagulation factor concentrates stored in the emergency department near the patient and immediately releases blood component therapy (platelets or fresh frozen plasma if needed) (Fig. 13.3).

In 2013 the Cesena Trauma Center adopted the ECS protocol [7, 8] from the Italian Trauma Update research group obtaining a statistically significant reduction of the transfusion of blood products in the first 24 h and during hospital stay (see Chap. 7).

After the positive experience in the setting of trauma, a second ROTEM instrument was introduced for the management of postpartum hemorrhage and perioperative bleeding with the same organization showed in Fig. 13.3.

The implementation of the goal-directed therapy by using ROTEM device has been useful not only for the reduction of transfusion therapy during critical bleeding but also to improve the multidisciplinary approach among different specialists.

13.3 POCT and Quality Assurance

Quality assurance (QA) for POCT is not less important than for conventional laboratory-based analysis and should incorporate both internal quality control (IQC) and external quality assessment (EQA) [3].

13.3.1 Internal Quality Control

IQC is used to establish whether the technique is performed consistently over a period of time and should be applied in order to obtain the immediate control of result generation [9].

IQC is extremely important in ensuring that precise and accurate results are provided.

The IQC is influenced by sample collection and handling, selection of right reagents when there is the choice, constant application of standard operational procedures (SOPs), training, and motivation of personnel involved in performing tests.

The manufacturers of viscoelastic device provide specific indications on how to perform the IQC and on the frequency of IQC.

IQC material is generally purchased from the manufacturers, who supply a normal control and a pathological control and target range for the material.

For ICQ the date of test, batch of reagents, acceptable range and operator identity should be recorded.

If an IQC result is outside the range, a second sample should be run, and if also the second control is outside the stated range, patient sample examination should be stopped until the resolution of the problem.

13.3.2 External Quality Assessment

Generally EQA exercises are distributed two to four times per year and measure the performance of the single center in comparison to that of other participants.

Whole-blood stable samples are not currently available to perform EQA exercises.

To date only the National External Quality Assessment Service (NEQAS) provides lyophilized plasma as test material for TEG and ROTEM [10]. Samples from normal control, factor VIII and IX deficiency plasma, and normal plasma spiked with heparin have been analyzed by TEG users and ROTEM users obtaining a wide range of coefficients of variance: 7.1–39.9 % for TEG and 7–83.6 % for ROTEM.

Conclusion

The last 10 years have seen an exponential increase in the utilization of viscoelastic tests such as rotational thromboelastometry and thromboelastography to support hemostasis during critical bleeding in different setting (perioperative bleeding, trauma-induced coagulopathy, postpartum hemorrhage).

Depending on local organization and human resources, POCT can be used at the bedside or in the central laboratory.

Different professional figures can perform the test: nurses, technicians, and physicians. This implies that in each hospital, a POCT team exists with the aim to disseminate the knowledge on coagulation monitoring during critical bleeding, to improve and maintain staff education, to organize the whole system from blood sample collection to the delivery of the results back to the clinicians, and finally to promote the quality assurance through the routine application of IQC and the participation to EQA.

References

1. Schochl H, Schlimp CJ (2014) Trauma bleeding management: the concept of goal-directed primary care. Anesth Analg 119:1064–1073
2. Inaba K, Rizoli S, Veigas PV et al (2015) 2014 Consensus conference on viscoelastic test-based transfusion guidelines for early trauma resuscitation: report of the panel. J Trauma Acute Care Surg 78:1220–1229
3. Device Bulletin (2010) Management and use of IVD point of care testing devices. Department of Health. Available at www.dhsspsni.gov.uk/db2010_02_ivd_poct.pdf
4. Chitlur M, Rivard GE, Lillicrap D et al (2014) Recommendations for performing thromboelastography/thromboelastometry in hemophilia: communication from the SSC of the ISTH. J Thromb Haemost 12:103–106
5. Perry DJ, Fitzmaurice DA, Kitchen S et al (2010) Point-of-care testing in haemostasis. Br J Haematol 150(5):501–514

6. Welsh KJ, Nedelcu E, Bai Y et al (2014) How do we manage cardiopulmonary bypass coagulopathy? Transfusion 54:2158–2166
7. Nardi G, Agostini V, Rondinelli MB et al (2013) Prevention and treatment of trauma induced coagulopathy (TIC). An intended protocol from the Italian trauma update research group. J Anesthesiol Clin Sci doi:10.7243/2049-9752-2-22
8. Nardi G, Agostini V, Rondinelli B et al (2015) Trauma-induced coagulopathy: impact of the early coagulation support protocol on blood product consumption, mortality and costs. Crit Care 19(1):83
9. Quarterman C, Shaw M, Johnson I et al (2014) Intra- and inter-centre standardisation of thromboelastography (TEG). Anaesthesia 69:883–890
10. Kitchen DP, Kitchen S, Jennings I et al (2010) Quality assurance and quality control of thromboelastography and rotational thromboelastometry: the UK NEQAS for blood coagulation experience. Semin Thromb Hemost 36:757–763

Clinical Cases 14

Daniele Penzo, Lesley De Pietri, Paolo Simioni, Luca Spiezia, Elena Campello, Sara Maggiolo, Marco Ranucci, Ekaterina Baryshnikova, Giuseppe Nardi, Alberto Grassetto, and Lucio Bucci

14.1 Introduction

This chapter integrates six clinical cases in different scenarios, where bleeding emergencies have been treated according to a coagulation point-of-care (POC) test-based strategy. All the cases come from the clinical experience of the authors of the present chapter.

14.2 Case 1: Maternal Cardiac Arrest Complicated by Acquired Hemophilia: Good Outcome after One of the Most Scary Clinical Conditions

The aim of this case report is to stress that cardiac arrest in a pregnant woman may be successfully treated with full recovery for both the patient and the baby by a well-trained multidisciplinary team. On June 3, 2014, at 16.42 a previously healthy 44-year-old patient on initial labor had a sudden loss of consciousness associated with diffuse cyanosis; congestion of the neck, the face, and the upper limbs; and tachypnea. She quickly developed severe hypotension with wide complex tachycardia, which rapidly evolved in pulseless electrical activity in spite of immediate resuscitation support. The patients were moved to the delivery room for Caesarean section. Surgery was started at 16.49 giving birth to a

D. Penzo, MD (✉)
2nd Service Anesthesia Critical Care Medicine, S. Chiara Hospital, Trento, Italy
e-mail: daniele.penzo@apss.tn.it

L. De Pietri, MD
Division of Anaesthesiology and Intensive Care Unit, Azienda Ospedaliero-Universitaria di Modena-Policlinico, Modena, Italy

P. Simioni, MD, PhD
Department of Medicine, Hemorrhagic and Thrombotic Diseases Unit, University of Padua Medical School, Padua, Italy

L. Spiezia, MD • E. Campello, MD • S. Maggiolo, MD
Department of Medicine, 5th Chair of Internal Medicine, University of Padua Medical School, Padua, Italy

M. Ranucci, MD, FESC • E. Baryshnikova, PhD
Department of Cardiothoracic-Vascular Anesthesia and ICU, IRCCS Policlinico San Donato, San Donato Milanese, Milan, Italy

G. Nardi, MD
Department of Shock and Trauma Center, S. Camillo-Forlanini Hospital, Rome, Italy

A. Grassetto, MD
UOC Anestesia e Rianimazione, Dipartimento Emergenza Urgenza, Ospedale dell'Angelo di Mestre, Venice, Italy

L. Bucci, MD
ICU "Bozza" – 1st Service Anesthesia and Intensive Care, A.O. Niguarda Ca' Granda Hospital, Milan, Italy

M. Ranucci, P. Simioni (eds.), *Point-of-Care Tests for Severe Hemorrhage: A Manual for Diagnosis and Treatment*, DOI 10.1007/978-3-319-24795-3_14

living child at 16.52. The mother was submitted to advanced life support resuscitation algorithm (external cardiac massage and adrenaline every 3–5 min) for over 40 min before obtaining a return of spontaneous circulation (ROSC). During the pulseless activity, no episodes of shockable rhythm were recorded. A transthoracic cardiac echography performed during cardiopulmonary resuscitation showed a picture of "plus" which was interpreted as a "floating thrombus" in the right ventricle. This suggested that the cardiac arrest might be caused by a pulmonary embolism. However, an angio-CT scan performed soon after hemodynamic stabilization could not confirm this diagnosis, and the finding of a normal PaO_2/FiO_2 (>500) was also not consistent with this hypothesis. Half an hour after ROSC, the patient showed a massive uncontrolled bleeding. She was immediately submitted to rescue hysterectomy, but hemorrhage could not be controlled. The massive transfusion protocol was started together with viscoelastic point-of-care monitoring (thromboelastometry – ROTEM). Data of the ROTEM suggested a severe coagulopathy. During the following 12 h, the patient was transfused with 26 units of blood (RBCs). She also received fibrinogen concentrate (4 g), tranexamic acid, fresh frozen plasma (FFP) (26 units), and platelet concentrates (12 units), but there was no way to stop the bleeding. At 5 AM, while the patients were still massively bleeding, the ROTEM showed a normal FIBTEM (suggesting normal level of fibrinogen), a nearly normal CT in the EXTEM test (suggesting normal thrombin generation in the extrinsic pathway), and a severely prolonged CT in INTEM (530 s), a pattern that suggests an elective impairment of the intrinsic pathway. An acquired hemophilia was therefore suspected. Acquired hemophilia is a rare but potentially life-threatening bleeding disorder caused by the development of autoantibodies directed against plasma coagulation factors, most frequently factor VIII. It has been described as a major complication of postpartum shock. The patient was therefore treated with activated recombinant Factor VII (rFVIIa) (100 μg/kg). Coagulation immediately normalized and bleeding stopped. She was admitted to the intensive care unit (ICU). She required treatment with vasoactive drugs and further volume loading with crystalloids. She also received subsequent doses of rFVIIa and high-dose steroids as part of the treatment of acquired hemophilia. During the next days, her coagulation pattern normalized and she did not require further transfusions. Factor VIII increased to 180 %. The patient was kept under deep sedation for several days and submitted to artificial ventilation through a percutaneous tracheostomy. Electroencephalography (EEG), magnetic nuclear resonance, and somatosensory evoked potentials were performed. Surprisingly these tests showed only little signs of brain damage. When sedation was discontinued, the patient progressively recovered. After 13 days since ICU admission, she was transferred to the ward. Although amnesic, she was fully awake and in good neurological condition. Her female baby was also doing well, and mother and child could finally join together. Investigations were made looking for the causes of cardiac arrest. At the beginning of her pregnancy, she performed an electrocardiogram and echocardiogram because of arrhythmias. Although the ECG showed a ventricular bigeminy and cardiac echography demonstrated a moderate mitral and tricuspid insufficiency, these findings were not further investigated. Moreover during the ICU stay, the patient had several similar episodes of ventricular bigeminy. She was therefore submitted to a full set of cardiologic investigations including transesophageal echocardiography and a coronary CT scan. The previous findings were confirmed, but these investigations were otherwise negative. Other investigations have been planned but not yet performed.

14.3 Case 2: Monitoring of Replacement Therapy for Intracranial Meningioma Resection in an End-Stage Cirrhotic Patient: A Possible Role for Thromboelastometry

The patient was a 59-year-old woman affected by end-stage liver cirrhosis due to HBV-HDV infection on a waiting list for liver transplantation. In August 2013 she was admitted to our hospital for slurred speech and slowed motility. A cerebral MRI showed a left frontal extra-axial expansive lesion of 3 cm in diameter, diffuse pachymeningeal thickening and enhancement, severe perilesional edema with distortion of anterior ventricular cavity, and right-sided shift of the median cerebral axis; the lesion was suggestive for atypical meningioma. Surgical resection of the intracranial neoplasm was necessary to allow liver transplantation. Laboratory tests were compatible with a severe coagulopathy (INR 2.18, aPTT 31 s, fibrinogen 1.10 g/L, platelet count 17 × 10^9/L). In order to guide replacement therapy for the surgical intervention, blood samples for ROTEM® and classical coagulation tests were planned before, during, and after the surgical intervention and then daily for 1 week.

ROTEM® performed the day before surgery (day 0) depicted a severe hypocoagulable profile (Fig. 14.1a) characterized by a prolongation of CT and CFT in INTEM (265 s and 832 s, respectively; reference ranges: CT 100–240 s, CFT 30–110 s) and EXTEM (142 s and 837 s, respectively; reference ranges: CT 38–79 s, CFT 34–159 s) and a reduction of MCF amplitude in INTEM (23 mm), EXTEM (22 mm), and FIBTEM (3 mm) (reference ranges: 50–72 mm in INTEM/EXTEM, 9–25 mm in FIBTEM). Platelet concentrates, FFP 10 ml/kg, fibrinogen concentrates 4 g (Haemocomplettan, CSL Behring GmbH, Marburg, Germany), prothrombin complex concentrates (PCC) 20 U/kg (Uman Complex-Kedrion S.p.A, Lucca, Italy), and tranexamic acid 1000 mg were administered immediately before surgery. The patient underwent surgical removal of the tumor through a standard craniotomy in general anesthesia. ROTEM® was performed during surgery and showed a stable profile (Fig. 14.1b) characterized by a prolongation of CT and CFT in INTEM (277 s and 1257 s, respectively), a normal CT and a prolonged CFT in EXTEM (52 s and 981 s, respectively), a stable reduction of MCF amplitude in INTEM (21 mm) and EXTEM (23 mm), and an amelioration of MCF in FIBTEM (7 mm).

After resection of tumor, an accurate hemostasis was pursued. Coagulation tests were repeated the day after the surgery (day 1), and they remained hypocoagulable (INR 1.50, aPTT 26 s, fibrinogen 1.10 g/L, platelet count 13 × 10^9/L). The corresponding ROTEM® profile is shown in Fig. 14.1c. In particular, a prolongation of CT and CFT in INTEM (298 s and 850 s, respectively), a normal CT and a prolonged CFT in EXTEM (53 s and 705 s, respectively), and a stable reduction of MCF amplitude in INTEM (23 mm) and EXTEM (26 mm) were demonstrated. MCF in FIBTEM (7 mm) was higher compared to basal MCF before surgery (3 mm). We decided to administer platelet concentrates, FFP 10 ml/kg, fibrinogen concentrates 2 g, PCC 20 U/kg, and tranexamic acid 1000 mg bid.

The coagulation monitoring was consecutively repeated daily after surgery for 7 days (days 2–7). ROTEM® (Fig. 14.1d) showed normalization of the activation phase (CT in INTEM and EXTEM) and less prolongation of the coagulation phase propagation (CFT in INTEM and EXTEM) associated with a lower reduction of MCF amplitude (6 mm in FIBTEM). Based on these findings, we decided to daily administer platelet concentrates, FFP 10 ml/kg, and fibrinogen concentrates 2 g until day 7 after surgery. No hemorrhagic episodes were observed during the following days. Two CT scans performed 7 and 30 days after surgery ruled out a cerebral hematoma occurrence.

14.3.1 Comment

Prompt availability of coagulation test results during surgery is mandatory for appropriate bleeding management, in particular for patients with severe bleeding for whom delays in the treatment must be minimized. The current solution to avoid unacceptable turnaround times, as recommended in European guidelines, is to implement viscoelastic devices to improve the management of hemostatic therapy.

In our patient, platelets concentrates, FFP, and PCC were given in order to ameliorate the severe coagulopathy detected by ROTEM® assay. In addition to platelets defect, decreased synthesis of clotting factors and inhibitors, and

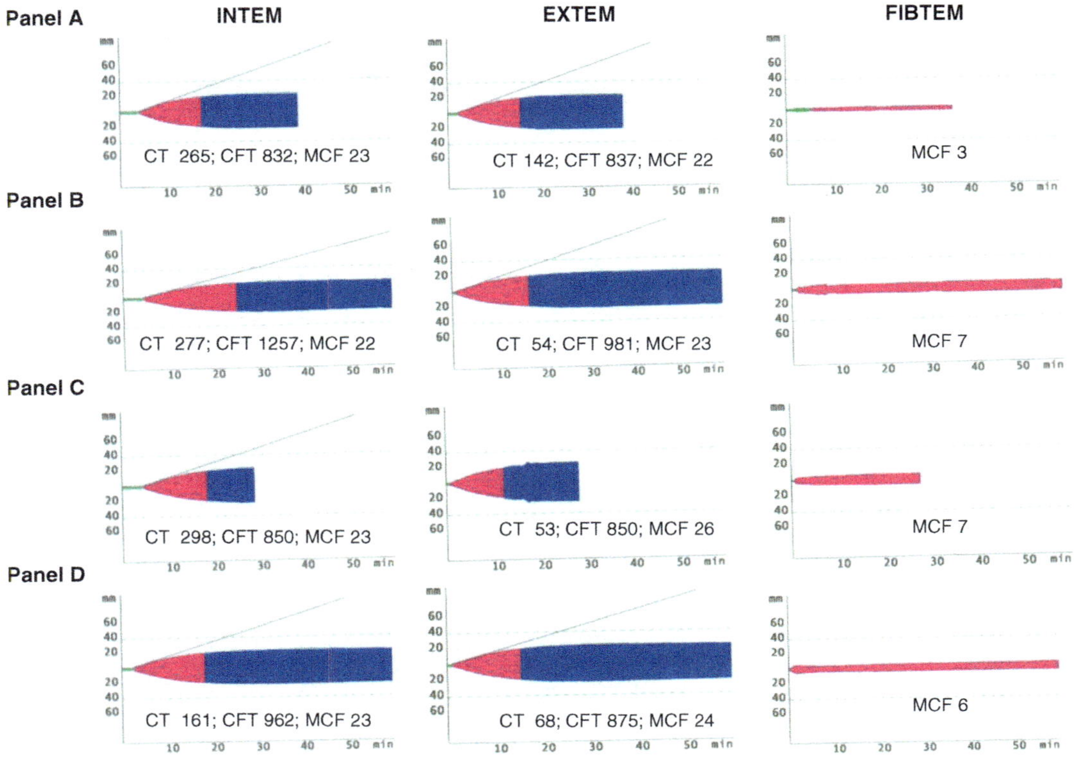

Fig. 14.1 ROTEM thromboelastometry profile performed before, during, and after the surgical intervention and then daily for 1 week. Reference values: INTEM CT 100–240 s, CFT 30–110 s, MCF 50–72 mm, EXTEM CT 38–79 s, CFT 34–159 s, MCF 50–72 mm, FIBTEM MCF 9–25 mm. (**a**) Before surgery: severe hypocoagulable profile characterized by a prolongation of CT and CFT in INTEM and EXTEM and severe reduction of MCF amplitude in INTEM, EXTEM, and FIBTEM. (**b**) Amelioration of hypocoagulable profile during neurosurgery after replacement therapy (FFP, platelets, and fibrinogen concentrates, PCC, tranexamic acid): stable prolongation of CT in INTEM, CFT in INTEM and EXTEM, and mild reduction of MCF amplitude in INTEM, EXTEM, and FIBTEM. (**c**) ROTEM profile 1 day after surgery before replacement therapy (FFP, platelets, and fibrinogen concentrates, PCC, tranexamic acid): prolongation of CT in INTEM and of CFT in INTEM and EXTEM and reduction of MCF amplitude in INTEM, EXTEM, and FIBTEM. (**d**) Stable hypocoagulable ROTEM profile on day 4 after neurosurgery: normalization of the activation phase (CT in INTEM and EXTEM) and less prolongation of the propagation phase (CFT in INTEM and EXTEM) associated with a lower reduction of MCF amplitude in FIBTEM. CT, clotting time; CFT, clot formation time; MCF, maximum clot firmness; FFP, fresh frozen plasma; PCC, prothrombin complex concentrates

hyperfibrinolysis, it is worth noting that coagulopathy-related bleeding in liver cirrhosis is also due to an abnormal fibrinogen synthesis/polymerization. This acquired dysfibrinogenemia is characterized by an increase in sialic acid content leading to an impaired fibrin monomer polymerization. It can be functionally detected by a prolongation of the thrombin time, which correlates with the increase in fibrinogen sialic acid content. In our case, ROTEM analysis was useful to demonstrate the presence of a dysfunctional fibrinogen through the measurement of MCF in FIBTEM, which showed a reduced fibrin clot formation despite plasma levels of fibrinogen measured by Clauss assay which were greater than 1 g/L and thus enough for hemostasis. Importantly, since FIBTEM is designed to measure elasticity of the fibrin clot under platelet inhibition by cytochalasin D, FIBTEM MCF should not be considered as a measurement of fibrinogen concentration, but mainly a measurement of mechanical properties of the fibrin clot which are only in part related to fibrinogen concentration. Low FIBTEM MCF may be interpreted as an indication for fibrinogen deficiency or fibrin polymerization disorders. Our findings confirm that the viscoelastic measure of the fibrinogen allows the evaluation of functional fibrinogen polymerization without platelet "noise" and may be a marker of a reduced fibrin polymerization and a bleeding tendency. These findings guided replacement therapy by fibrinogen concentrates in our patient and the use of antifibrinolytic agents to stabilize fibrin clot.

Fibrinogen plays an important role in the coagulation process and clot stabilization binding of FXIII. In addition, it plays a central role in platelet activation and aggregation by binding to the platelet glycoprotein receptor GPIIb/IIIa. Interestingly, in experimental studies it has been shown that fibrinogen administration counteracts the effects of low platelet count and improves platelet aggregation. In our thromboelastometry whole blood analysis, the decrease in platelets could be offset by an increase in fibrinogen/fibrin polymerization, which results in the restoration of MCF in FIBTEM compared to baseline levels following administration of fibrinogen concentrate. It seems that the amelioration of fibrinogen concentration would improve clot formation and platelets aggregation and allows for a safe surgery despite the low platelets count.

Our experience suggests that a ROTEM®-based approach could be helpful in identifying the blood components necessary to restore coagulation. In fact, no intracranial bleeding complications occurred either during the intervention or in the whole postoperative course. Thromboelastometry is able to optimize the choice of replacement therapy with hemostatic products, thus preventing hemorrhagic complications. Another considerable advantage is the short time required to use the algorithm approach, which makes it possible to obtain a rapid and focused intervention. Larger and prospective studies are needed to validate the use of ROTEM "theragnostic" approach in the management of neurosurgery or invasive procedures in coagulopathic population.

14.4 Case 3: Postoperative Bleeding Management in a Liver Transplant Patient

A 63-year-old male underwent liver transplantation for HBV-related cirrhosis. The preoperative laboratory profile is reported below:

- Hemoglobin, 7.9 g/dL; hematocrit, 24 %; platelet count, 94 × 10^6/L
- Bilirubin, 2.85 mg/dL; creatinine, 2.14 mg/dL; albumin, 3.2 g/dL
- PT, 22 %; INR, 2.98; aPTT, 1.82; fibrinogen, 119 mg/dL

During surgery, the following blood products and substitutes were administered: red blood cells (RBCs), 3876 mL; platelet concentrate, 1 U; and fibrinogen concentrate (Haemocomplettan® P, CSL Behring, Marburg, Germany), 4 g. Additionally, 1 g of tranexamic acid was administered.

Post-surgery, a native thromboelastographic (TEG) test was done, without showing significant alterations (Fig. 14.2). The corresponding standard laboratory data are reported below:

- Hemoglobin, 10.1 g/dL; hematocrit, 29.2 %; platelet count, 52 × 10^6/L
- Bilirubin, 4.36 mg/dL; creatinine, 1.84 mg/dL; albumin, 1.2 g/dL
- PT, 16 %; INR, 3.96; aPTT, 3.64; fibrinogen, 109 mg/dL

Two hours after extubation, a moderate bleeding from the abdominal drains starts, without hemodynamic compromise. After one hour of ongoing bleeding, a moderate hypotension appears (systemic blood pressure 95/50 mmHg, heart rate 100 beats/min). Lactated Ringer's solution (500 mL) and 2 units of fresh frozen plasma (FFP) were infused. The surgeon in charge is alerted but did not judge that the patient merits further surgery. A second TEG test is performed, highlighting a worsened coagulation status (Fig. 14.3). The blood loss from the drains became more evident in the subsequent hours, and the patient developed signs of shock. The circulating volume is replaced with an additional 2 units of RBCs, 1100 mL of

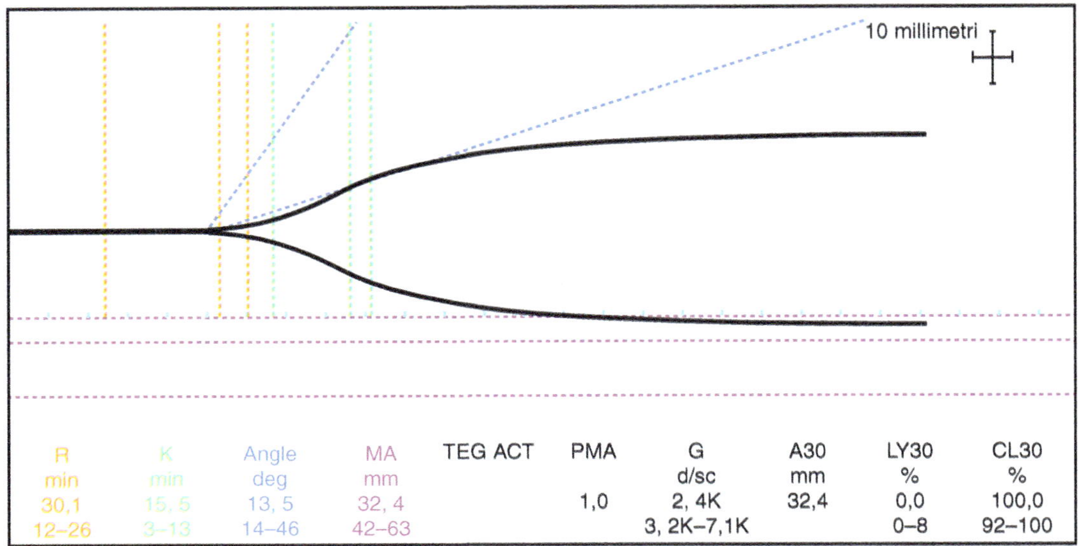

Fig. 14.2 1st postoperative TEG

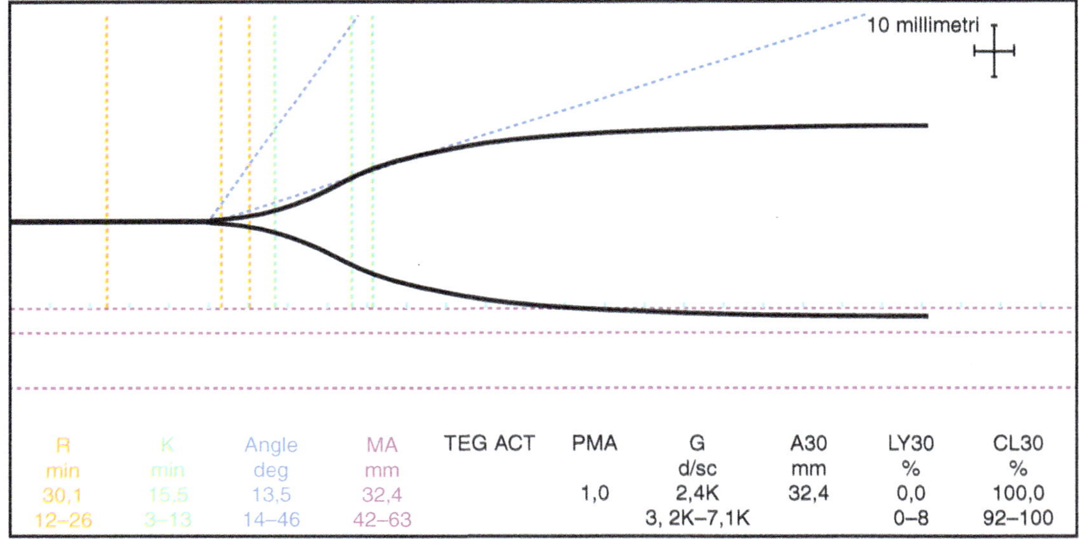

Fig. 14.3 2nd postoperative TEG at the initial stage of bleeding

FFP, 500 mL crystalloid, and 500 mL colloid fluids for a total of 2 l of hemo-derivatives and 1 l of colloids/crystalloids. A blood sample is taken for laboratory tests and TEG analysis. TEG with heparinase is severely impaired (Fig. 14.4). The laboratory data are as follows:

- Hemoglobin, 7.2 g/dL; hematocrit, 20.9 %; platelet count, 33 × 10^6/L
- Bilirubin, 3.0 mg/dL; creatinine, 2.0 mg/dL; albumin, 1.3 g/dL
- PT, 42 %; INR, 1.77; aPTT, 1.74; fibrinogen, 100 mg/dL

The patient was then transferred to the operating room and treated with 1500 IU of prothrombin complex concentrate (PCC, Uman Complex DI, Kedrion, Castelvecchio Pascoli, Italy), 4 g of

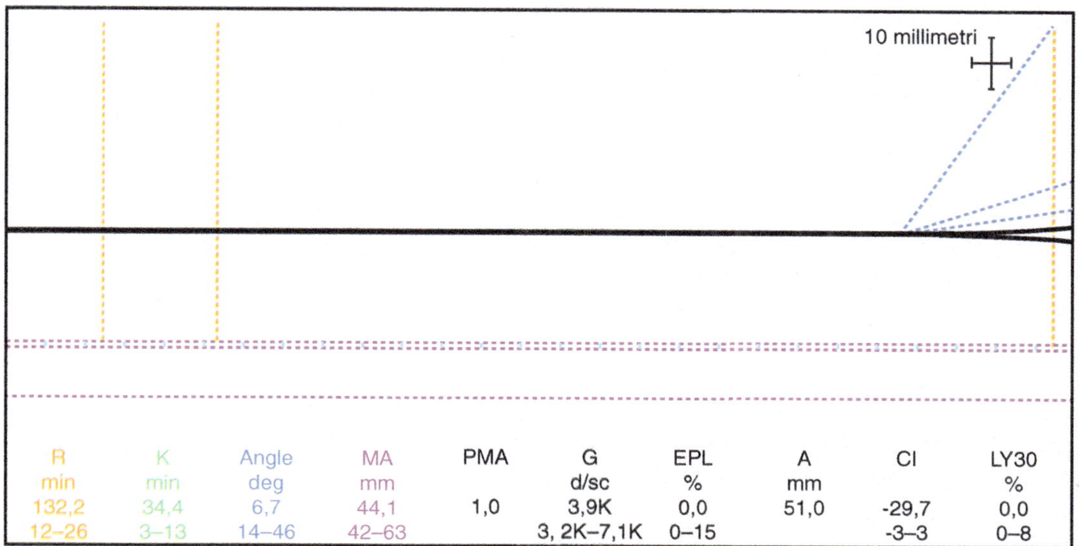

Fig. 14.4 Severe impairment of coagulation before hemostatic drug administration

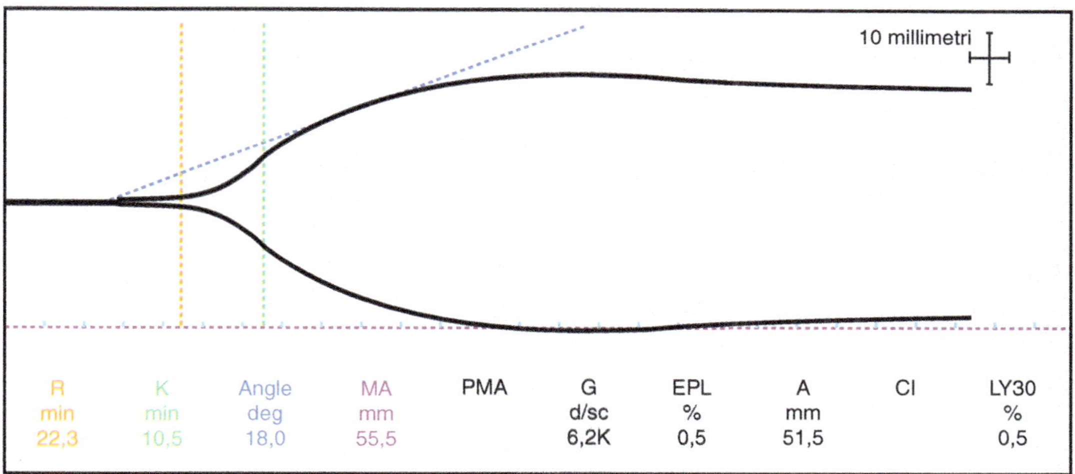

Fig. 14.5 Hemostasis improvement after pharmacological treatment of bleeding

fibrinogen (Haemocompletta® P, CSL Behring, Marburg, Germany), 1 g of tranexamic acid, and 3 units of RBCs.

The improvement of hemostasis allows the surgeon to identify the source of bleeding. The TEG is now almost normalized (Fig. 14.5). The patient is then transferred to the intensive care unit where the laboratory data are as follows:

- Hemoglobin, 10.2 g/dL; hematocrit, 30.2 %; platelet count, 34 × 10^6/L
- Bilirubin, 3.0 mg/dL; creatinine, 1.89 mg/dL; albumin, 1.3 g/dL
- PT, 53 %; INR, 1.49; aPTT, 1.44; fibrinogen, 231 mg/dL

The rest of the clinical course was uneventful.

14.4.1 Comment

A case of coagulopathy triggered by surgical bleeding is resolved with substitution therapy based on PCC and fibrinogen concentrate.

14.5 Case 4: ROTEM-Directed Therapy in Craniofacial Injury

A 68-year-old male cyclist sustained serious craniofacial trauma through collision with a car at 16:30. He was intubated by the on-call anesthesiologist, and blood analyses and a full-body computed tomography scan were performed. Multiple fractures were observed in the frontal, orbital, zygomatic, ethmoid, and nasal processes of the maxilla and the pterygoid process of the sphenoid, and the patient's right leg was heavily contused. The patient became severely anemic (hemoglobin [Hb] = 4.7 g/dL) with ongoing facial bleeding, and 4 U red blood cells (RBCs), 3 U FFP, and 3000 mL colloid (Amidolite, B. Braun, Italy) were transfused. Following posterior nasal and oral cavity packing, the patient was still bleeding with continued anemia (Hb = 6.4 g/dL).

At 20:30, signs of shock were still present (blood pressure = 85/55 mmHg, heart rate = 110 bpm, base excess = −10.4 mEq/L). These signs prompted the team leader to activate our massive hemorrhage protocol. The maxillofacial surgeon reported great difficulty in achieving hemostasis. Multifocal bleeding from soft tissues was still present, and although packing of the oral cavity was repeated, bleeding continued, and the Hb level was 5.8 g/dL. RBCs (4 units) were transfused, and norepinephrine infusion was started at 0.1 mg/kg/min.

A blood sample was taken for ROTEM analysis (Fig. 14.6). In the EXTEM assay both clotting time and clot formation time (CFT) were pro-

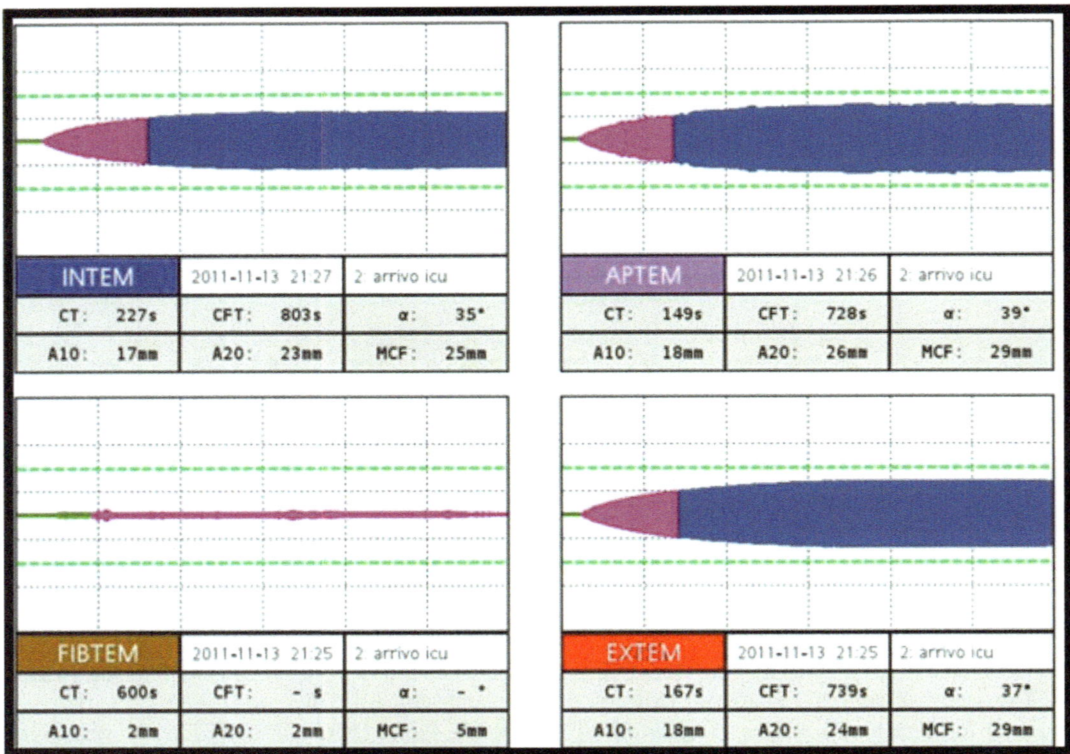

Fig. 14.6 First ROTEM analysis for severe multifocal bleeding

longed (167 s and 739 s, respectively), and maximum clot firmness (MCF) was below normal (29 mm). In addition, the amplitude 10 min after clotting time (A10) in the FIBTEM assay was only 2 mm, and a shorter clotting time was observed in the APTEM assay than in the EXTEM assay. These results indicated that the patient was severely coagulopathic. Tranexamic acid (2 g) was administered to correct fibrinolysis. The patient was then treated with 1000 IU PCC (Uman Complex DI, Kedrion, Castelvecchio Pascoli, Italy), 5 g fibrinogen (Haemocomplettan® P, CSL Behring, Marburg, Germany), and 2 U platelet concentrate.

A second ROTEM analysis was performed 2 h after administration of hemostatic therapy. This showed normalization of coagulation, in terms of clotting time in the EXTEM assay (62 s) and MCF in both the EXTEM (50 mm) and FIBTEM (10 mm) assays (Fig. 14.7). A further 3 units of RBCs were administered to correct anemia.

14.5.1 Comment

In this case, ROTEM-guided administration of PCC and fibrinogen concentrate was effective in correcting coagulopathy in a patient with craniofacial trauma and massive hemorrhage. The first ROTEM analysis revealed specific hemostatic defects that were treated successfully using a targeted approach. We administered fibrinogen concentrate in response to a low FIBTEM MCF. This approach is supported by the fact that fibrinogen is the first coagulation factor to reach a critically low level upon blood loss and that adequate fibrinogen levels are essential for hemostasis [1, 2]. Moreover, in a study of patients with severe traumatic brain injury, low FIBTEM MCF was associated with an increase in mortality and RBC transfusion [3]. Low EXTEM MCF was corrected by also administering platelet concentrate; fibrinogen, platelets, and activated factor XIII all contribute to clot strength in the EXTEM assay. MCF in the EXTEM, INTEM, and FIBTEM assays is predictive of increased risk of massive transfusion [4, 5], demonstrating the importance of this parameter in the diagnosis of coagulopathy in massive bleeding.

Tranexamic acid was given because of a longer clotting time in the EXTEM assay than in the APTEM assay, suggesting the presence of hyperfibrinolysis. Such comparison of EXTEM and APTEM clotting times is used in a number of European trauma centers as a criterion for diagnosing hyperfibrinolysis, although there is currently little published data to support this practice. However, recent evidence from the CRASH-2 trial has shown that early treatment with tranexamic acid is beneficial for survival [6]. Although we were unable to administer tranexamic acid until more than 3 h after the accident, we considered that the evidence of fibrinolysis in the bleeding patient warranted rapid, targeted treatment. PCC was admin-

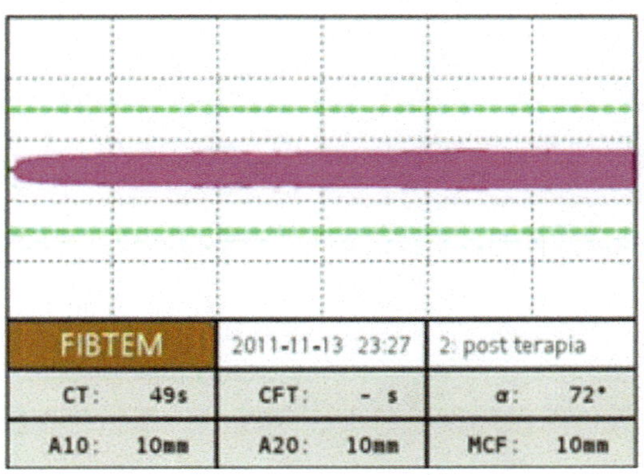

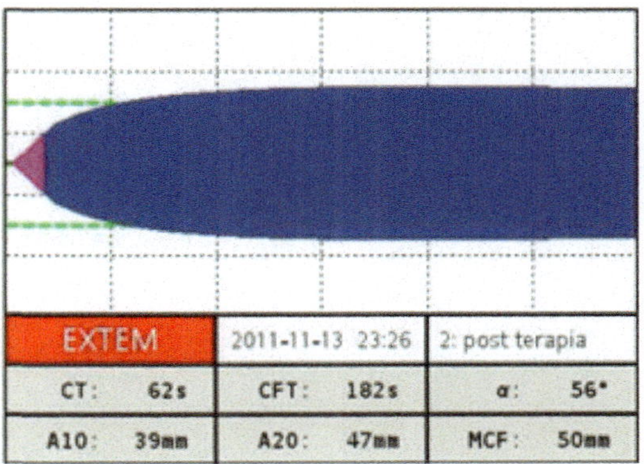

Fig. 14.7 ROTEM analysis after hemostatic treatment administration

istered because clotting time was prolonged in the APTEM as well as the EXTEM assay. Coagulation factor concentrates appear to minimize risks of complications such as transfusion-related acute lung injury or virus transmission. In addition, small volumes mean that concentrates are quick to administer, without causing hemodilution or volume overload.

Viscoelastic methods such as ROTEM or thromboelastography (TEG) allow drug therapy to be tailored to the patient's actual needs with a feedback loop to monitor and optimize treatment effectiveness and to minimize side effects.

14.6 Case 5: A 79-Year-Old Lady Admitted to the ICU With a Hemorrhagic Shock

Medical history: atrial fibrillation (no oral anticoagulants) and hypothyroidism. Previous hip replacement (2 years before).

Admitted to the ICU after elective surgery (removal of the infected hip prosthesis). During surgery, extensive blood loss (estimated at 2000 mL) treated with 5000 mL of crystalloids, 1500 mL of colloids, 5 units of red blood cells, and 3 units of fresh frozen plasma (FFP). The patient is hemodynamically unstable, with signs of hemorrhagic shock.

Laboratory Assays Are as Follows

- Hemoglobin 8 g/dL, hematocrit 23 %
- Platelet count 45,000/μL
- INR 3.6, aPTT ratio 3.8, d-dimer 0,5
- ph 7.05
- Base Excess -11, lactates 10 mMol/L
- Body temperature: 34 °C

A thromboelastographic (TEG) test is run and reveals a severe coagulopathy with prolonged R time (12.8 min), decreased maximum amplitude (MA, 20.7 mm), and severe primary hyperfibrinolysis (LY30 40.7 %) (Fig. 14.8).

A goal-directed, TEG-based therapeutic treatment is established, including 6 units of FFP.

8 units of cryoprecipitate, 2 units of platelet concentrates, and tranexamic acid (15 mg/kg bolus dose, followed by a continuous infusion of 2 mg kg^{-1} h^{-1}).

After this treatment, the bleeding stopped. The second TEG tests showed a complete recovery of the hemostatic process (Fig. 14.9).

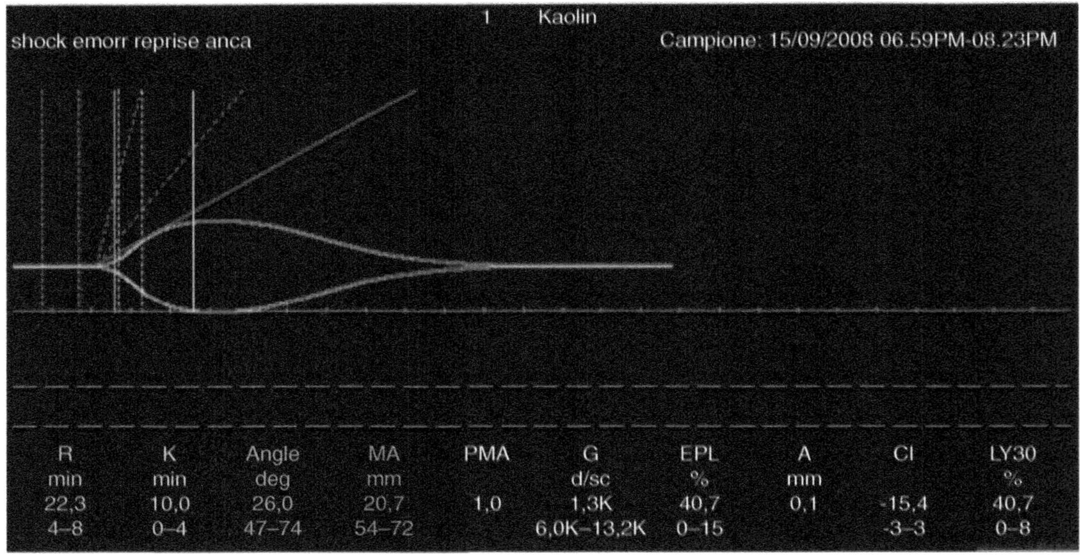

Fig. 14.8 First TEG analysis for hemorrhagic shock with signs of primary hyperfibrinolysis

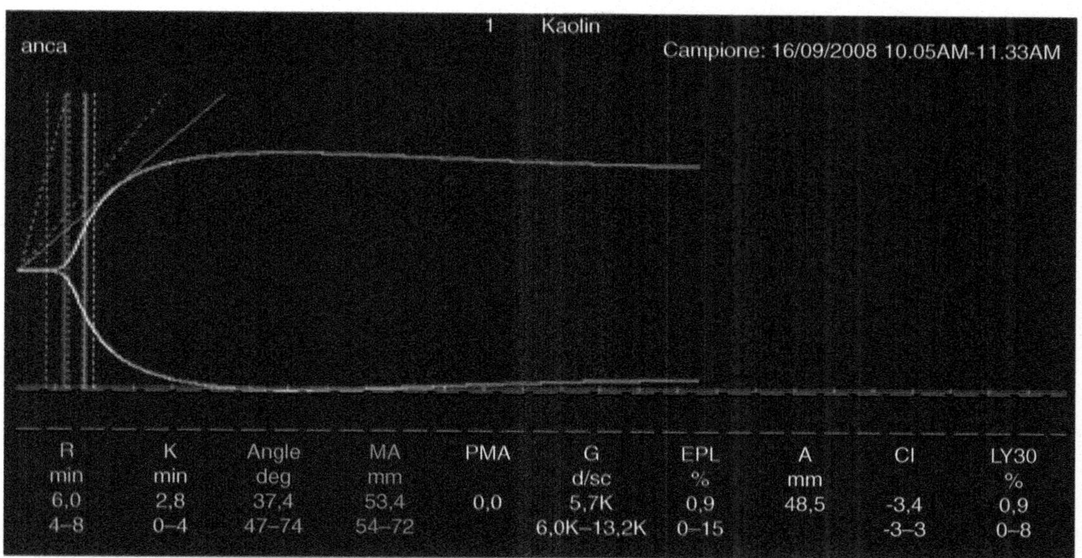

Fig. 14.9 Complete recovery of TEG parameters after hemostatic treatment

14.7 Case 6: Massive Postoperative Bleeding Refractory to Late Prohemostatic Treatment

A 42-year-old female presenting a thoracoabdominal aortic aneurysm was admitted to vascular surgery for reconstruction. Anamnestic data included hemoglobin C disease, Takayasu arteritis with associated renovascular hypertension (obstruction of renal arteries), obstruction of the right carotid artery, and history of meningoencephalitis. Coagulation values at admission were prothrombin time (PT) 77 %, international normalized ratio (INR) 1.18, activated partial thromboplastin time (aPTT) 34.9 s, and platelets 138,000 cells/μL. Surgery was carried out uneventfully with aortic clamp duration of 42 min. However, intraoperative blood loss was considerable, and cell saver was extensively used.

At the intensive care unit, admission standard coagulation parameters were PT 43 %, INR 1.87, aPTT 46.4 s, fibrinogen 190 mg/dL, and platelets 69,000 cells/μL. The first postoperative 12 h was complicated by a cardiac arrest treated with resuscitation maneuvers and inotropic drugs, acute renal failure, and massive bleeding (1250 ml) with no specific hemostatic treatment. At that point, coagulation was severely impaired: PT 14 %, INR 5.86, aPTT >300 s, antithrombin III 9 %, fibrinogen 60 mg/dL, and platelets 34,000 cells/μL. Prohemostatic therapy included FFP, platelet concentrate, human fibrinogen concentrate, and PCC. TEG analysis showed no curve at kaolin alone and an R time 24.0 min and MA 16.6 mm at kaolin with heparinase (Fig. 14.10). Protamine was administered, and kaolin curve was now present and almost comparable with the heparinase one (Fig. 14.11). However, given that a very severe bleeding was still ongoing, a surgical re-exploration was settled. After surgical re-exploration bleeding was almost ceased, but TEG analysis still presented signs of severe coagulopathy – R time 26.2 min, MA 12.5 mm (Fig. 14.12), and the following coagulation parameters: PT 21 %, INR 3.64, aPTT 111.0 s, and fibrinogen 77 mg/dL. Fibrinogen and platelet concentrates, together with PCC, continued to be administered with almost no effect. Twelve hours after the previous TEG, the coagulopathy was not improved – kaolin and heparinase showing R time 27.7 min and MA 27.0 mm with no curve at kaolin channel (Fig. 14.13) associated to PT 19 %, INR 4.18, aPTT 80.8, and platelets 19,000 cells/μL. A few hours later, the clinical conditions further aggravated and the patient died.

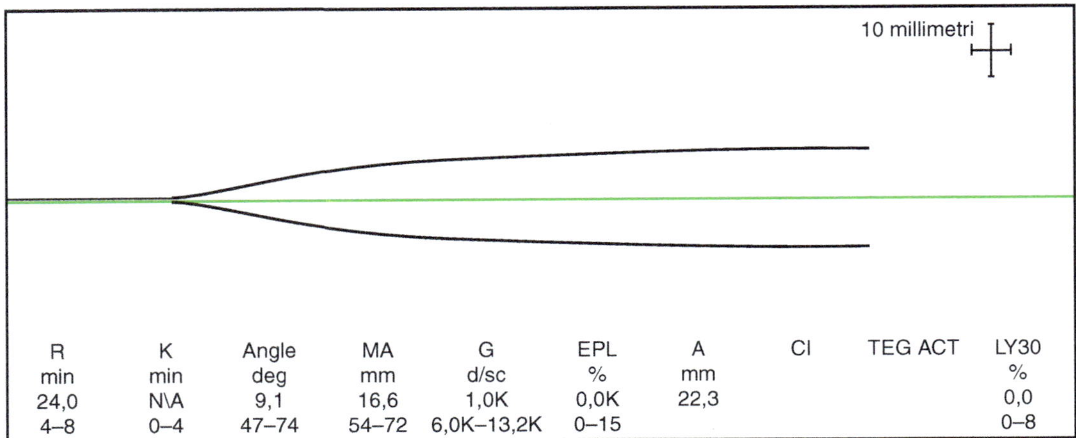

Fig. 14.10 First control at TEG showing extensive residual heparin

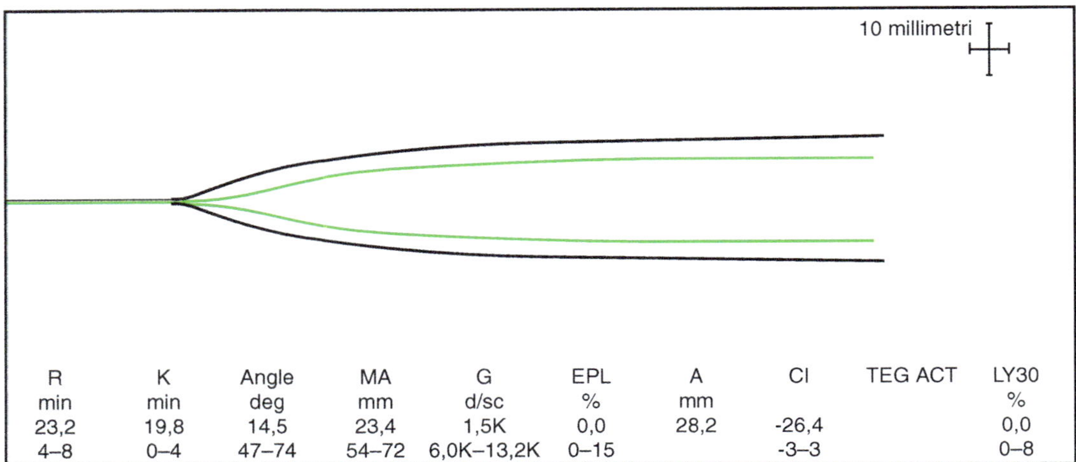

Fig. 14.11 Recovery of the residual heparinization by protamine

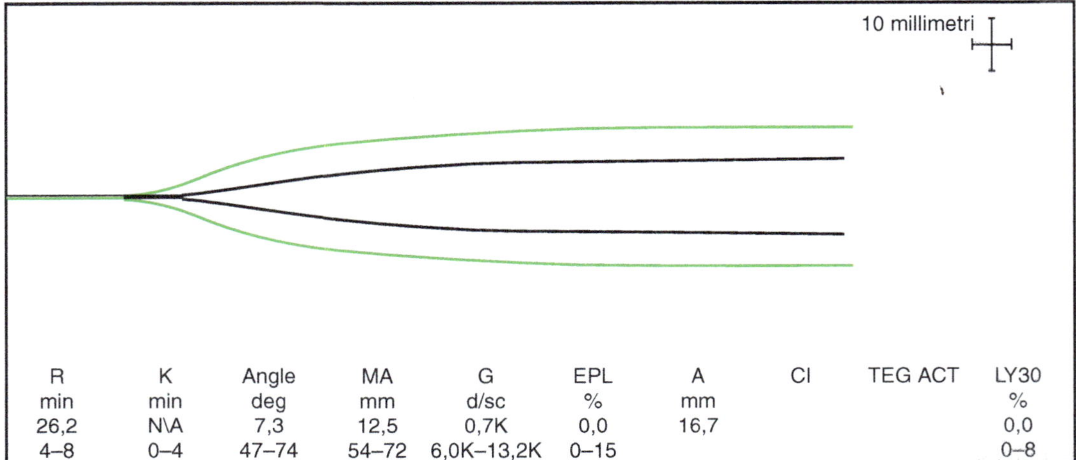

Fig. 14.12 Severe coagulopathy after surgical reexploration

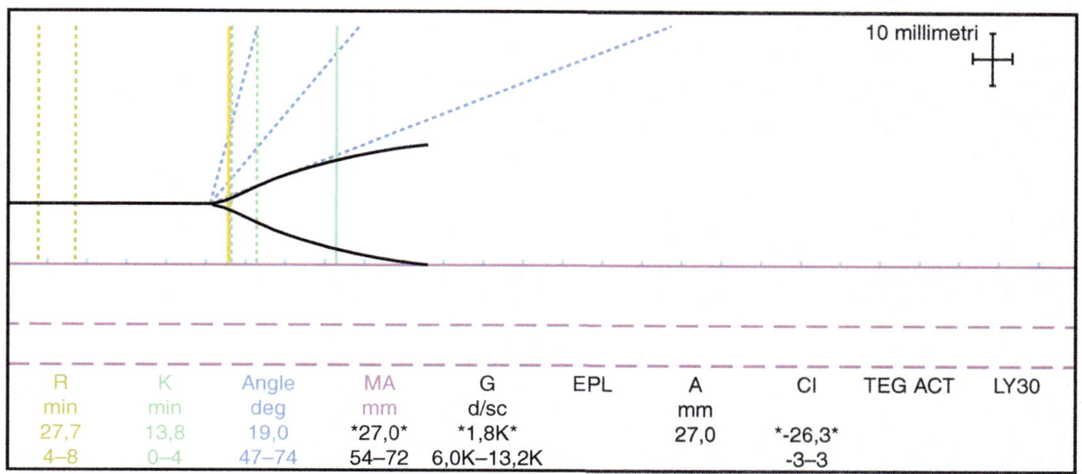

Fig. 14.13 Coagulopathy refractive to hemostatic treatment with PCC, fibrinogen and platelet concentrates

14.7.1 Comment

Failure to treat the initial coagulopathy led to an irreversible hemorrhagic complication.

It is likely that the patient suffered from a combination of severe coagulation factors and platelet consumption, exacerbated by the extensive use of the cell saver. An initial aggressive treatment based on TEG tests would have probably prevented the final pattern of disseminated intravascular coagulopathy.

References

1. Fries D, Martini WZ (2010) Role of fibrinogen in trauma-induced coagulopathy. Br J Anaesth 105:116–121
2. Levy JH, Szlam F, Tanaka KA, Sniecienski RM (2012) Review article: fibrinogen and hemostasis: a primary hemostatic target for the management of acquired bleeding. Anesth Analg 114:261–274
3. Schöchl H, Solomon C, Traintinger S, Nienaber U, Tacacs-Tolnai A, Windhofer C et al (2011) Thromboelastometric (ROTEM) findings in patients suffering from isolated severe traumatic brain injury. J Neurotrauma 28:2033–2041
4. Schöchl H, Cotton B, Inaba K, Nienaber U, Fischer H, Voelckel W et al (2011) FIBTEM provides early prediction of massive transfusion in trauma. Crit Care 15:R265
5. Leemann H, Lustenberger T, Talving P, Kobayashi L, Bukur M, Brenni M et al (2010) The role of rotation thromboelastometry in early prediction of massive transfusion. J Trauma 69:1403–1408
6. Roberts I, Shakur H, Afolabi A, Brohi K, Coats T, Dewan Y et al (2011) The importance of early treatment with tranexamic acid in bleeding trauma patients: an exploratory analysis of the CRASH-2 randomised controlled trial. Lancet 377:1096–1101

The manufacturer's authorised representative in the EU is Springer Nature Customer Service Centre GmbH, Europaplatz 3, 69115 Heidelberg, Germany. If you have any concerns regarding our products, please contact ProductSafety@springernature.com

Printed and bound by CPI Group (UK) Ltd, Croydon, CR0 4YY
15/07/2026
02167638-0001